Alzheimer Disease

SOURCEBOOK

SEVENTH EDITION

Alzheimer Disease
SOURCEBOOK

SEVENTH EDITION

Basic Consumer Health Information about Alzheimer Disease and Other Forms of Dementia, Including Mild Cognitive Impairment, Corticobasal Degeneration, Dementia with Lewy Bodies, Frontotemporal Dementia, Huntington Disease, Parkinson Disease, and Vascular Dementia

Along with Information about Recent Research on the Diagnosis and Prevention of Alzheimer Disease and Genetic Testing, Tips for Maintaining Cognitive Functioning, Strategies for Long-Term Planning, Advice for Caregivers, a Glossary of Related Terms, and Directories of Resources for Additional Help and Information

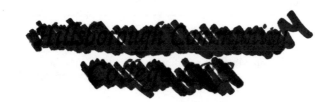

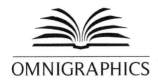

OMNIGRAPHICS

615 Griswold, Ste. 901, Detroit, MI 48226

Bibliographic Note
Because this page cannot legibly accommodate all the copyright notices, the Bibliographic Note portion of the Preface constitutes an extension of the copyright notice.

* * *

OMNIGRAPHICS
Angela L. Williams, *Managing Editor*
* * *

Copyright © 2019 Omnigraphics

ISBN 978-0-7808-1677-0
E-ISBN 978-0-7808-1678-7

Library of Congress Cataloging-in-Publication Data

Names: Omnigraphics, Inc., issuing body.

Title: Alzheimer disease sourcebook: basic consumer health information about alzheimer disease and other forms of dementia, including mild cognitive impairment, corticobasal degeneration, dementia with lewy bodies, frontotemporal dementia, huntington disease, parkinson disease, and vascular dementia; along with information about recent research on the diagnosis and prevention of alzheimer disease and genetic testing, tips for maintaining cognitive functioning, strategies for long-term planning, advice for caregivers, a glossary of related terms, and directories of resources for additional help and information.

Description: Seventh edition. | Detroit, MI: Omnigraphics, Inc., [2019] | Series: Health reference series | "Angela L. Williams, editorial manager." | Includes bibliographical references and index.

Identifiers: LCCN 2018053288 | ISBN 9780780816770 (hard cover: alk. paper) | ISBN 9780780816787 (ebook)

Subjects: LCSH: Alzheimer's disease--Popular works. | Dementia--Popular works.

Classification: LCC RC523.2.A45 2019 | DDC 616.8/311--dc23

LC record available at https://lccn.loc.gov/2018053288

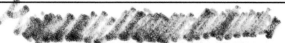

Table of Contents

Part III: Other Dementia Disorders

Part IV: Recognizing, Diagnosing, and Treating Symptoms of Alzheimer Disease and Dementias

Part V: Living with Alzheimer Disease and Dementias

Part VI: Caregiver Concerns

Part VII: Additional Help and Information

Preface

About This Book

Approximately 5 million Americans are estimated to be living with the progressive, incurable, fatal brain disorder known as Alzheimer disease (AD). By 2050, this number is projected to quadruple and affect 14 million U.S. adults aged 65 years of age or older. AD, which accounts for between 60 percent and 80 percent of all cases of dementia, destroys brain cells, causes memory loss and confusion, and worsens over time until patients eventually lose the ability to work, walk, and communicate.

Alzheimer Disease Sourcebook, Seventh Edition provides updated information about the causes, symptoms, and stages of AD and other forms of dementia, including mild cognitive impairment, corticobasal degeneration, dementia with Lewy bodies, frontotemporal dementia, Huntington disease, Parkinson disease, and dementia caused by infections. It discusses the structure of the brain, how it changes with age, and the cognitive decline and degeneration that occur in dementia. Facts about genetic testing, cognitive and behavioral symptoms, AD clinical trials, and recent research efforts are also included, along with information about legal, financial, and medical planning and coping strategies for caregivers. The book concludes with a glossary of related terms and directories of resources.

How to Use This Book

This book is divided into parts and chapters. Parts focus on broad areas of interest. Chapters are devoted to single topics within a part.

Part One: Facts about the Brain and Cognitive Decline provides information about healthy brain function and examines changes in cognitive functions and memory that occur during the typical aging process. Facts about the types, symptoms, causes, risk factors, and prevalence of dementia—a brain disorder that significantly impairs intellectual functions—are also included.

Part Two: Alzheimer Disease: The Most Common Type of Dementia discusses Alzheimer disease (AD), an irreversible and progressive brain disease and identifies the signs, symptoms, and diagnostic stages of this disorder. Information about the role that genetics, brain injuries, weight, and injuries play in the development of AD is also presented, along with facts about early-onset AD, a form of the disease that affects people under the age of 65. It also discusses the factors that influence AD risk, such as alcohol, nicotine, and sleep deprivation.

Part Three: Other Dementia Disorders identifies types, signs, and symptoms of dementia other than AD, including cognitive impairment, corticobasal degeneration, dementia with Lewy bodies, frontotemporal disorders, Huntington disease, Parkinson disease, and vascular dementia. It details various causes of dementia, such as AIDS, cancer, delirium, and other diseases.

Part Four: Recognizing, Diagnosing, and Treating Symptoms of Alzheimer Disease and Dementias explains neurocognitive and imaging tools used to assess and diagnose dementia, such as positron emission tomography, single photon emission computed tomography, magnetic resonance imaging, and biomarker testing. Medications used manage AD and other dementias, are identified, and information about participating in AD clinical trials and studies is included. An explanation of recent developments in AD research is also provided.

Part Five: Living with Alzheimer Disease and Dementias describes strategies for maintaining health and wellness after a dementia diagnosis. Patients and caregivers will find information about nutrition, exercises, and dental care for dementia patients, tips on telling someone about the diagnosis, strategies for slowing the rate of cognitive decline, and advice on pain, sleep problems, and sexuality in people with dementia. Information about Medicare and financial, legal, and healthcare planning is included.

Part Six: Caregiver Concerns offers advice to those who care for people with AD or dementia. Strategies for coping with challenging behaviors, communicating, and planning daily activities for someone with dementia are discussed, along with tips on creating a safe environment at home. Caregivers struggling to control frustration and cope with fatigue will find information about respite, home health, and nursing home care, as well as suggestions on evaluating difficult health decisions near the end of life.

Part Seven: Additional Help and Information provides a glossary of terms related to AD and dementia and a directory of organizations that provide health information about AD and dementia.

Bibliographic Note

This volume contains documents and excerpts from publications issued by the following U.S. government agencies: Administration for Community Living (ACL); Agency for Healthcare Research and Quality (AHRQ); Centers for Disease Control and Prevention (CDC); Centers for Medicare & Medicaid Services (CMS); National Cancer Institute (NCI); National Center for Biotechnology Information (NCBI); National Center for Complementary and Integrative Health (NCCIH); National Heart, Lung, and Blood Institute (NHLBI); National Institute of Biomedical Imaging and Bioengineering (NIBIB); National Institute of Diabetes and Digestive and Kidney Diseases (NIDDK); National Institute of Neurological Disorders and Stroke (NINDS); National Institute on Aging (NIA); National Institute on Alcohol Abuse and Alcoholism (NIAAA); National Institutes of Health (NIH); *NIH News in Health*; Office of the Assistant Secretary for Planning and Evaluation (ASPE); Office of the Surgeon General (OSG); U.S. Department of Veterans Affairs (VA); and U.S. Social Security Administration (SSA).

About the Health Reference Series

The *Health Reference Series* is designed to provide basic medical information for patients, families, caregivers, and the general public. Each volume takes a particular topic and provides comprehensive coverage. This is especially important for people who may be dealing with a newly diagnosed disease or a chronic disorder in themselves or in a family member. People looking for preventive guidance, information about disease warning signs, medical statistics, and risk factors for health problems will also find answers to their questions in the *Health Reference Series*. The *Series*, however, is not intended to serve as a tool for diagnosing illness, in prescribing treatments, or as a substitute for the physician/patient relationship. All people concerned about medical symptoms or the possibility of disease are encouraged to seek professional care from an appropriate healthcare provider.

A Note about Spelling and Style

Health Reference Series editors use *Stedman's Medical Dictionary* as an authority for questions related to the spelling of medical terms and the *Chicago Manual of Style* for questions related to grammatical structures, punctuation, and other editorial concerns. Consistent adherence is not always possible, however, because the individual volumes within the *Series* include many documents from a wide variety of different producers, and the editor's primary goal is to present material from each source as accurately as is possible. This sometimes means that information in different chapters or sections may follow other guidelines and alternate spelling authorities. For example, occasionally a copyright holder may require that eponymous terms be shown in possessive forms (Crohn's disease vs. Crohn disease) or that British spelling norms be retained (leukaemia vs. leukemia).

Medical Review

Omnigraphics contracts with a team of qualified, senior medical professionals who serve as medical consultants for the *Health Reference Series*. As necessary, medical consultants review reprinted material for currency and accuracy. Citations including the phrase "Reviewed (month, year)" indicate material reviewed by this team. Medical consultation services are provided to the *Health Reference Series* editors by:

Dr. Vijayalakshmi, MBBS, DGO, MD
Dr. Senthil Selvan, MBBS, DCH, MD
Dr. K. Sivanandham, MBBS, DCH, MS (Research), PhD

Our Advisory Board

We would like to thank the following board members for providing initial guidance on the development of this series:

- Dr. Lynda Baker, Associate Professor of Library and Information Science, Wayne State University, Detroit, MI

- Nancy Bulgarelli, William Beaumont Hospital Library, Royal Oak, MI

- Karen Imarisio, Bloomfield Township Public Library, Bloomfield Township, MI

- Karen Morgan, Mardigian Library, University of Michigan-Dearborn, Dearborn, MI

- Rosemary Orlando, St. Clair Shores Public Library, St. Clair Shores, MI

Health Reference Series *Update Policy*

The inaugural book in the *Health Reference Series* was the first edition of *Cancer Sourcebook* published in 1989. Since then, the *Series* has been enthusiastically received by librarians and in the medical community. In order to maintain the standard of providing high-quality health information for the layperson the editorial staff at Omnigraphics felt it was necessary to implement a policy of updating volumes when warranted.

Medical researchers have been making tremendous strides, and it is the purpose of the *Health Reference Series* to stay current with the most recent advances. Each decision to update a volume is made on an individual basis. Some of the considerations include how much new information is available and the feedback we receive from people who use the books. If there is a topic you would like to see added to the update list, or an area of medical concern you feel has not been adequately addressed, please write to:

Managing Editor
Health Reference Series
Omnigraphics
615 Griswold, Ste. 901
Detroit, MI 48226

Part One

Facts about the Brain and Cognitive Decline

Chapter 1

The Basics of a Healthy Brain

The brain is the most complex part of the human body. This three-pound organ is the seat of intelligence, interpreter of the senses, initiator of body movement, and controller of behavior. Lying in its bony shell and washed by protective fluid, the brain is the source of all the qualities that define our humanity. The brain is the crown jewel of the human body.

For centuries, scientists and philosophers have been fascinated by the brain, but until recently they viewed the brain as nearly incomprehensible. Now, however, the brain is beginning to relinquish its secrets. Scientists have learned more about the brain in the last few years than in all previous centuries because of the accelerating pace of research in neurological and behavioral science and the development of new research techniques. As a result, Congress named the 1990s the Decade of the Brain. At the forefront of research on the brain and other elements of the nervous system is the National Institute of Neurological Disorders and Stroke (NINDS), which conducts and supports scientific studies in the United States and around the world.

This chapter is a basic introduction to the human brain. It may help you understand how the healthy brain works, how to keep it healthy, and what happens when the brain is diseased or dysfunctional.

This chapter includes text excerpted from "Brain Basics: Know Your Brain," National Institute of Neurological Disorders and Stroke (NINDS), October 28, 2018.

The Architecture of the Brain

The brain is like a committee of experts. All the parts of the brain work together, but each part has its own special properties. The brain can be divided into three basic units: the forebrain, the midbrain, and the hindbrain.

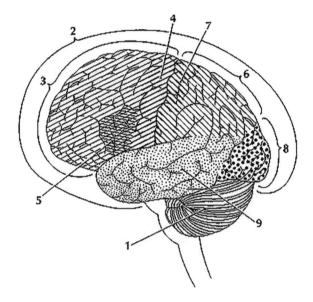

Figure 1.1. *The Human Brain*

The hindbrain includes the upper part of the spinal cord, the brain stem, and a wrinkled ball of tissue called the **cerebellum (1)**. The hindbrain controls the body's vital functions such as respiration and heart rate. The cerebellum coordinates movement and is involved in learned rote movements. When you play the piano or hit a tennis ball you are activating the cerebellum. The uppermost part of the brainstem is the midbrain, which controls some reflex actions and is part of the circuit involved in the control of eye movements and other voluntary movements. The forebrain is the largest and most highly developed part of the human brain: it consists primarily of the **cerebrum (2)** and the structures are hidden beneath it.

When people see pictures of the brain it is usually the cerebrum that they notice. The cerebrum sits at the topmost part of the brain and is the source of intellectual activities. It holds your memories, allows you to plan, enables you to imagine and think. It allows you to recognize friends, read books, and play games.

The cerebrum is split into two halves (hemispheres) by a deep fissure. Despite the split, the two cerebral hemispheres communicate with each other through a thick tract of nerve fibers that lies at the base of this fissure. Although the two hemispheres seem to be mirror images of each other, they are different. For instance, the ability to form words seems to lie primarily in the left hemisphere, while the right hemisphere seems to control many abstract reasoning skills.

For some as-yet-unknown reason, nearly all of the signals from the brain to the body and vice versa crossover on their way to and from the brain. This means that the right cerebral hemisphere primarily controls the left side of the body and the left hemisphere primarily controls the right side. When one side of the brain is damaged, the opposite side of the body is affected. For example, a stroke in the right hemisphere of the brain can leave the left arm and leg paralyzed.

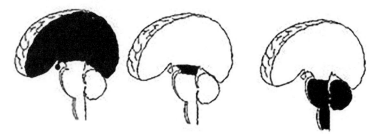

Figure 1.2. *Forebrain, Midbrain, and Hindbrain*

The Geography of Thought

Each cerebral hemisphere can be divided into sections, or lobes, each of which specializes in different functions. To understand each lobe and its specialty we will take a tour of the cerebral hemispheres, starting with the two **frontal lobes (3)**, which lie directly behind the forehead. When you plan a schedule, imagine the future, or use reasoned arguments, these two lobes do much of the work. One of the ways the frontal lobes seem to do these things is by acting as short-term storage sites, allowing one idea to be kept in mind while other ideas are considered. In the rearmost portion of each frontal lobe is a **motor area (4)**, which helps control voluntary movement. A nearby place on the left frontal lobe called **Broca area (5)** allows thoughts to be transformed into words.

When you enjoy a good meal—the taste, aroma, and texture of the food—two sections behind the frontal lobes called the **parietal lobes**

(**6**) are at work. The forward parts of these lobes, just behind the motor areas, are the primary **sensory areas (7)**. These areas receive information about temperature, taste, touch, and movement from the rest of the body. Reading and arithmetic are also functions in the repertoire of each parietal lobe.

As you look at the words and pictures on this page, two areas at the back of the brain are at work. These lobes, called the **occipital lobes (8)**, process images from the eyes and link that information with images stored in memory. Damage to the occipital lobes can cause blindness.

The last lobes on our tour of the cerebral hemispheres are the **temporal lobes (9)**, which lie in front of the visual areas and nest under the parietal and frontal lobes. Whether you appreciate symphonies or rock music, your brain responds through the activity of these lobes. At the top of each temporal lobe is an area responsible for receiving information from the ears. The underside of each temporal lobe plays a crucial role in forming and retrieving memories, including those associated with music. Other parts of this lobe seem to integrate memories and sensations of taste, sound, sight, and touch.

The Cerebral Cortex

Coating the surface of the cerebrum and the cerebellum is a vital layer of tissue the thickness of a stack of two or three dimes. It is called the cortex, from the Latin word for bark. Most of the actual information processing in the brain takes place in the cerebral cortex. When people talk about "gray matter" in the brain they are talking about this thin rind. The cortex is gray because nerves in this area lack the insulation that makes most other parts of the brain appear to be white. The folds in the brain add to its surface area, and therefore, increase the amount of gray matter and the quantity of information that can be processed.

The Inner Brain

Deep within the brain, hidden from view, lie structures that are the gatekeepers between the spinal cord and the cerebral hemispheres. These structures not only determine our emotional state, they also modify our perceptions and responses depending on that state, and allow us to initiate movements that you make without thinking about them. Like the lobes in the cerebral hemispheres, the structures described below come in pairs: each is duplicated in the opposite half of the brain.

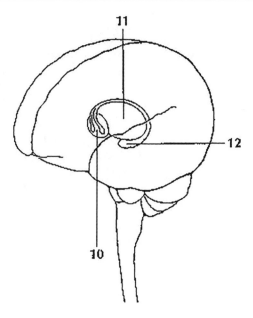

Figure 1.3. *Inner Brain*

The **hypothalamus (10)**, about the size of a pearl, directs a multitude of important functions. It wakes you up in the morning, and gets the adrenaline flowing during a test or job interview. The hypothalamus is also an important emotional center, controlling the molecules that make you feel exhilarated, angry, or unhappy. Near the hypothalamus lies the **thalamus (11)**, a major clearinghouse for information going to and from the spinal cord and the cerebrum.

An arching tract of nerve cells leads from the hypothalamus and the thalamus to the **hippocampus (12)**. This tiny nub acts as a memory indexer—sending memories out to the appropriate part of the cerebral hemisphere for long-term storage and retrieving them when necessary. The basal ganglia are clusters of nerve cells surrounding the thalamus. They are responsible for initiating and integrating movements. Parkinson disease (PD), which results in tremors, rigidity, and a stiff, shuffling walk, is a disease of nerve cells that lead into the basal ganglia.

Making Connections

The brain and the rest of the nervous system are composed of many different types of cells, but the primary functional unit is a cell called the neuron. All sensations, movements, thoughts, memories, and feelings are the result of signals that pass through neurons. Neurons consist of three parts. The **cell body (13)** contains the nucleus, where most of the molecules that the neuron needs to survive and function are manufactured. **Dendrites (14)** extend out from the cell body like the branches of a tree and receive messages from other nerve cells. Signals then pass from the dendrites through the cell body and may travel away from the cell body down an **axon (15)** to another neuron, a muscle cell, or cells in some other organ. The neuron is usually surrounded by many support cells. Some types of cells wrap around the axon to form an insulating **sheath (16)**. This sheath can include a fatty molecule called myelin, which provides insulation for the axon and helps nerve signals travel faster and farther. Axons may be very short, such as those that carry signals from one cell in the cortex to another cell less than a hair's width away. Or axons may be very long, such as those that carry messages from the brain all the way down the spinal cord.

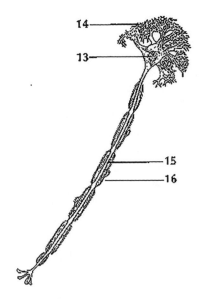
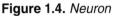
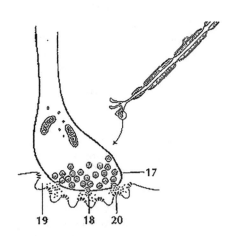

Figure 1.4. *Neuron*   **Figure 1.5.** *Synapse*

Scientists have learned a great deal about neurons by studying the synapse—the place where a signal passes from the neuron to another cell. When the signal reaches the end of the axon it stimulates the release of **tiny sacs (17)**. These sacs release chemicals known as **neurotransmitters (18)** into the **synapse (19)**. The neurotransmitters cross the synapse and attach to **receptors (20)** on the neighboring cell. These receptors can change the properties of the receiving cell. If the receiving cell is also a neuron, the signal can continue the transmission to the next cell.

Some Key Neurotransmitters at Work

Acetylcholine is called an excitatory neurotransmitter because it generally makes cells more excitable. It governs muscle contractions and causes glands to secrete hormones. Alzheimer disease (AD), which initially affects memory formation, is associated with a shortage of acetylcholine.

Gamma-aminobutyric acid (GABA) is called an inhibitory neurotransmitter because it tends to make cells less excitable. It helps control muscle activity and is an important part of the visual system. Drugs that increase GABA levels in the brain are used to treat epileptic seizures and tremors in patients with Huntington disease (HD).

Serotonin is a neurotransmitter that constricts blood vessels and brings on sleep. It is also involved in temperature regulation. Dopamine is an inhibitory neurotransmitter involved in mood and the control of complex movements. The loss of dopamine activity in some portions of the brain leads to the muscular rigidity of Parkinson disease. Many medications used to treat behavioral disorders work by modifying the action of dopamine in the brain.

Neurological Disorders

When the brain is healthy it functions quickly and automatically. But when problems occur, the results can be devastating. Some 50 million people in this country—one in five—suffer from damage to the nervous system. The NINDS supports research on more than 600 neurological diseases. Some of the major types of disorders include: neurogenetic diseases (such as Huntington disease and muscular dystrophy (MD)), developmental disorders (such as cerebral palsy (CP)), degenerative diseases of adult life (such as Parkinson disease and Alzheimer disease), metabolic diseases (such as Gaucher disease), cerebrovascular diseases (such as stroke and vascular dementia), trauma (such as spinal cord and head injury), convulsive disorders (such as epilepsy), infectious diseases (such as acquired immunodeficiency syndrome (AIDS) dementia), and brain tumors.

Chapter 2

The Changing Brain in Healthy Aging

The brain controls many aspects of thinking—remembering, planning and organizing, making decisions, and much more. These cognitive abilities can decline with age. Exactly what controls aging in the brain, however, is not clear.

You naturally lose brain cells with age. Certain regions of the brain have cells called neural stem cells that can regenerate. These stem cells serve as a sort of internal repair system, dividing to replenish other cells. They have only been found in a few brain regions, including the hypothalamus. The hypothalamus is critical for regulating the endocrine system—the glands and hormones throughout the body. The region is known to play a role in development, reproduction, and metabolism. It has also been implicated in aging.

To investigate whether stem cells in the hypothalamus influence the aging process, a team of scientists led by Dr. Dongsheng Cai at Albert Einstein College of Medicine examined these cells in mice. The study was funded by National Institutes of Health's (NIH) National Institute on Aging (NIA), National Institute of Diabetes and Digestive and Kidney Diseases (NIDDK), and National Heart, Lung, and Blood

This chapter contains text excerpted from the following sources: Text in this chapter begins with excerpts from "Brain Cells That Influence Aging," National Institutes of Health (NIH), August 15, 2017; Text beginning with the heading "How the Aging Brain Affects Thinking" is excerpted from "How the Aging Brain Affects Thinking," National Institute on Aging (NIA), National Institutes of Health (NIH), May 17, 2017.

11

Institute (NHLBI). Results were published in the August 3, 2017, issue of *Nature*.

The researchers first observed what happens to stem cells in the hypothalamus as healthy mice age. They found that the number of stem cells gradually diminished in early to middle-aged mice and were almost completely absent in older mice. They then experimentally disrupted these stem cells in middle-aged mice and examined the effects on aging over three to four months. Mice with the disrupted stem cells showed signs of cognitive impairment and other signs of aging earlier than control mice. Mice with the disrupted stem cells also had a shortened lifespan.

The researchers were able to slow these signs of aging by implanting hypothalamic stem cells harvested from newborn mice into the brains of middle-aged mice. The mice also lived longer than control mice. These antiaging effects could be replicated by injecting the tiny fluid-filled sacs, called exosomes, that are secreted by hypothalamic neural stem cells. Exosomes circulate in blood and carry genetic material called microRNA (miRNA), which regulates genes in tissues throughout the body.

These results suggest that it's the endocrine function of the hypothalamic stem cells that essentially controls the aging process. It remains to be seen what role the cells' regenerative properties play in the long-term control of aging.

"Our research shows that the number of hypothalamic neural stem cells naturally declines over the life of the animal, and this decline accelerates aging," Cai says. "But we also found that the effects of this loss are not irreversible. By replenishing these stem cells or the molecules they produce, it's possible to slow and even reverse various aspects of aging throughout the body."

How the Aging Brain Affects Thinking

Some changes in thinking are common as people get older. For example, older adults may have:

- Increased difficulty finding words and recalling names
- More problems with multitasking
- Mild decreases in the ability to pay attention

Aging may also bring positive cognitive changes. People often have more knowledge and insight from a lifetime of experiences. Research shows that older adults can still:

- Learn new things

- Create new memories
- Improve vocabulary and language skills

The Older, Healthy Brain

As a person gets older, changes occur in all parts of the body, including the brain.

- Certain parts of the brain shrink, especially those important to learning and other complex mental activities.
- In certain brain regions, communication between neurons (nerve cells) can be reduced.
- Blood flow in the brain may also decrease.
- Inflammation, which occurs when the body responds to an injury or disease, may increase.

These changes in the brain can affect mental function, even in healthy older people. For example, some older adults find that they don't do as well as younger people on complex memory or learning tests. Given enough time, though, they can do as well. There is growing evidence that the brain remains "plastic"—able to adapt to new challenges and tasks—as people age.

It is not clear why some people think well as they get older while others do not. One possible reason is "cognitive reserve," the brain's ability to work well even when some part of it is disrupted. People with more education seem to have more cognitive reserve than others.

Some brain changes, like those associated with Alzheimer disease (AD), are NOT a normal part of aging. Talk with your healthcare provider if you are concerned.

Brain Regions

The brain is complex and has many specialized parts. For example, the two halves of the brain, called cerebral hemispheres, are responsible for intelligence.

The cerebral hemispheres have an outer layer called the cerebral cortex. This region, the brain's "gray matter," is where the brain processes sensory information, such as what we see and hear. The cerebral cortex also controls movement and regulates functions such as thinking, learning, and remembering.

How Brain Cells Work

The healthy human brain contains many different types of cells. Neurons are nerve cells that process and send information throughout the brain, and from the brain to the muscles and organs of the body.

The ability of neurons to function and survive depends on three important processes:

- **Communication.** When a neuron receives signals from other neurons, it generates an electrical charge. This charge travels to the synapse, a tiny gap where chemicals called neurotransmitters are released and move across to another neuron.

- **Metabolism.** This process involves all chemical reactions that take place in a cell to support its survival and function. These reactions require oxygen and glucose, which are carried in blood flowing through the brain.

- **Repair, remodeling, and regeneration.** Neurons live a long time—more than 100 years in humans. As a result, they must constantly maintain and repair themselves. In addition, some brain regions continue to make new neurons.

Other types of brain cells, called glial cells, play critical roles in supporting neurons. In addition, the brain has an enormous network of blood vessels. Although the brain is only 2 percent of the body's weight, it receives 20 percent of the body's blood supply.

Chapter 3

Understanding Memory Loss

Memory and Thinking: What's Normal and What's Not?

Many older people worry about their memory and other thinking abilities. For example, they might be concerned about taking longer than before to learn new things, or they might sometimes forget to pay a bill. These changes are usually signs of mild forgetfulness—often a normal part of aging—not serious memory problems.

Talk with your doctor to determine if memory and other thinking problems are normal or not, and what is causing them.

What's Normal and What's Not?

What's the difference between normal, age-related forgetfulness and a serious memory problem? Serious memory problems make it

This chapter contains text excerpted from the following sources: Text under the heading "Memory and Thinking: What's Normal and What's Not?" is excerpted from "Memory and Thinking: What's Normal and What's Not?" National Institute on Aging (NIA), National Institutes of Health (NIH), May 17, 2017; Text beginning with the heading "Differences between Mild Forgetfulness and More Serious Memory Problems" is excerpted from "Understanding Memory Loss," National Institute on Aging (NIA), National Institutes of Health (NIH), January 2018; Text under the heading "Noticing Memory Problems? What to Do Next" is excerpted from "Noticing Memory Problems? What to Do Next," National Institute on Aging (NIA), National Institutes of Health (NIH), May 17, 2017.

hard to do everyday things like driving and shopping. Signs may include:

- Asking the same questions over and over again
- Getting lost in familiar places
- Not being able to follow instructions
- Becoming confused about time, people, and places

Differences between Mild Forgetfulness and More Serious Memory Problems

What Is Mild Forgetfulness?

It is true that some of us get more forgetful as we age. It may take longer to learn new things, remember certain words, or find our glasses. These changes are often signs of mild forgetfulness, not serious memory problems.

See your doctor if you're worried about your forgetfulness. Tell him or her about your concerns. Be sure to make a follow-up appointment to check your memory in the next six months to a year. If you think you might forget, ask a family member, friend, or the doctor's office to remind you.

What Can I Do about Mild Forgetfulness?

You can do many things to help your memory. Here are some ways to help your memory:

- Learn a new skill
- Volunteer in your community, at a school, or at your place of worship
- Spend time with friends and family
- Use memory tools such as big calendars, to-do lists, and notes to yourself
- Put your wallet or purse, keys, and glasses in the same place each day
- Get lots of rest
- Exercise and eat well
- Don't drink a lot of alcohol
- Get help if you feel depressed for weeks at a time

What Is a Serious Memory Problem?

Serious memory problems make it hard to do everyday things. For example, you may find it hard to drive, shop, or even talk with a friend. Signs of serious memory problems may include:

- Asking the same questions over and over again
- Getting lost in places you know well
- Not being able to follow directions
- Becoming more confused about time, people, and places
- Not taking care of yourself—eating poorly, not bathing
- Being unsafe

What Can I Do about Serious Memory Problems?

See your doctor if you are having any of the problems listed above. It's important to find out what might be causing a serious memory problem. Once you know the cause, you can get the right treatment.

Causes of Serious Memory Problems

Many things can cause serious memory problems, such as blood clots, depression, and Alzheimer disease (AD).

Medical Conditions

Certain medical conditions can cause serious memory problems. These problems should go away once you get treatment. Some medical conditions that may cause memory problems are:

- Bad reaction to certain medicines
- Depression
- Not eating enough healthy foods, or too few vitamins and minerals in your body
- Drinking too much alcohol
- Blood clots or tumors in the brain
- Head injury, such as a concussion from a fall or accident
- Thyroid, kidney, or liver problems.

17

Emotional Problems

Some emotional problems in older people can cause serious memory problems. Feeling sad, lonely, worried, or bored can cause you to be confused or forgetful.

Mild Cognitive Impairment

As some people grow older, they have more memory problems than other people their age. This condition is called mild cognitive impairment, or MCI. People with MCI can take care of themselves and do their normal activities. MCI memory problems may include:

- Losing things often

- Forgetting to go to events or appointments

- Having more trouble coming up with words than other people of the same age

Your doctor can do thinking, memory, and language tests to see if you have MCI. She or he also may suggest that you see a specialist for more tests. Because MCI may be an early sign of Alzheimer disease, it's important to see your doctor or specialist every 6–12 months.

Alzheimer Disease

Alzheimer disease causes serious memory problems. The signs of Alzheimer disease begin slowly and get worse over time. This is because changes in the brain cause large numbers of brain cells to die. It may look like simple forgetfulness at first, but over time, people with Alzheimer disease have trouble thinking clearly. They find it hard to do everyday things like shopping, driving, and cooking. As the illness gets worse, people with Alzheimer disease may need someone to take care of all their needs at home or in a nursing home. These needs may include feeding, bathing, and dressing.

Vascular Dementia

Many people have never heard of vascular dementia. Like Alzheimer disease, it is a medical condition that causes serious memory problems. Unlike Alzheimer disease, signs of vascular dementia may appear suddenly. This is because the memory loss and confusion are caused by changes in the blood supply to the brain, often after a stroke.

If the strokes stop, you may get better or stay the same for a long time. If you have more strokes, you may get worse.

Noticing Memory Problems? What to Do Next

We've all forgotten a name, where we put our keys, or if we locked the front door. It's normal to forget things once in a while. But serious memory problems make it hard to do everyday things. Forgetting how to make change, use the telephone, or find your way home may be signs of a more serious memory problem.

For some older people, memory problems are a sign of mild cognitive impairment, Alzheimer disease, or a related dementia. People who are worried about memory problems should see a doctor. Signs that it might be time to talk to a doctor include:

- Asking the same questions over and over again
- Getting lost in places a person knows well
- Not being able to follow directions
- Becoming more confused about time, people, and places
- Not taking care of oneself—eating poorly, not bathing, or being unsafe

People with memory complaints should make a follow-up appointment to check their memory after six months to a year. They can ask a family member, friend, or the doctor's office to remind them if they're worried they'll forget.

Chapter 4

What Is Dementia?

Dementia is the loss of cognitive functioning—the ability to think, remember, problem solve or reason—to such an extent that it interferes with a person's daily life and activities. Dementia ranges in severity from the mildest stage, when it is just beginning to affect a person's functioning, to the most severe stage, when the person must depend completely on others for basic activities of daily living. Functions affected include memory, language skills, visual perception, problem-solving, self-management, and the ability to focus and pay attention. Some people with dementia cannot control their emotions, and their personalities may change.

Symptoms

Signs and symptoms of dementia result when once-healthy neurons (nerve cells) in the brain stop working, lose connections with other brain cells, and die. While everyone loses some neurons as they age, people with dementia experience far greater loss. Unlike dementia, age-related memory loss isn't disabling. While dementia is more common with advanced age (as many as half of all people age 85 or older may have some form of dementia), it is not normal part of aging. Many people live into their 90s and beyond without any signs of dementia. The causes of dementia can vary. Many people with dementia have

This chapter includes text excerpted from "Dementia Information Page," National Institute of Neurological Disorders and Stroke (NINDS), June 12, 2018.

both Alzheimer disease (AD) and one or more closely related disorders that share brain scanning or clinical (and sometimes both) features with Alzheimer disease. When a person is affected by more than one dementia disorder, the dementia can be referred to as a mixed dementia. Some people may have mixed dementia caused by Alzheimer-related neurodegenerative processes, vascular disease-related processes, or another neurodegenerative condition. Many other conditions such as Creutzfeldt-Jakob disease (CJD), Huntington disease (HD), and chronic traumatic encephalopathy (CTE) can cause dementia or dementia-like symptoms. Risk factors for dementia include advancing age, stroke, high blood pressure, poorly controlled diabetes, and a thickening of blood vessel walls (atherosclerosis). Other dementias include frontotemporal disorders (FTD), vascular dementia, and Lewy body dementia (LBD).

Treatment

No treatments currently exist to stop or slow dementia caused by neurodegenerative diseases (ND) or progressive dementias. Drugs such as donepezil, rivastigmine, and galantamine can temporarily improve or stabilize memory and thinking skills in some people. Some studies suggest that drugs that improve memory in AD might benefit people with early vascular dementia. Some diseases that occur at the same time as dementia, such as diabetes and depression, can be treated. Other drugs may help manage certain symptoms and behavioral problems associated with the disorders. Some symptoms that may occur in dementia-like conditions can also be treated, although some symptoms may only respond to treatment for a period of time. A team of specialists—doctors, nurses, and speech, physical, and other therapists—familiar with these disorders can help guide patient care.

Prognosis

Many disorders can cause dementia or dementia-like symptoms. Some, such as Alzheimer disease or Huntington disease, lead to a progressive loss of mental functions. Many conditions that cause dementia-like symptoms can be halted or even reversed with the appropriate treatment. Individuals with dementia and caregivers can face challenges including the person's ability to handle tasks, changes in family relationships, loss of work, and long-term care. Individuals may need assistance with daily activities. People with advanced dementia may need constant care and supervision. Dementia disorders are not easy to live with, but with help, people can meet the challenges and prepare for the future. Getting an early accurate diagnosis and the right medical team are crucial first steps.

Chapter 5

Dementia: Causes and Risk Factors

Doctors have identified many other conditions that can cause dementia or dementia-like symptoms. The diseases have different symptoms that involve body and brain functions, and affect mental health and cognition.

Argyrophilic grain disease (AGD) is a common, late-onset degenerative disease that affects brain regions involved in memory and emotion. It causes cognitive decline and changes in memory and behavior, with difficulty finding words. The disease's signs and symptoms are indistinguishable from late-onset Alzheimer disease (LOAD). Confirmation of the diagnosis can be made only at autopsy.

Creutzfeldt-Jakob disease (CJD) is a rare brain disorder that is characterized by rapidly progressing dementia. Scientists found that infectious proteins called prions become misfolded and tend to clump together, causing the brain damage. Initial symptoms include impaired memory, judgment, and thinking, along with loss of muscle coordination and impaired vision. Some symptoms of CJD can be similar to symptoms of other progressive neurological diseases (PND), such as Alzheimer disease.

This chapter includes text excerpted from "The Dementias: Hope through Research," National Institute of Neurological Disorders and Stroke (NINDS), July 23, 2018.

Chronic traumatic encephalopathy (CTE) is caused by repeated traumatic brain injury (TBI) in some people who suffered multiple concussions. People with CTE may develop dementia, poor coordination, slurred speech, and other symptoms similar to those seen in Parkinson disease (PD) twenty years or more after the injury. Late-stage CTE is also characterized by brain atrophy and widespread deposits of tau in nerve cells. In some people, even just 5–10 years beyond the traumatic brain injury, behavioral and mood changes may occur. Dementia may not yet be present and the brain may not have started to shrink, but small deposits of tau are seen in specific brain regions at autopsy.

Huntington disease (HD) is an inherited, progressive brain disease that affects a person's judgment, memory, ability to plan and organize, and other cognitive functions. Symptoms typically begin around age 30–40 years and include abnormal and uncontrollable movements called chorea, as well as problems with walking and lack of coordination. Cognitive problems worsen as the disease progresses, and problems controlling movement lead to complete loss of ability for self-care.

HIV-associated dementia (HAD) can occur in people who have human immunodeficiency virus (HIV), the virus that causes acquired immunodeficiency syndrome (AIDS). HAD damages the brain's white matter and leads to a type of dementia associated with memory problems, social withdrawal, and trouble concentrating. People with HAD may develop movement problems as well. The incidence of HAD has dropped dramatically with the availability of effective antiviral therapies for managing the underlying HIV infections.

Secondary dementias occur in people with disorders that damage brain tissue. Such disorders may include multiple sclerosis, meningitis, and encephalitis, as well as Wilson disease (in which excessive amounts of copper build up to cause brain damage). People with malignant brain tumors may develop dementia or dementia-like symptoms because of damage to their brain circuits or a buildup of pressure inside the skull.

Risk Factors for Dementia and Vascular Cognitive Impairment

The following risk factors may increase a person's chance of developing one or more kinds of dementia. Some of these factors can be modified, while others cannot.

- **Age.** Advancing age is the best-known risk factor for developing dementia.

- **Hypertension.** High blood pressure has been linked to cognitive decline, stroke, and types of dementia that damage the white matter regions of the brain. High blood pressure causes "wear-and-tear" to brain blood vessel walls called arteriosclerosis.

- **Stroke.** A single major stroke or a series of smaller strokes increases a person's risk of developing vascular dementia. A person who has had a stroke is at an increased risk of having additional strokes, which further increases the risk of developing dementia.

- **Alcohol use.** Most studies suggest that regularly drinking large amounts of alcohol increases the risk of dementia. Specific dementias are associated with alcohol abuse, such as Wernicke-Korsakoff syndrome (WKS).

- **Atherosclerosis.** The accumulation of fats and cholesterol in the lining of arteries, coupled with an inflammatory process that leads to a thickening of the vessel walls (known as atherosclerosis), can lead to stroke, which raises the risk for vascular dementia.

- **Diabetes.** People with diabetes appear to have a higher risk for dementia. Poorly controlled diabetes is a risk factor for stroke and cardiovascular disease (CVD), which in turn increase the risk for vascular dementia.

- **Down syndrome (DS).** Many people with Down syndrome develop symptoms of Alzheimer disease by the time they reach middle age.

- **Genetics.** The chance of developing a genetically linked form of dementia increases when more than one family member has the disorder. In many dementias, there can be a family history of a similar disease. In some cases, such as with the frontotemporal dementias (FTD), having just one parent who carries a mutation increases the risk of inheriting the condition. A very small proportion of dementia is inherited.

- **Head injury.** An impact to the head can cause a traumatic brain injury or TBI. Certain types of TBI, or repeated TBIs, can cause dementia and other severe cognitive problems.

- **Parkinson disease.** The degeneration and death of nerve cells in the brain in people with Parkinson disease can cause dementia and significant memory loss.

- **Smoking.** Smoking increases the risk of developing cardiovascular diseases that slow or stop blood from getting to the brain.

Chapter 6

Statistics on Dementia Prevalence and Mortality

What Is Alzheimer Disease?

Alzheimer disease (AD), a fatal form of dementia, is a public health problem. Alzheimer disease-related deaths have increased over the past 16 years in every race, sex, and ethnicity category, and will most likely continue to increase as the population continues to age. More persons with Alzheimer disease are dying at home, and this means more caregivers are needed to care in the final stages of Alzheimer disease is very great.

- The most common form of dementia, which is a general term for a decline in mental ability severe enough to interfere with daily life

- A progressive disease beginning with mild memory loss possibly leading to loss of the ability to carry on a conversation and respond to the environment

---

This chapter contains text excerpted from the following sources: Text beginning with the heading "What Is Alzheimer Disease?" is excerpted from "Deaths from Alzheimer's Disease," Centers for Disease Control and Prevention (CDC), May 26, 2017; Text beginning with the heading "Percentage of Long-Term Care Services Users Diagnosed with Alzheimer Disease" is excerpted from "FastStats— Alzheimer's Disease," Centers for Disease Control and Prevention (CDC), March 11, 2016.

- Involves parts of the brain that control thought, memory, and language
- Can seriously affect a person's ability to carry out daily activities

Who Has Alzheimer Disease?

Scientists do not yet fully understand what causes Alzheimer disease. There probably is not one single cause, but several factors that affect each person differently.

- Five million Americans are estimated to be living with Alzheimer disease
- The symptoms of the disease usually appear after age 60 and the risk increases with age
- Younger people may get Alzheimer disease, but it is less common
- By 2050, this number is projected to quadruple this affect 14 million U.S. adults aged $\geq$ 65 years

Deaths from Alzheimer Disease in the United States

Alzheimer disease is ultimately a fatal form of dementia. It is the sixth leading cause of death in the United States, accounting for almost 4 percent of all deaths in 2014. The number of Alzheimer disease deaths has increased, in part, because of a growing population of older adults.

- The death rate due to Alzheimer disease has increased 55 percent from 1999 to 2014.
- In 2014, over 93,500 deaths across all 50 states and the District of Columbia occurred due to Alzheimer disease.
- The number of deaths in medical facilities has declined from 15 to 7 percent in the same period.
- The number of Alzheimer disease deaths at home has increased from 14 to 25 percent.
- Deaths attributed to Alzheimer disease increased among adults 75 years or older.
- Counties with the highest death rates from Alzheimer disease were primarily in the southeast with some additional areas in the Midwest and West.

The Burden on Caregivers

The increase of Alzheimer disease deaths and those deaths occurring at home has increased the burden on caregivers. In the final stages of Alzheimer disease, people with the disease require constant care regardless of the setting due to declines in memory, thinking, and the ability to solve problems as well as difficulties with everyday activities like bathing, feeding, and moving around the house. This means that both paid and unpaid (i.e., friends and family members) caregivers are likely faced with increased burden and strains. Therefore, there is a large need for education programs, breaks for caregivers, and case management services, to help caregivers. These activities, programs and services can lessen the potential burden of caregiving and improve the care for those with Alzheimer disease.

What Does This Mean?

While there is currently no cure for Alzheimer disease, people should see a doctor if they experience symptoms such as memory loss affecting their daily life, difficulties with problem-solving, or misplacing objects. Early diagnosis is important to allow patients and their families to begin planning for medical and caregiving needs at all stages. These findings highlight the escalating demand for in-home care and the need to prepare and provide support to caregivers.

Percentage of Long-Term Care Services Users Diagnosed with Alzheimer Disease

Percent of long-term care services users diagnosed with Alzheimer disease or other dementias:

- Percent of adult day services center participants: 29.9 percent (2014)
- Percent of residential care community residents: 39.6 percent (2014)
- Percent of home health agency patients: 31.4 percent (2013)
- Percent of hospice patients: 44.7 percent (2013)
- Percent of nursing home residents: 50.4 percent (2014)

Mortality

- Number of deaths: 110,561
- Deaths per 100,000 population: 34.4
- Cause of death rank: 6

Chapter 7

National Plan to Address Alzheimer Disease: 2017 Update

National Alzheimer Project Act

On January 4, 2011, the National Alzheimer Project Act (NAPA) (Public Law 111-375) was signed into law. The Act defines "Alzheimer" as Alzheimer disease and related dementias (AD/ADRD) and requires the Secretary of the United States. U.S. Department of Health and Human Services (HHS) to establish the National Alzheimer Project to:

- Create and maintain an integrated National Plan to overcome Alzheimer disease;

- Coordinate Alzheimer disease research and services across all federal agencies;

- Accelerate the development of treatments that would prevent, halt, or reverse the course of Alzheimer disease;

- Improve early diagnosis and coordination of care and treatment of Alzheimer disease;

This chapter includes text excerpted from "National Plan to Address Alzheimer's Disease: 2017 Update," Office of the Assistant Secretary for Planning and Evaluation (ASPE), September 15, 2017.

- Decrease disparities in Alzheimer disease for ethnic and racial minority populations that are at higher risk for Alzheimer disease; and

- Coordinate with international bodies to fight Alzheimer disease globally.

The law also establishes the Advisory Council on Alzheimer Research, Care, and Services (Advisory Council) and requires the Secretary of HHS, in collaboration with the Advisory Council, to create and maintain a National Plan to overcome AD/ADRD. NAPA offers a historic opportunity to address the many challenges facing people with AD/ADRD and their families. Given the great demographic shifts that will occur over the next thirty years, including the doubling of the population of older adults, the success of this effort is of great importance to people with AD/ADRD and their family members, caregivers, public policymakers, and health and social service providers.

The Challenges

The National Plan was designed to address the major challenges presented by AD/ADRD:

1. While research on AD/ADRD has made steady progress, there are no pharmacological or other interventions to definitively prevent, treat, or cure the diseases.

2. While HHS and other groups have taken steps to develop quality measures to assess dementia care and to improve the training of the health and long-term care workforce—for both paid and unpaid caregivers—there is room for improvement.

3. Family members and other unpaid caregivers, who take on the responsibility of caring for a loved one with AD/ADRD, also need services and supports. The majority of people with AD/ADRD live in the community, where their families provide most of their care. The toll of caregiving can have major implications for caregivers and families as well as population health, with about one-third of caregivers reporting symptoms of depression.

4. Stigmas and misconceptions associated with AD/ADRD are widespread and profoundly impact the care provided to and the isolation felt by people with AD/ADRD and their families and caregivers.

5. Public and private sector progress is significant but should be coordinated and tracked. In addition, data to track the incidence, prevalence, trajectory, and costs of AD/ADRD are limited.

Framework and Guiding Principles

The enactment of NAPA provided an opportunity to focus the Nation's attention on the challenges of AD/ADRD. In consultation with stakeholders both inside and outside of the federal government, this National Plan represents the blueprint for achieving the vision of a nation free of AD/ADRD.

Central to and guiding the National Plan are the people most intimately impacted by AD/ADRD—those who have the diseases and their families and other caregivers. Individuals with AD/ADRD and their caregivers receive assistance from both the clinical healthcare system and long-term care including home and community-based services (HCBS), legal services, and other social services. Both the clinical care and community/support environments need better tools to serve people with AD/ADRD and their unpaid caregivers. Ongoing and future research seeks to identify interventions to assist clinicians, supportive service providers, HCBS providers, persons living with dementia, and caregivers. All of these efforts must occur in the context of improved awareness of the diseases and its impacts, and the opportunities for improvement. The Plan aims to address these key needs. Health and Human Services (HHS) is committed to tracking and coordinating the implementation of NAPA and making improvements aimed at achieving its ambitious vision.

The National Plan continues to be guided by three principles:

1. **Optimize existing resources, and improve and coordinate ongoing activities.** The first step in developing the National Plan was to set up a federal interagency working group and conduct an inventory of all federal activities involving AD/ADRD. In creating the Plan, HHS and its partners sought to leverage these resources and activities, improve coordination, and reduce duplication of efforts to better meet the challenges of AD/ADRD. The activities included in the inventory comprise ongoing work and new opportunities created legislation and authority. The federal working group process continues to improve coordination and awareness throughout the federal government and set

in motion commitments for further collaboration. Further, this process has allowed for identification of non-AD-specific programs and resources that may be leveraged to advance AD/ADRD care and prevention.

2. **Support public-private partnerships.** The scope of the problem of AD/ADRD is so great that partnerships with a multitude of public and private stakeholders are essential to making progress. The original National Plan began the partnership process by identifying areas of need and opportunity. The plan continues to rely on the Advisory Council in particular to identify key areas where public-private partnerships can improve outcomes.

3. **Transform the way we approach Alzheimer disease and related dementias.** The National Plan recognizes that this undertaking will require continued, large-scale, coordinated efforts across the public and private sectors. With principles 1–2 above, as well as the ambitious vision that the federal government has committed to through this plan, HHS and its federal partners seek to take the first of many transformative actions that will be needed to address these diseases. Through an ongoing dialogue with the Advisory Council, the federal government continues to identify the most promising areas for progress and marshal resources from both within and outside the government to act on these opportunities.

Goals as Building Blocks for Transformation

Achieving the vision of eliminating the burden of AD/ADRD starts with concrete goals. Below are the five that form the foundation of the National Plan:

1. Prevent and effectively treat Alzheimer disease and related dementias by 2025.

2. Enhance care quality and efficiency.

3. Expand supports for people with Alzheimer disease and related dementias and their families.

4. Enhance public awareness and engagement.

5. Track progress and drive improvement.

2017 Update

This is the 2017 Update to the National Plan. In order to create a focused and accessible document, agencies have provided narrative descriptions of activities that were completed in 2016, as well as some which are ongoing and have updates. This provides a clear report of progress that was made since the last plan update in August 2016.

The activities outlined in this National Plan update vary in scope and impact, and include:

- Immediate actions that the federal government has taken and will take;

- Actions toward the goals that can be initiated by the federal government or its public and private partners in the near term; and

- Longer-range activities that will require numerous actions by federal and nonfederal partners to achieve.

The National Plan was never designed to be a "Federal Plan." The 2017 Plan Update includes a number of activities and projects submitted by nonfederal partners. These items have been organized according to the Goals and Strategies in the Plan. Active engagement of public and private sector stakeholders is critical to achieving these national goals. In the case of many of the long-range activities, the path forward will be contingent upon resources, scientific progress, and focused collaborations across many partners. Over time, HHS will work with the Advisory Council and stakeholders to incorporate and update additional transformative actions.

Additionally, in an effort to clearly respond to the annual recommendations made by the nonfederal members of the Advisory Council, the 2017 National Plan update includes an appendix in which relevant federal agencies have briefly responded to the recommendations made by the Advisory Council. Fulfilling the recommendations is contingent on limitations on legislative authority, resources, and data among the federal agencies and the federal government, and this appendix makes clear which recommendations have been addressed and which would require congressional authority or additional resources.

Goal 1: Prevent and Effectively Treat Alzheimer Disease and Related Dementias by 2025

Research continues to expand HHS's understanding of the causes of, treatments for, and prevention of AD/ADRD. Goal 1 seeks to develop effective prevention and treatment modalities by 2025. Ongoing research and clinical inquiry can inform HHS's ability to delay onset of AD/ADRD, minimize its symptoms, and delay its progression. Under this goal, HHS will prioritize and accelerate the pace of scientific research and ensure that as evidence-based solutions are identified and quickly translated, put into practice, and brought to scale so that individuals with AD/ADRD can benefit from increases in scientific knowledge. HHS will identify interim milestones and set ambitious deadlines for achieving these milestones in order to meet this goal.

In 2016/2017, Goal 1 showed substantial progress across a spectrum of research areas, thanks to the continued support from the national leadership and the American public, the dedication of study volunteers and their families and caregivers, and the valued work of clinicians and scientists.

Federal funding devoted to AD/ADRD research has expanded over the past several years, reflecting intensified national interest in finding ways to treat these devastating diseases. The National Institutes of Health (NIH) played a lead role by redirecting $50 million in funding in fiscal year (FY) 2012 and allocating $40 million in FY 2013 to promising avenues of AD/ADRD research. Federal appropriations increases to the NIH budget by $100 million in FY 2014 and $25 million in FY 2015, primarily directed toward AD/ADRD research, were also approved.

However, the biggest increases in funding came in FY 2016 and FY 2017, following Congressional passage of the Consolidated Appropriations Act 2016 (P.L. 114-113) and the Consolidated Appropriations Act, 2017 (P.L. 115-31). The FY 2016 appropriations directed an unprecedented additional $350 million toward AD/ADRD research, with an additional $400 million provided for this research in FY 2017; increasing overall NIH funding from Congress for AD/ADRD research by $912 million from FY 2012 to FY 2017. In FY 2017 alone, NIH estimates spending $1.4 billion on AD/ADRD research. This enormous infusion of resources enabled the launch and expansion of research programs and invigorated investigator-initiated research, further accelerating progress towards the Plan's ultimate research goal: finding effective interventions to treat or prevent AD/ADRD by 2025. NIH was already poised to integrate the extraordinary new funds into its research portfolio. In July 2015, NIH released the first of what is now an annual professional judgment budget for Congress—and the American people—estimating the costs of accomplishing the research goals of the National Plan to Address Alzheimer's Disease. This report is known as a "bypass budget" because of its direct transmission to the President and subsequently to Congress without modification through the normal federal budget process. The most recent estimate, submitted in July 2017, outlines funding needs for the most promising research approaches for FY 2019.

The NIH will continue to prepare these estimates through FY 2025. Only two other areas of biomedical research have previously been the subject of this special budget approach: cancer and HIV/AIDS.

Planning for the annual bypass budget and NIH's current AD/ADRD research portfolio are informed by research implementation milestones based on recommendations for AD/ADRD developed at a series of the NIH-convened research summits.

Goal 2: Enhance Care Quality and Efficiency

High-quality care for people with AD/ADRD requires an adequate supply of culturally-competent professionals with appropriate skills, ranging from direct care workers to community health and social workers, to HCBS providers, to primary care providers and specialists. High-quality care should be provided from the point of diagnosis onward in settings including doctor's offices, hospitals, people's homes, and nursing homes. Person-centered quality should be measured accurately and inter-operably across all settings of care, coupled with quality improvement tools.

Further, care should address the complex care needs that persons with AD/ADRD have due to the physical, cognitive, emotional, and behavioral symptoms of the disease and any co-occurring chronic conditions.

High-quality and efficient care often depends on:

1. Smooth transitions between care settings

2. Coordination among healthcare and long-term services and supports (LTSS) providers

3. Dementia-capable healthcare

Goal 3: Expand Supports for People with Alzheimer Disease and Related Dementias and Their Families

Families and other unpaid caregivers play a central role in caring for people with AD/ADRD and may need supports beyond the care provided in settings such as doctors' offices, hospitals, and nursing homes. Supporting people with AD/ADRD and their families and caregivers include providing access to tools that they need and helping to plan for future needs with the goal of maintaining safety and dignity. Under this goal, the federal government and partners will undertake strategies and actions that will support people with the disease and their families and caregivers.

Goal 4: Enhance Public Awareness and Engagement

Most of the public is aware of AD/ADRD; more than 85 percent of people surveyed can identify the disease and its symptoms. AD/ADRD is also one of the most feared health conditions. Yet there are widespread and significant public misperceptions about diagnosis and clinical management. These issues can lead to delayed diagnosis, and to people with the disease and their caregivers feeling isolated and stigmatized. Enhancing public awareness and engagement is an essential goal because it forms the basis for advancing the subsequent goals of the National Plan. A better understanding of AD/ADRD will help engage stakeholders who can help address the challenges faced by people with the disease and their families and caregivers. These stakeholders include a range of groups such as healthcare providers who care for people with AD/ADRD and their caregivers, employers whose employees request flexibility to care for a loved one with the disease, groups whose members are caregivers, and broader aging organizations. The strategies and actions under this goal are designed to educate these and other groups about the disease.

Goal 5: Improve Data to Track Progress

The federal government is committed to better understanding AD/ADRD and its impact on individuals, families, the health and long-term care systems, and society as a whole. Data and surveillance efforts are paramount to tracking the burden of AD/ADRD on individual and population health, and will be used to identify and monitor trends in risk factors associated with AD/ADRD, and assist with understanding health disparities among populations such as racial and ethnic minorities. HHS will make efforts to expand and enhance data infrastructure and make data easily accessible to federal agencies and other researchers. This data infrastructure will help HHS in its multi-level monitoring and evaluation of progress on the National Plan.

Part Two

Alzheimer Disease: The Most Common Type of Dementia

Chapter 8

Facts about Alzheimer Disease

Alzheimer disease (AD) is an irreversible, progressive brain disorder that slowly destroys memory and thinking skills, and eventually the ability to carry out the simplest tasks. In most people with AD, symptoms first appear in their mid-60s. Estimates vary, but experts suggest that more than 5.5 million Americans may have AD.

Alzheimer disease is ranked as the sixth leading cause of death in the United States, but some estimates indicate that the disorder may rank third, just behind heart disease and cancer, as a cause of death for older people.

AD is the most common cause of dementia among older adults. Dementia is the loss of cognitive functioning—thinking, remembering, and reasoning—and behavioral abilities to such an extent that it interferes with a person's daily life and activities. Dementia ranges in severity from the mildest stage, when it is just beginning to affect a person's functioning, to the most severe stage, when the person must depend completely on others for basic activities of daily living.

The causes of dementia can vary, depending on the types of brain changes that may be taking place. Other dementias include "Lewy body dementia (LBD)," frontotemporal disorders (FTD), and vascular dementia. It is common for people to have mixed dementia—a

This chapter includes text excerpted from "Alzheimer's Disease Fact Sheet," National Institute on Aging (NIA), National Institutes of Health (NIH), August 17, 2016.

combination of two or more disorders, at least one of which is dementia. For example, some people have both Alzheimer disease and vascular dementia.

Alzheimer disease is named after Dr. Alois Alzheimer. In 1906, Dr. Alzheimer noticed changes in the brain tissue of a woman who had died of an unusual mental illness. Her symptoms included memory loss, language problems, and unpredictable behavior. After she died, he examined her brain and found many abnormal clumps (now called amyloid plaques) and tangled bundles of fibers (now called neurofibrillary, or tau, tangles).

These plaques and tangles in the brain are still considered some of the main features of Alzheimer disease. Another feature is the loss of connections between nerve cells (neurons) in the brain. Neurons transmit messages between different parts of the brain, and from the brain to muscles and organs in the body.

Changes in the Brain

Scientists continue to unravel the complex brain changes involved in the onset and progression of Alzheimer disease. It seems likely that damage to the brain starts a decade or more before memory and other cognitive problems appear. During this preclinical stage of Alzheimer disease, people seem to be symptom-free, but toxic changes are taking place in the brain. Abnormal deposits of proteins form amyloid plaques and tau tangles throughout the brain, and once-healthy neurons stop functioning, lose connections with other neurons, and die.

The damage initially appears to take place in the hippocampus, the part of the brain essential in forming memories. As more neurons die, additional parts of the brain are affected, and they begin to shrink. By the final stage of AD, damage is widespread, and brain tissue has shrunk significantly.

Signs and Symptoms

Memory problems are typically one of the first signs of cognitive impairment related to Alzheimer disease. Some people with memory problems have a condition called mild cognitive impairment (MCI). In MCI, people have more memory problems than normal for their age, but their symptoms do not interfere with their everyday lives. Movement difficulties and problems with the sense of smell have also been linked to MCI. Older people with MCI are at greater risk for developing AD, but not all of them do. Some may even go back to normal cognition.

The first symptoms of AD vary from person to person. For many, decline in nonmemory aspects of cognition, such as word-finding, vision/spatial issues, and impaired reasoning or judgment, may signal the very early stages of Alzheimer disease. Researchers are studying biomarkers (biological signs of disease found in brain images, cerebrospinal fluid (CSF), and blood) to see if they can detect early changes in the brains of people with MCI and in cognitively normal people who may be at greater risk for AD. Studies indicate that such early detection may be possible, but more research is needed before these techniques can be relied upon to diagnose Alzheimer disease in everyday medical practice.

Healthy Brain   Severe Alzheimer's

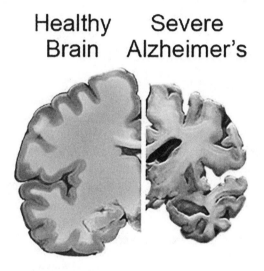

Figure 8.1. *Changes in the Brain*

Mild Alzheimer Disease

As Alzheimer disease progresses, people experience greater memory loss and other cognitive difficulties. Problems can include wandering and getting lost, trouble handling money and paying bills, repeating questions, taking longer to complete normal daily tasks, and personality and behavior changes. People are often diagnosed in this stage.

Moderate Alzheimer Disease

In this stage, damage occurs in areas of the brain that control language, reasoning, sensory processing, and conscious thought. Memory loss and confusion grow worse, and people begin to have problems recognizing family and friends. They may be unable to learn new things, carry out multistep tasks such as getting dressed, or cope with new situations. In addition, people at this stage may have hallucinations, delusions, and paranoia and may behave impulsively.

Severe Alzheimer Disease

Ultimately, plaques and tangles spread throughout the brain, and brain tissue shrinks significantly. People with severe AD cannot communicate and are completely dependent on others for their care. Near the end, the person may be in bed most or all of the time as the body shuts down.

What Causes Alzheimer Disease

Scientists don't yet fully understand what causes Alzheimer disease in most people. There is a genetic component to some cases of early-onset Alzheimer disease (EOAD). Late-onset Alzheimer disease arises from a complex series of brain changes that occur over decades. The causes probably include a combination of genetic, environmental, and lifestyle factors. The importance of any one of these factors in increasing or decreasing the risk of developing Alzheimer disease may differ from person to person.

The Basics of Alzheimer Disease

Scientists are conducting studies to learn more about plaques, tangles, and other biological features of Alzheimer disease. Advances in brain imaging techniques allow researchers to see the development and spread of abnormal amyloid and tau proteins in the living brain, as well as changes in brain structure and function. Scientists are also exploring the very earliest steps in the disease process by studying changes in the brain and body fluids that can be detected years before Alzheimer disease symptoms appear. Findings from these studies will help in understanding the causes of Alzheimer disease and make diagnosis easier.

One of the great mysteries of Alzheimer disease is why it largely strikes older adults. Research on normal brain aging is shedding light on this question. For example, scientists are learning how age-related changes in the brain may harm neurons and contribute to AD damage. These age-related changes include atrophy (shrinking) of certain parts of the brain, inflammation, production of unstable molecules called free radicals, and mitochondrial dysfunction (a breakdown of energy production within a cell).

Genetics

Most people with Alzheimer disease have the late-onset form of the disease, in which symptoms become apparent in their mid-60s. The apolipoprotein E (APOE) gene is involved in late-onset Alzheimer disease. This gene has several forms. One of them, APOE ε4, increases a person's risk of developing the disease and is also associated with an earlier age of disease onset. However, carrying the APOE ε4 form of the gene does not mean that a person will definitely develop Alzheimer disease, and some people with no APOE ε4 may also develop the disease.

Also, scientists have identified a number of regions of interest in the genome (an organism's complete set of "deoxyribonucleic acid (DNA)" that may increase a person's risk for late-onset Alzheimer disease to varying degrees.

Early-onset Alzheimer disease (EOAD) occurs between a person's thirties to mid-sixties and represents less than ten percent of all people with AD. Some cases are caused by an inherited change in one of three genes, resulting in a type known as early-onset familial Alzheimer disease, or FAD. For other cases of early-onset Alzheimer disease, research suggests there may be a genetic component related to factors other than these three genes.

Most people with Down syndrome (DS) develop AD. This may be because people with Down syndrome have an extra copy of chromosome 21, which contains the gene that generates harmful amyloid.

Health, Environmental, and Lifestyle Factors

Research suggests that a host of factors beyond genetics may play a role in the development and course of Alzheimer disease. There is a great deal of interest, for example, in the relationship between cognitive decline and vascular conditions such as heart disease, stroke, and high blood pressure, as well as metabolic conditions such as diabetes and obesity. Ongoing research will help understand whether and how reducing risk factors for these conditions may also reduce the risk of Alzheimer disease.

A nutritious diet, physical activity, social engagement, and mentally stimulating pursuits have all been associated with helping people stay healthy as they age. These factors might also help reduce the risk of cognitive decline and Alzheimer disease. Clinical trials are testing some of these possibilities.

Diagnosis of Alzheimer Disease

Doctors use several methods and tools to help determine whether a person who is having memory problems has "possible Alzheimer dementia" (dementia may be due to another cause) or "probable Alzheimer dementia" (no other cause for dementia can be found).

To diagnose AD, doctors may:

- Ask the person and a family member or friend questions about overall health, past medical problems, ability to carry out daily activities, and changes in behavior and personality

- Conduct tests of memory, problem-solving, attention, counting, and language

- Carry out standard medical tests, such as blood and urine tests, to identify other possible causes of the problem

- Perform brain scans, such as computed tomography (CT), magnetic resonance imaging (MRI), or positron emission tomography (PET), to rule out other possible causes for symptoms.

These tests may be repeated to give doctors information about how the person's memory and other cognitive functions are changing over time.

Alzheimer disease can be definitely diagnosed only after death, by linking clinical measures with an examination of brain tissue in an autopsy.

People with memory and thinking concerns should talk to their doctor to find out whether their symptoms are due to AD or another cause, such as stroke, tumor, Parkinson disease (PD), sleep disturbances, side effects of medication, an infection, or a non-Alzheimer dementia. Some of these conditions may be treatable and possibly reversible.

If the diagnosis is Alzheimer disease, beginning treatment early in the disease process may help preserve daily functioning for some time, even though the underlying disease process cannot be stopped or reversed. An early diagnosis also helps families plan for the future. They can take care of financial and legal matters, address potential safety issues, learn about living arrangements, and develop support networks.

In addition, an early diagnosis gives people greater opportunities to participate in clinical trials that are testing possible new treatments for Alzheimer disease or other research studies.

Treatment of Alzheimer Disease

Alzheimer disease is complex, and it is unlikely that any one drug or other intervention can successfully treat it. Current approaches focus on helping people maintain mental function, manage behavioral symptoms, and slow down certain problems, such as memory loss. Researchers hope to develop therapies targeting specific genetic, molecular, and cellular mechanisms so that the actual underlying cause of the disease can be stopped or prevented.

Maintaining Mental Function

Several medications are approved by the U.S. Food and Drug Administration (FDA) to treat symptoms of AD. Donepezil (Aricept®), rivastigmine (Exelon®), and galantamine (Razadyne®) are used to treat mild to moderate Alzheimer disease (donepezil can be used for severe Alzheimer disease as well). Memantine (Namenda®) is used to treat moderate to severe AD. These drugs work by regulating neurotransmitters, the chemicals that transmit messages between neurons. They may help reduce symptoms and help with certain behavioral problems. However, these drugs don't change the underlying disease process. They are effective for some but not all people, and may help only for a limited time. The FDA has also approved Aricept® and Namzaric®, a combination of Namenda® and Aricept®, for the treatment of moderate to severe Alzheimer disease.

Managing Behavior

Common behavioral symptoms of Alzheimer disease include sleeplessness, wandering, agitation, anxiety, and aggression. Scientists are learning why these symptoms occur and are studying new treatments—drug and nondrug—to manage them. Research has shown that treating behavioral symptoms can make people with Alzheimer disease more comfortable and makes things easier for caregivers.

Looking for New Treatments

Alzheimer disease research has developed to a point where scientists can look beyond treating symptoms to think about addressing underlying disease processes. In ongoing clinical trials, scientists are developing and testing several possible interventions, including immunization therapy, drug therapies, cognitive training, physical activity, and treatments used for cardiovascular disease and diabetes.

Support for Families and Caregivers

Caring for a person with Alzheimer disease can have high physical, emotional, and financial costs. The demands of day-to-day care, changes in family roles, and decisions about placement in a care facility can be difficult. There are several evidence-based approaches and programs that can help, and researchers are continuing to look for new and better ways to support caregivers.

Becoming well-informed about the disease is one important long-term strategy. Programs that teach families about the various stages of Alzheimer disease and about ways to deal with difficult behaviors and other caregiving challenges can help.

Good coping skills, a strong support network, and respite care are other ways that help caregivers handle the stress of caring for a loved one with Alzheimer disease. For example, staying physically active provides physical and emotional benefits.

Some caregivers have found that joining a support group is a critical lifeline. These support groups allow caregivers to find respite, express concerns, share experiences, get tips, and receive emotional comfort. Many organizations sponsor in-person and online support groups, including groups for people with early-stage Alzheimer disease and their families.

Chapter 9

What Happens to the Brain in Alzheimer Disease

The healthy human brain contains tens of billions of neurons—specialized cells that process and transmit information via electrical and chemical signals. They send messages between different parts of the brain, and from the brain to the muscles and organs of the body. Alzheimer disease (AD) disrupts this communication among neurons, resulting in loss of function and cell death.

Key Biological Processes in the Brain

Most neurons have three basic parts: a cell body, multiple dendrites, and an axon.

- The cell body contains the nucleus, which houses the genetic blueprint that directs and regulates the cell's activities.

- Dendrites are branch-like structures that extend from the cell body and collect information from other neurons.

- The axon is a cable-like structure at the end of the cell body opposite the dendrites and transmits messages to other neurons.

This chapter includes text excerpted from "What Happens to the Brain in Alzheimer's Disease?" National Institute on Aging (NIA), National Institutes of Health (NIH), May 16, 2017.

The function and survival of neurons depend on several key biological processes:

- **Communication.** Neurons are constantly in touch with neighboring brain cells. When a neuron receives signals from other neurons, it generates an electrical charge that travels down the length of its axon and releases neurotransmitter chemicals across a tiny gap, called a synapse. Like a key fitting into a lock, each neurotransmitter molecule then binds to specific receptor sites on a dendrite of a nearby neuron. This process triggers chemical or electrical signals that either stimulate or inhibit activity in the neuron receiving the signal. Communication often occurs across networks of brain cells. In fact, scientists estimate that in the brain's communications network, one neuron may have as many as 7,000 synaptic connections with other neurons.

- **Metabolism.** Metabolism—the breaking down of chemicals and nutrients within a cell—is critical to healthy cell function and survival. To perform this function, cells require energy in the form of oxygen and glucose, which are supplied by blood circulating through the brain. The brain has one of the richest blood supplies of any organ and consumes up to 20 percent of the energy used by the human body—more than any other organ.

- **Repair, remodeling, and regeneration.** Unlike many cells in the body, which are relatively short-lived, neurons have evolved to live a long time—more than 100 years in humans. As a result, neurons must constantly maintain and repair themselves. Neurons also continuously adjust, or "remodel," their synaptic connections depending on how much stimulation they receive from other neurons. For example, they may strengthen or weaken synaptic connections, or even break down connections with one group of neurons and build new connections with a different group. Adult brains may even generate new neurons—a process called neurogenesis. Remodeling of synaptic connections and neurogenesis are important for learning, memory, and possibly brain repair.

Neurons are a major player in the central nervous system, but other cell types are also key to healthy brain function. In fact, glial cells are by far the most numerous cells in the brain, outnumbering neurons by about 10 to 1. These cells, which come in various forms— such as microglia, astrocytes, and oligodendrocytes—surround and support the function and health of neurons. For example, microglia protect neurons from physical and chemical damage and are responsible for clearing foreign substances and cellular debris from the brain. To carry out these functions, glial cells often collaborate with blood vessels in the brain. Together, glial and blood vessel cells regulate the delicate balance within the brain to ensure that it functions at its best.

How Does Alzheimer Disease Affect the Brain?

The brain typically shrinks to some degree in healthy aging but, surprisingly, does not lose neurons in large numbers. In Alzheimer disease, however, damage is widespread, as many neurons stop functioning, lose connections with other neurons, and die. AD disrupts processes vital to neurons and their networks, including communication, metabolism, and repair.

At first, Alzheimer disease typically destroys neurons and their connections in parts of the brain involved in memory, including the entorhinal cortex and hippocampus. It later affects areas in the cerebral cortex responsible for language, reasoning, and social behavior. Eventually, many other areas of the brain are damaged. Over time, a person with Alzheimer disease gradually loses his or her ability to live and function independently. Ultimately, the disease is fatal.

What Are the Main Characteristics of the Brain with Alzheimer Disease?

Many molecular and cellular changes take place in the brain of a person with Alzheimer disease. These changes can be observed in brain tissue under the microscope after death. Investigations are underway to determine which changes may cause Alzheimer disease and which may be a result of the disease.

Amyloid Plaques

The beta-amyloid (Aβ) protein involved in Alzheimer disease comes in several different molecular forms that collect between neurons. It is formed from the breakdown of a larger protein, called amyloid precursor protein (APP). One form, beta-amyloid 42, is thought to be especially toxic. In the Alzheimer disease brain, abnormal levels of this naturally occurring protein clump together to form plaques that collect between neurons and disrupt cell function. Research is ongoing to better understand how, and at what stage of the disease, the various forms of beta-amyloid influence Alzheimer disease.

Neurofibrillary Tangles

Neurofibrillary tangles are abnormal accumulations of a protein called tau that collects inside neurons. Healthy neurons, in part, are supported internally by structures called microtubules, which help guide nutrients and molecules from the cell body to the axon and dendrites. In healthy neurons, tau normally binds to and stabilizes microtubules. In Alzheimer disease, however, abnormal chemical changes cause tau to detach from microtubules and stick to other tau molecules, forming threads that eventually join to form tangles inside neurons. These tangles block the neuron's transport system, which harms the synaptic communication between neurons.

Emerging evidence suggests that Alzheimer disease-related brain changes may result from a complex interplay among abnormal tau and beta-amyloid proteins and several other factors. It appears that abnormal tau accumulates in specific brain regions involved in memory. Beta-amyloid clumps into plaques between neurons. As the level of beta-amyloid reaches a tipping point, there is a rapid spread of tau throughout the brain.

Chronic Inflammation

Research suggests that chronic inflammation may be caused by the buildup of glial cells normally meant to help keep the brain free of debris. One type of glial cell, microglia, engulfs and destroys waste and toxins in a healthy brain. In Alzheimer disease, microglia fail to clear away waste, debris, and protein collections, including beta-amyloid plaques. Researchers are trying to find out why microglia fail to perform this vital function in Alzheimer disease.

One focus of study is a gene called *TREM2*. Normally, *TREM2* tells the microglia cells to clear beta-amyloid plaques from the brain and helps fight inflammation in the brain. In the brains of people where this gene does not function normally, plaques build up between neurons. Astrocytes—another type of glial cell—are signaled to help clear the buildup of plaques and other cellular debris left behind. These microglia and astrocytes collect around the neurons but fail to perform their debris-clearing function. In addition, they release chemicals that cause chronic inflammation and further damage the neurons they are meant to protect.

Vascular Contributions to Alzheimer Disease

People with dementia seldom have only Alzheimer disease-related changes in their brains. Any number of vascular issues—problems that affect blood vessels, such as beta-amyloid deposits in brain arteries, atherosclerosis (hardening of the arteries), and ministrokes—may also be at play.

Vascular problems may lead to reduced blood flow and oxygen to the brain, as well as a breakdown of the blood–brain barrier (BBB), which usually protects the brain from harmful agents while allowing in glucose and other necessary factors. In a person with Alzheimer disease, a faulty blood–brain barrier (BBB), prevents glucose from reaching the brain and prevents the clearing away of toxic beta-amyloid and tau proteins. This results in inflammation, which adds to vascular problems in the brain. Because it appears that Alzheimer disease is both a cause and consequence of vascular problems in the brain, researchers are seeking interventions to disrupt this complicated and destructive cycle.

Loss of Neuronal Connections and Cell Death

In Alzheimer disease, as neurons are injured and die throughout the brain, connections between networks of neurons may break down, and many brain regions begin to shrink. By the final stages of Alzheimer disease, this process—called brain atrophy—is widespread, causing significant loss of brain volume.

Chapter 10

Signs and Symptoms of Alzheimer Disease

Scientists continue to unravel the complex brain changes involved in the onset and progression of Alzheimer disease (AD). It seems likely that damage to the brain starts a decade or more before memory and other cognitive problems appear. During this preclinical stage of Alzheimer disease, people seem to be symptom-free, but toxic changes are taking place in the brain.

Damage occurring in the brain of someone with Alzheimer disease begins to show itself in very early clinical signs and symptoms. For most people with AD—those who have the late-onset variety—symptoms first appear in their mid-sixties. Signs of early-onset AD begin between a person's thirties and mid-sixties.

The first symptoms of AD vary from person to person. Memory problems are typically one of the first signs of cognitive impairment related to Alzheimer disease. Decline in nonmemory aspects of cognition, such as word-finding, vision/spatial issues, and impaired reasoning or judgment, may also signal the very early stages of Alzheimer disease. And some people may be diagnosed with mild cognitive impairment (MCI). As the disease progresses, people experience greater memory loss and other cognitive difficulties.

This chapter includes text excerpted from "What Are the Signs of Alzheimer's Disease?" National Institute on Aging (NIA), National Institutes of Health (NIH), May 16, 2017.

Alzheimer disease progresses in several stages: preclinical, mild (sometimes called early-stage), moderate, and severe (sometimes called late-stage).

Signs of Mild Alzheimer Disease

In mild Alzheimer disease, a person may seem to be healthy but has more and more trouble making sense of the world around him or her. The realization that something is wrong often comes gradually to the person and his or her family. Problems can include:

- Memory loss
- Poor judgment leading to bad decisions
- Loss of spontaneity and sense of initiative
- Taking longer to complete normal daily tasks
- Repeating questions
- Trouble handling money and paying bills
- Wandering and getting lost
- Losing things or misplacing them in odd places
- Mood and personality changes
- Increased anxiety and/or aggression
- Alzheimer disease is often diagnosed at this stage

Signs of Moderate Alzheimer Disease

In this stage, more intensive supervision and care become necessary, which can be difficult for many spouses and families. Symptoms may include:

- Increased memory loss and confusion
- Inability to learn new things
- Difficulty with language and problems with reading, writing, and working with numbers
- Difficulty organizing thoughts and thinking logically
- Shortened attention span
- Problems coping with new situations

- Difficulty carrying out multistep tasks, such as getting dressed
- Problems recognizing family and friends
- Hallucinations, delusions, and paranoia
- Impulsive behavior such as undressing at inappropriate times or places or using vulgar language
- Inappropriate outbursts of anger
- Restlessness, agitation, anxiety, tearfulness, wandering—especially in the late afternoon or evening
- Repetitive statements or movement, occasional muscle twitches

Signs of Severe Alzheimer Disease

People with severe AD cannot communicate and are completely dependent on others for their care. Near the end, the person may be in bed most or all of the time as the body shuts down. Their symptoms often include:

- Inability to communicate
- Weight loss
- Seizures
- Skin infections
- Difficulty swallowing
- Groaning, moaning, or grunting
- Increased sleeping
- Loss of bowel and bladder control

A common cause of death for people with Alzheimer disease is aspiration pneumonia. This type of pneumonia develops when a person cannot swallow properly and takes food or liquids into the lungs instead of air.

There is currently no cure for AD, though there are medicines that can treat the symptoms of the disease.

Chapter 11

The Connection between Alzheimer Disease and Genes

Alzheimer disease (AD) is an illness of the brain. It breaks down connections among brain cells and causes these cells to die. Over time, this affects how well a person can remember, think clearly, and use good judgment. AD begins slowly and gets worse over time. Many people wonder if AD runs in the family. Your chance of having the disease may be higher if you have certain genes passed down from a parent. However, having a parent with AD does not always mean that you will develop it.

What Are Genes?

Genes are found in every cell in every person's body (except red blood cells (RBCs)). They are passed down from a person's birth parents. They carry information that defines traits such as eye color and height.

Genes also play a role in keeping the body's cells healthy. Problems with genes—even small changes to a gene—can cause diseases like Alzheimer disease.

This chapter includes text excerpted from "Understanding Alzheimer's Genes," National Institute on Aging (NIA), National Institutes of Health (NIH), August 2016.

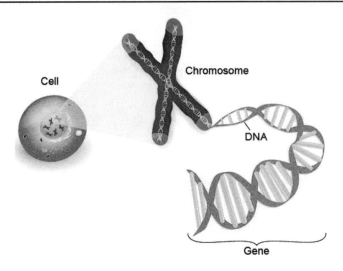

Figure 11.1. *Gene*

Each human cell contains the instructions a cell needs to do its job. These instructions are made up of deoxyribonucleic acid (DNA), which is packed tightly into structures called chromosomes. Each chromosome has thousands of segments called genes. Parents pass down genes to their children.

Do Genes Cause Alzheimer Disease?

AD is a complex disease. Doctors and scientists don't know yet exactly what causes it. But we do know that a person's genes can affect how likely they are to develop the disease. Having certain genes is a risk factor for Alzheimer disease.

A risk factor is something that increases the chance of getting a disease. For example, smoking is a risk factor for cancer. High blood pressure is a risk factor for stroke.

Risk factors can include:

- Genes passed down from a parent to a child

- A person's health habits, like eating unhealthy food or being inactive

- Something in a person's surroundings, like in the air or water

Genetic risk factors are changes or differences in genes that can influence the chance of getting a disease. These risk factors are the reason some diseases run in families.

There are two types of Alzheimer disease—late-onset and early-onset. They have different genetic risk factors.

Late-Onset Alzheimer Disease

Most people with Alzheimer disease first show signs of the disease when they are in their mid-60s or later. The risk for late-onset Alzheimer disease increases as a person gets older. The causes of late-onset Alzheimer disease are not fully known. They likely involve a mix of genes, lifestyle, and environment. A gene called APOE is often involved in Alzheimer disease. Genes can have multiple forms. One form of APOE, called APOE e4, increases the risk for late-onset Alzheimer disease. But, not everyone with APOE e4 will develop Alzheimer disease. Also, people without this gene form can still develop the disease.

Early-Onset Alzheimer Disease

Early-onset Alzheimer disease is another type of the disease. People with this type start to show signs between age 30 and age 60. It is very rare. Most people with early-onset Alzheimer disease have familial Alzheimer disease, or FAD. Some types of FAD are caused by a permanent change in one or more genes. The genetic change is passed down from a parent to a child. Some people with early-onset Alzheimer disease do not have FAD. The reason they get the disease is not known.

Some differences between late-onset and early-onset Alzheimer disease

Table 11.1. Differences between Late-Onset and Early-Onset Alzheimer Disease

Late-Onset Alzheimer Disease	Early-Onset Alzheimer Disease
Signs first appear in a person's mid-60s	Signs first appear between a person's 30s and mid-60s
Most common type	Very rare
May involve a gene called APOE ε4	Usually caused by gene changes passed down from parent to child

Down Syndrome and Alzheimer Disease

Many, but not all, people with Down syndrome develop Alzheimer disease as they get older. People with Down syndrome are born with an extra copy of chromosome 21. This chromosome carries a gene that increases the risk of Alzheimer disease. This type of Alzheimer disease is not passed down from a parent to a child.

If Someone in My Family Has Had Alzheimer Disease, Will I Have It, Too?

Many people worry about developing Alzheimer disease, especially if a family member has had it. Having a family history of the disease does not mean for sure that you'll have it, too. But, it may mean you are more likely to develop it.

Late-Onset Alzheimer Disease

No one can yet predict if you will develop late-onset Alzheimer disease, even if it runs in your family. Late-onset Alzheimer disease (LOAD) has been linked to APOE e4. But, having this gene form does not always mean a person will develop the disease.

Early-Onset Alzheimer Disease

Familial Alzheimer disease, or FAD—the most common type of early-onset Alzheimer disease—is inherited. If a parent has a gene for FAD, there is a 50/50 chance that a child will inherit the gene. If the gene is passed down, the child will usually—but not always—have FAD. Doctors and scientists don't yet know if other types of early-onset Alzheimer disease can be passed down.

How Can I Know If I'm at Increased Risk for Alzheimer Disease?

Families have many things in common, including their genes, environment, and lifestyle. Together, these things may offer clues to diseases, like Alzheimer disease, that can run in a family.

Late-Onset Alzheimer Disease

There is no test yet to predict if someone will get late-onset Alzheimer disease. If you are worried about changes in your memory or other problems with your thinking, talk with your doctor. Let him or her know if one or more close relatives has had the disease. Your doctor can suggest ways to stay healthy and watch for changes in your memory and thinking.

Early-Onset Alzheimer Disease

There is a test to learn if you have the gene changes that cause familial Alzheimer disease, or FAD.

If you have a family history of FAD, talk with your doctor about getting tested. It's your choice to get tested or not.

Your doctor may suggest meeting first with a genetic counselor. This type of counselor helps people learn the risk of getting genetic conditions. They also help people make decisions about testing and what comes next.

What Can I Do If I'm at Increased Risk for Alzheimer Disease?

No medicine or other treatment is currently known to prevent or delay Alzheimer disease. But, you can take steps to keep your brain and body as healthy as possible.

These steps included are as follows:

- Exercise regularly

- Eat a healthy diet that is rich in fruits and vegetables

- Spend time with family and friends

- Keep your mind active

- Control type 2 diabetes

- Keep blood pressure and cholesterol at healthy levels

- Maintain a healthy weight

- Stop smoking

- Get help for depression

- Avoid drinking a lot of alcohol

- Get plenty of sleep

Talk with your doctor if you or someone close to you sees changes in your memory or thinking.

Learn about Clinical Trials and Studies

Joining a clinical trial or other research study is a way to help fight Alzheimer disease. Some studies need people with a family history of Alzheimer disease, and some seek families with early-onset Alzheimer disease, or FAD. Other studies need healthy people with no history of the disease. To find out more about clinical trials and studies:

- Call the Alzheimer Disease Education and Referral (ADEAR) Center at 800-438-4380. It's a free call.

- Visit the ADEAR Center website at www.nia.nih.gov/alzheimers/ volunteer

- Contact an Alzheimer Disease Research Center. All Centers are listed at www.nia.nih.gov/alzheimers/ alzheimers-disease-research-centers.

- See "NIH Clinical Research Trials and You" at www.nih.gov/ health/clinicaltrials

What Do I Need to Know?

- Genes are passed down from a person's birth parents. They carry information that determines a person's traits. They also play a role in keeping a body's cells healthy.

- Small changes or differences in a gene can lead to some diseases, such as Alzheimer disease.

- A family history of Alzheimer disease may mean a person is more likely to develop the disease. But, it does not mean she or he will get Alzheimer disease for sure.

- People can take steps to keep their brains and bodies as healthy as possible.

- Joining a clinical trial or signing up for a registry is a way to help fight Alzheimer disease.

Talk with your doctor if you or someone close to you has changes in memory or thinking. Your doctor can help find out what might be causing the problems. Many things that cause memory or thinking problems can be treated.

Chapter 12

Clinical Stages of Alzheimer Disease

Preclinical Alzheimer Disease

Alzheimer disease (AD) begins deep in the brain, in the entorhinal cortex, a brain region that is near the hippocampus and has direct connections to it. Healthy neurons in this region begin to work less efficiently, lose their ability to communicate, and ultimately die. is process gradually spreads to the hippocampus, the brain region that plays a major role in learning and is involved in converting short-term memories to long-term memories. Affected regions begin to atrophy. Ventricles, the fluid-filled spaces inside the brain, begin to enlarge as the process continues. Scientists believe that these brain changes begin 10 to 20 years before any clinically detectable signs or symptoms of forgetfulness appear. That's why they are increasingly interested in the very early stages of the disease process. They hope to learn more about what happens in the brain that sets a person on the path to developing AD. By knowing more about the early stages, they also hope to be able to develop drugs or other treatments that will slow or stop the disease process before significant impairment occurs.

This chapter includes text excerpted from "Alzheimer's Disease: Unraveling the Mystery," National Institute on Aging (NIA), National Institutes of Health (NIH), September 2008. Reviewed December 2018.

Very Early Signs and Symptoms

At some point, the damage occurring in the brain begins to show itself in very early clinical signs and symptoms. Much research is being done to identify these early changes, which may be useful in predicting dementia or AD. An important part of this research effort is the development of increasingly sophisticated neuroimaging techniques and the use of biomarkers. Biomarkers are indicators, such as changes in sensory abilities, or substances that appear in body fluids, such as blood, cerebrospinal fluid (CSF), or urine. Biomarkers can indicate exposure to a substance, the presence of a disease, or the progression over time of a disease. For example, high blood cholesterol is a biomarker for risk of heart disease. Such tools are critical to helping scientists detect and understand the very early signs and symptoms of AD.

Mild Cognitive Impairment

As some people grow older, they develop memory problems greater than those expected for their age. But they do not experience the personality changes or other problems that are characteristic of AD. These people may have a condition called mild cognitive impairment (MCI). MCI has several subtypes. The type most associated with memory loss is called amnestic MCI. People with MCI are a critically important group for research because a much higher percentage of them go on to develop AD than do people without these memory problems. About 8 of every 10 people who fit the definition of amnestic MCI go on to develop AD within seven years. In contrast, 1 to 3 percent of people older than 65 who have normal cognition will develop AD in any one year. However, researchers are not yet able to say definitively why some people with amnestic MCI do not progress to AD, nor can they say who will or will not go on to develop AD. is raises pressing questions, such as: In cases when MCI progresses to AD, what was happening in the brain that made that transition possible? Can MCI be prevented or its progress to AD delayed? Scientists also have found that genetic factors may play a role in MCI, as they do in AD. And, they have found that different brain regions appear to be activated during certain mental activities in cognitively healthy people and those with MCI. These changes appear to be related to the early stages of cognitive impairment.

Other Signs of Early Alzheimer Disease Development

- As scientists have sharpened their focus on the early stages of AD, they have begun to see hints of other changes that may signal a developing disease process. For example, in the Religious Orders Study, a large AD research effort that involves older nuns, priests, and religious brothers, investigators have explored whether changes in older adults' ability to move about and use their bodies might be a sign of early AD. The researchers found that participants with MCI had more movement difficulties than the cognitively healthy participants but less than those with AD. Moreover, those with MCI who had lots of trouble moving their legs and feet were more than twice as likely to develop AD as those with good lower body function.

- It is not yet clear why people with MCI might have these motor function problems, but the scientists who conducted the study speculate that they may be a sign that damage to blood vessels in the brain or damage from AD is accumulating in areas of the brain responsible for motor function. If further research shows that some people with MCI do have motor function problems in addition to memory problems, the degree of difficulty, especially with walking, may help identify those at risk of progressing to AD.

- Other scientists have focused on changes in sensory abilities as possible indicators of early cognitive problems. For example, in one study they found associations between a decline in the ability to detect odors and cognitive problems or dementia.

- These findings are tentative, but they are promising because they suggest that, someday, it may be possible to develop ways to improve early detection of MCI or AD. These tools also will help scientists answer questions about causes and very early development of AD, track changes in brain and cognitive function over time, and ultimately track a person's response to treatment for AD.

Mild Alzheimer Disease

As AD spreads through the brain, the number of plaques and tangles grows, shrinkage progresses, and more and more of the cerebral cortex is affected. Memory loss continues and changes in other cognitive abilities begin to emerge. The clinical diagnosis of AD is usually made during this stage. Signs of mild AD can include:

- Memory loss
- Confusion about the location of familiar places (getting lost begins to occur)

- Taking longer than before to accomplish normal daily tasks
- Trouble handling money and paying bills
- Poor judgment leading to bad decisions
- Loss of spontaneity and sense of initiative
- Mood and personality changes, increased anxiety and/or aggression

In mild AD, a person may seem to be healthy but is actually having more and more trouble making sense of the world around him or her. The realization that something is wrong often comes gradually to the person and his or her family.

Accepting these signs as something other than normal and deciding to go for diagnostic tests can be a big hurdle for people and families. Once this hurdle is overcome, many families are relieved to know what is causing the problems. They also can take comfort in the fact that despite a diagnosis of MCI or early AD, a person can still make meaningful contributions to his or her family and to society for a time.

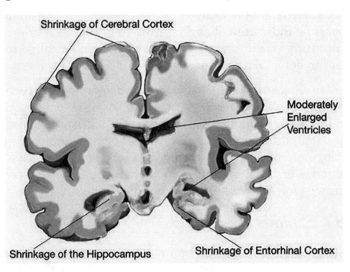

Figure 12.1. *Mild to Moderate Alzheimer Disease*

Moderate Alzheimer Disease

By this stage, AD damage has spread to the areas of the cerebral cortex that control language, reasoning, sensory processing, and conscious thought. Affected regions continue to shrink, ventricles enlarge, and signs and symptoms of the disease become more pronounced and widespread. Behavioral problems, such as wandering and agitation, can occur. More intensive supervision and care become necessary, which can be difficult for many spouses and families. The symptoms of this stage can include:

- Increasing memory loss and confusion
- Shortened attention span
- Inappropriate outbursts of anger
- Problems recognizing friends and family members
- Difficulty with language and problems with reading, writing, and working with numbers
- Difficulty organizing thoughts and thinking logically
- Inability to learn new things or to cope with new or unexpected situations
- Restlessness, agitation, anxiety, tearfulness, wandering— especially in the late afternoon or at night
- Repetitive statements or movement, occasional muscle twitches
- Hallucinations, delusions, suspiciousness or paranoia, irritability
- Loss of impulse control (shown through undressing at inappropriate times or places or vulgar language)
- An inability to carry out activities that involve multiple steps in sequence, such as dressing, making a pot of coffee, or setting the table

Behavior is the result of complex brain processes, all of which take place in a fraction of a second in the healthy brain. In AD, many of those processes are disturbed, and these disrupted communications between neurons are the basis for many distressing or inappropriate behaviors.

For example, a person may angrily refuse to take a bath or get dressed because he does not understand what his caregiver has asked him to do. If The does understand, he may not remember how to do it. The anger can be a mask for his confusion and anxiety. Or, a person with AD may constantly follow her husband or caregiver and fret when the person is out of sight. To a person who cannot remember the past or anticipate the future, the world can be strange and frightening.

Sticking close to a trusted and familiar caregiver may be the only thing that makes sense and provides security.

Severe Alzheimer Disease

In the last stage of AD, plaques and tangles are widespread throughout the brain, most areas of the brain have shrunk further, and ventricles have enlarged even more. People with AD cannot recognize family and loved ones or communicate in any way. They are completely dependent on others for care. Other symptoms can include:

- Weight loss

- Seizures

- Skin infections

- Difficulty swallowing

- Groaning, moaning, or grunting

- Increased sleeping

- Lack of bladder and bowel control

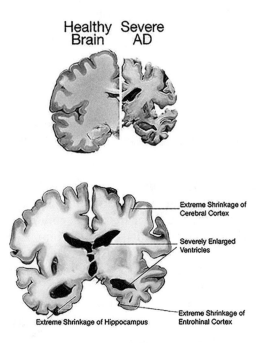

Figure 12.2. *Severe Alzheimer Disease*

Near the end, the person may be in bed much or all of the time. The most frequent cause of death for people with AD is aspiration pneumonia. This type of pneumonia develops when a person is not able to swallow properly and takes food or liquids into the lungs instead of air.

Chapter 13

Early-Onset Alzheimer Disease

Early-onset Alzheimer disease (EOAD) occurs between a person's thirties to mid-sixties. It is rare, representing less than 10 percent of all people who have Alzheimer disease. People with this disorder are younger than those with late-onset Alzheimer disease and face different issues, such as dealing with disability at work, raising children, and finding the right support groups.

The Genetics of Early-Onset Alzheimer Disease

Some cases of EOAD are caused by an inherited change in one of three genes, resulting in a type known as early-onset familial Alzheimer disease, or FAD. For other cases of early-onset Alzheimer disease,

This chapter contains text excerpted from the following sources: Text in this chapter begins with excerpts from "Early-Onset Alzheimer's Disease: A Resource List," National Institute on Aging (NIA), National Institutes of Health (NIH), June 27, 2017; Text under the heading "The Genetics of Early-Onset Alzheimer Disease" is excerpted from "Alzheimer's Disease Genetics Fact Sheet," National Institute on Aging (NIA), National Institutes of Health (NIH), August 30, 2015. Reviewed December 2018; Text beginning with the heading "Onset and Progression of EOAD" is excerpted from "Early-Onset Alzheimer's Disease," U.S. Social Security Administration (SSA), March 28, 2018; Text under the heading "Early-Onset Alzheimer and Disability Benefits" is excerpted from "Relief for Thousands Suffering from Alzheimer's Disease," U.S. Social Security Administration (SSA), November 29, 2016.

research suggests there may be a genetic component related to factors other than these three genes.

A child whose biological mother or father carries a genetic mutation for early-onset FAD has a 50/50 chance of inheriting that mutation. If the mutation is in fact inherited, the child has a very strong probability of developing early-onset FAD.

Early-onset FAD is caused by any one of a number of different single-gene mutations on chromosomes 21, 14, and 1. Each of these mutations causes abnormal proteins to be formed. Mutations on chromosome 21 cause the formation of abnormal amyloid precursor protein (APP). A mutation on chromosome 14 causes abnormal presenilin 1 (a protein that processes amyloid β-protein from the amyloid protein precursor) to be made, and a mutation on chromosome 1 leads to abnormal presenilin 2.

Each of these mutations plays a role in the breakdown of APP, a protein whose precise function is not yet fully understood. This breakdown is part of a process that generates harmful forms of amyloid plaques, a hallmark of the disease.

Critical research findings about EOAD have helped identify key steps in the formation of brain abnormalities typical of the more common late-onset form of Alzheimer disease. Genetics studies have helped explain why the disease develops in people at various ages.

National Institute on Aging (NIA)-supported scientists are continuing research into early-onset disease through the Dominantly Inherited Alzheimer Network (DIAN), an international partnership to study families with early-onset FAD. By observing the Alzheimer disease-related brain changes that occur in these families long before symptoms of memory loss or cognitive issues appear, scientists hope to gain insight into how and why the disease develops in both its early- and late-onset forms.

In addition, an NIA-supported clinical trial in Colombia, South America, is testing the effectiveness of an amyloid-clearing drug in symptom-free volunteers at high risk of developing early-onset FAD.

Onset and Progression of Early-Onset Alzheimer Disease

Early-onset Alzheimer disease is the diagnosis of AD for a person younger than age 65 years. AD is a degenerative, irreversible brain disease that usually affects older people and causes a dementia characterized by the gradual loss of previously attained cognitive abilities, such as memory, language, judgment, and the ability to function.

Physiological changes in the brain include the rampant growth of two abnormal structures, amyloid plaques and neurofibrillary tangles, which interrupt normal brain activity. The onset of AD is subtle; memory impairment is frequently its earliest manifestation, quickly followed by learning and language impairments. Because people with early-onset AD are often in the workforce, it is not uncommon for the disease to first manifest as a decline or loss in their ability to perform work-related activities. In the earlier stages of AD, depression is a common complaint. In later stages, agitation, changes in personality and behavior, restlessness, and withdrawal become evident. People with early-onset AD decline possibly at a faster rate than those with late-onset AD.

Diagnosis of Early-Onset Alzheimer Disease

The diagnosis of early-onset AD is based on the combination of clinical and family history; neurological, cognitive, or neuropsychological examination; and neuroimaging. Pertinent clinical information includes history of onset and description of cognitive and functional impairments at home and at work. Currently, there is no specific clinical or laboratory diagnostic test for early-onset (or late-onset) AD and at present, the diagnosis can only be confirmed by brain biopsy or postmortem examination of the brain. A decline in Mini-Mental Status Examination (MMSE) scores over time is a likely indicator of possible dementia. Neuroimaging, such as computerized tomography (CT) or magnetic resonance imaging (MRI) is useful to demonstrate changes in the brain and to exclude other causes of dementia.

Treatment and Prognosis of Early-Onset Alzheimer Disease

People diagnosed with early-onset AD experience gradual cognitive decline until death. Death usually results from pneumonia, malnutrition, or general body wasting. The average time of survival after diagnosis of early-onset AD varies but generally is 8 to 10 years, and many people with early-onset AD require institutionalization.

Currently, there is no treatment to cure or slow the progression of early-onset AD. Treatment for the symptoms of early-onset AD may include drugs such as cholinesterase inhibitors (galantamine, rivastigmine, or donepezil) and an N-methyl D-aspartate (NMDA) antagonist (memantine).

Early-Onset Alzheimer Disease and Disability Benefits

Early onset Alzheimer disease is a progressive, terminal disease, which cannot be prevented, cured or even slowed. Since the onset can occur in people as early as their thirties and forties, it often strikes during an individual's prime working years, and as the disease progresses it prevents gainful employment. As a result, individuals are coming to grips with a devastating diagnosis all while losing employment and the salary and benefits that come with being employed. These individuals and their caregivers then must figure out how they will pay for their care.

Thankfully, since 2010 Social Security has helped by adding Alzheimer disease to its Compassionate Allowances Initiative. The initiative identifies debilitating diseases and medical conditions so severe they obviously meet Social Security's disability standards. Compassionate Allowances allow for faster payment of Social Security benefits to individuals with Alzheimer disease.

Chapter 14

The Genetics of
Alzheimer Disease

Chapter Contents

Section 14.1

Alzheimer Disease Genetics Fact Sheet

This section includes text excerpted from "Alzheimer's Disease
Genetics Fact Sheet," National Institute on Aging (NIA),
National Institutes of Health (NIH), August 30, 2015.
Reviewed December 2018.

Scientists believe that many factors influence when Alzheimer
disease (AD) begins and how it progresses. The more they study this
devastating disease, the more they realize that genes play an important role. Research conducted and funded by the National Institute on
Aging (NIA) at the National Institutes of Health (NIH) and others is
advancing the understanding of Alzheimer disease genetics.

The Genetics of Disease

Some diseases are caused by a genetic mutation, or permanent
change in one or more specific genes. If a person inherits from a parent a genetic mutation that causes a certain disease, then she or he
will usually get the disease. Sickle cell anemia, cystic fibrosis (CF),
and early-onset familial Alzheimer disease (eFAD) are examples of
inherited genetic disorders.

In other diseases, a genetic variant may occur. A single gene can
have many variants. Sometimes, this difference in a gene can cause
a disease directly. More often, a variant plays a role in increasing or
decreasing a person's risk of developing a disease or condition. When
a genetic variant increases disease risk but does not directly cause a
disease, it is called a genetic risk factor.

Identifying genetic variants may help researchers find the most
effective ways to treat or prevent diseases such as Alzheimer disease
in an individual. This approach, called precision medicine, takes into
account individual variability in genes, environment, and lifestyle for
each person.

Alzheimer Disease Genetics

Alzheimer disease (AD) is an irreversible, progressive brain disease. It is characterized by the development of amyloid plaques and
neurofibrillary, or tau, tangles; the loss of connections between nerve
cells (neurons) in the brain; and the death of these nerve cells. There

are two types of Alzheimer disease—early-onset and late-onset. Both types have a genetic component.

Early-Onset Alzheimer Disease

Early-onset Alzheimer disease occurs between a person's thirties to mid-sixties and represents less than 10 percent of all people with Alzheimer disease. Some cases are caused by an inherited change in one of three genes, resulting in a type known as early-onset familial Alzheimer disease, or FAD. For other cases of early-onset Alzheimer disease, research suggests there may be a genetic component related to factors other than these three genes.

A child whose biological mother or father carries a genetic mutation for early-onset FAD has a 50/50 chance of inheriting that mutation. If the mutation is in fact inherited, the child has a very strong probability of developing early-onset FAD.

Early-onset FAD is caused by any one of a number of different single-gene mutations on chromosomes 21, 14, and 1. Each of these mutations causes abnormal proteins to be formed. Mutations on chromosome 21 cause the formation of abnormal amyloid precursor protein (APP). A mutation on chromosome 14 causes abnormal presenilin 1 to be made, and a mutation on chromosome 1 leads to abnormal presenilin 2.

Each of these mutations plays a role in the breakdown of APP, a protein whose precise function is not yet fully understood. This breakdown is part of a process that generates harmful forms of amyloid plaques, a hallmark of the disease.

Critical research findings about early-onset Alzheimer disease have helped identify key steps in the formation of brain abnormalities typical of the more common late-onset form of Alzheimer disease. Genetics studies have helped explain why the disease develops in people at various ages.

NIA-supported scientists are continuing research into early-onset disease through the Dominantly Inherited Alzheimer Network (DIAN) (dian.wustl.edu), an international partnership to study families with early-onset FAD. By observing the Alzheimer disease-related brain changes that occur in these families long before symptoms of memory loss or cognitive issues appear, scientists hope to gain insight into how and why the disease develops in both its early- and late-onset forms.

In addition, an NIA-supported clinical trial in Colombia, South America, is testing the effectiveness of an amyloid-clearing drug in symptom-free volunteers at high risk of developing early-onset FAD.

Late-Onset Alzheimer Disease

Most people with Alzheimer disease have the late-onset form of the disease, in which symptoms become apparent in the mid-60s and later. The causes of late-onset Alzheimer disease are not yet completely understood, but they likely include a combination of genetic, environmental, and lifestyle factors that affect a person's risk for developing the disease.

Researchers have not found a specific gene that directly causes the late-onset form of the disease. However, one genetic risk factor—having one form of the apolipoprotein E (APOE) gene on chromosome 19—does increase a person's risk. APOE comes in several different forms, or alleles:

APOE ε2 is relatively rare and may provide some protection against the disease. If Alzheimer disease occurs in a person with this allele, it usually develops later in life than it would in someone with the APOE ε4 gene.

APOE ε3, the most common allele, is believed to play a neutral role in the disease—neither decreasing nor increasing risk.

APOE ε4 increases risk for Alzheimer disease and is also associated with an earlier age of disease onset. A person has zero, one, or two APOE ε4 alleles. Having more APOE ε4 alleles increases the risk of developing Alzheimer disease.

APOE ε4 is called a risk-factor gene because it increases a person's risk of developing the disease. However, inheriting an APOE ε4 allele does not mean that a person will definitely develop Alzheimer disease. Some people with an APOE ε4 allele never get the disease, and others who develop Alzheimer disease do not have any APOE ε4 alleles.

Using a relatively new approach called genome-wide association study (GWAS), researchers have identified a number of regions of interest in the genome (an organism's complete set of deoxyribonucleic acid (DNA), including all of its genes) that may increase a person's risk for late-onset Alzheimer disease to varying degrees. By 2015, they had confirmed 33 regions of interest in the Alzheimer disease genome.

A method called whole genome sequencing determines the complete DNA sequence of a person's genome at a single time. Another method called whole exome sequencing looks at the parts of the genome that directly code for the proteins. Using these two approaches, researchers can identify new genes that contribute to or protect against disease risk. Some discoveries have led to new insights about biological pathways involved in Alzheimer disease and may one day lead to effective interventions.

Genetic Testing

A blood test can identify which APOE alleles a person has, but results cannot predict who will or will not develop Alzheimer disease. It is unlikely that genetic testing will ever be able to predict the disease with 100 percent accuracy, researchers believe, because too many other factors may influence its development and progression.

At present, APOE testing is used in research settings to identify study participants who may have an increased risk of developing Alzheimer disease. This knowledge helps scientists look for early brain changes in participants and compare the effectiveness of treatments for people with different APOE profiles. Most researchers believe that APOE testing is useful for studying Alzheimer disease risk in large groups of people but not for determining any one person's risk.

Genetic testing is used by researchers conducting clinical trials and by physicians to help diagnose early-onset Alzheimer disease. However, genetic testing is not otherwise recommended.

Research Questions

Discovering the role of Alzheimer disease genetic risk and protective factors is an important area of research. Understanding more about the genetic basis of the disease will help researchers to:

- Answer a number of basic questions—What makes the disease process begin? Why do some people with memory and other thinking problems develop Alzheimer disease while others do not?

- Determine how genetic risk and protective factors may interact with other genes and lifestyle or environmental factors to affect Alzheimer disease risk in any one person.

- Identify people who are at high risk for developing Alzheimer disease so they can benefit from new interventions and treatments as soon as possible.

- Focus on new prevention and treatment approaches.

Section 14.2

Gene Linked to Alzheimer Disease Plays Key Role in Cell Survival

This section includes text excerpted from "Gene Linked to Alzheimer's Disease Plays Key Role in Cell Survival," National Institutes of Health (NIH), June 10, 2010. Reviewed December 2018.

Scientists have discovered that a gene linked to Alzheimer disease may play a beneficial role in cell survival by enabling neurons to clear away toxic proteins. A study funded by the National Institute on Aging (NIA), part of the National Institutes of Health (NIH), shows the presenilin 1 (*PS1*) gene is essential to the function of lysosomes, the cell component that digests and recycles unwanted proteins. However, mutations in the PS1 gene—a known risk factor for a rare, early onset form of Alzheimer disease (AD)—disrupt this crucial process.

Ralph Nixon, M.D., Ph.D., of the Nathan Kline Institute (NKI), Orangeburg, N.Y., and New York University (NYU) Langone Medical Center, directed the study involving researchers from the United States, Europe, Japan, and Canada. Also supported in part by the Alzheimer Association, the study appears in the June 10, 2010, online issue of *Cell*.

Researchers have theorized for more than a decade that *PS1* mutations linked to early-onset Alzheimer disease, a rare form of the disease that usually affects people between ages 30 and 60, may trigger abnormally high levels of beta-amyloid protein to clump together in the brain.

Amyloid deposits and tau protein tangles are hallmarks of both early-onset and the sporadic, more common form of the disease found in people aged 60 and older. These new findings, however, suggest *PS1* mutations may play a more general role in the development of early-onset Alzheimer disease.

"This study expands our understanding of the role presenilin 1 mutations may play in Alzheimer pathology," said NIA Director Richard J. Hodes, M.D. "While more research is needed, lysosome disruption may be worth exploring as a potential target for new therapeutics to treat, prevent or delay this progressive and debilitating disease."

Working in cells from Alzheimer disease mouse models and in skin cells from Alzheimer disease patients with the mutated gene, the researchers found:

- The *PS1* gene activates lysosome enzymes that digest waste proteins during a process called autophagy. This is the cell's main method of recycling unwanted proteins and other cellular debris. While these waste proteins occur naturally, they are overproduced in neurological disorders like Alzheimer and Parkinson disease, and can be toxic to brain cells.

- Mutations in the *PS1* gene disrupt autophagy. This impairs the ability of neurons to remove waste proteins and other debris. Neurons then may fill with sacs containing potentially toxic amyloid fragments and other unwanted proteins.

- Other genetic mutations may be risk factors for similar disruptions to autophagy found in the more common, sporadic form of the disease in people age 60 and older, and in other neurological disorders like Parkinson disease.

"It has become increasingly clear that many factors may drive the development and progression of this very complex disease," said Nixon, the principal investigator. "I believe we will need to explore an array of therapeutic targets, including ones to normalize or moderate disrupted autophagy."

Section 14.3

Genetic Risk Variants Linked to Alzheimer Disease Amyloid Brain Changes

This section includes text excerpted from "Genetic Risk Variants Linked to Alzheimer's Amyloid Brain Changes at Different Stages of Disease," National Institute on Aging (NIA), National Institutes of Health (NIH), May 30, 2018.

New National Institute on Aging (NIA)-supported research ties several genetic risk variants for late-onset Alzheimer disease (LOAD) to levels of amyloid at different disease stages. The results, published online January 16, 2018, in *JAMA Neurology*, provide insight into the genetic influences on Alzheimer disease-related brain changes, namely, buildup of amyloid, a protein that turns toxic and accumulates in the brains of people with Alzheimer disease (AD).

There is growing evidence that there is a strong genetic component to Alzheimer disease. In this study, researchers sought to better understand the genetic contributions to late-onset Alzheimer disease, beyond those related to APOE4, the strongest known genetic risk factor for the disease.

Researchers from the Indiana University School of Medicine, Indianapolis, and the David Geffen School of Medicine at the University of California, Los Angeles, analyzed associations between the top 20 Alzheimer disease genetic risk variants, as well as other variants previously associated with amyloid deposition, and amyloid levels measured by brain imaging. The study included 977 participants (average age, 74 years) from the NIA-supported Alzheimer Disease Neuroimaging Initiative (ADNI) (www.nia.nih.gov/research/dn/alzheimers-disease-neuroimaging-initiative-adni): 322 who were cognitively normal, 496 who were in the mild cognitive impairment stage, and 159 who were in the dementia stage.

Findings showed that after APOE4, the gene with the strongest association with amyloid deposits was ABCA7, especially in the asymptomatic and early symptomatic disease stages. Studies have previously connected ABCA7 with Alzheimer disease processes in the brain; these findings provide further evidence of its role. Research has also shown that African Americans are more likely than whites to have a variant of the ABCA7 gene, with almost double the risk of developing Alzheimer disease.

Other Alzheimer disease risk genes found to be associated with amyloid buildup at different disease stages included FERMT2, which was most pronounced in people with mild cognitive impairment; SORL1 and EPHA1, which were associated with both the mild cognitive impairment and dementia stages; and CLU, DSG2, and ZCWPWI, which were linked to the dementia stage. Results suggest genetic variants might affect Alzheimer disease processes differently across disease stages.

Researchers noted that improved understanding of these genetic risk factors could help predict which people are most at risk of developing dementia due to Alzheimer disease and identify gene-specific drug targets.

Chapter 15

Health Conditions Linked to Alzheimer Disease

Chapter Contents

Section 15.1

Down Syndrome and Alzheimer Disease

This section includes text excerpted from "Alzheimer's Disease in People with Down Syndrome," National Institute on Aging (NIA), National Institutes of Health (NIH), May 19, 2017.

Many, but not all, people with Down syndrome (DS), develop Alzheimer disease (AD) when they get older.

People with Down syndrome are born with an extra copy of chromosome 21, which carries the *APP* gene. This gene produces a specific protein called amyloid precursor protein (APP). Too much APP protein leads to a buildup of protein clumps called beta-amyloid (Aβ) plaques in the brain. By age 40, almost all people with Down syndrome have these plaques, along with other protein deposits, called tau tangles, which cause problems with how brain cells function and increase the risk of developing Alzheimer dementia.

However, not all people with these brain plaques will develop the symptoms of Alzheimer disease. Estimates suggest that 50 percent or more of people with Down syndrome will develop dementia due to Alzheimer disease as they age. People with Down syndrome begin to show symptoms of Alzheimer disease in their fifties or sixties.

This type of Alzheimer disease is not passed down from a parent to a child.

Down Syndrome and Alzheimer Disease Research

Scientists are working hard to understand why some people with Down syndrome develop dementia while others do not. They want to know how Alzheimer disease begins and progresses, so they can develop drugs or other treatments that can stop, delay, or even prevent the disease process.

Research in this area includes:

- Basic studies to improve the understanding of the genetic and biological causes of brain abnormalities that lead to Alzheimer disease

- Observational research to measure cognitive changes in people over time

- Studies of biomarkers (biological signs of disease), brain scans, and other tests that may help diagnose Alzheimer disease—even

before symptoms appear—and show brain changes as people
with Down syndrome age

- Clinical trials to test treatments for dementia in adults with
Down syndrome

Section 15.2

Obesity May Raise Risk of Alzheimer Disease and Dementia

This section includes text excerpted from "Adults Obese or
Overweight at Midlife May Be at Risk for Earlier Onset of
Alzheimer's Disease," National Institute on Aging (NIA),
National Institutes of Health (NIH), September 1, 2015.
Reviewed December 2018.

Being obese or overweight in middle age has been linked to increased
risk of dementia. To learn more, researchers at the National Institute
on Aging (NIA), part of the National Institutes of Health (NIH), further
explored the relationship between weight at midlife and Alzheimer
disease among volunteers participating in the Baltimore Longitudinal
Study of Aging (BLSA), one of the longest running studies of human
aging in North America. They found that being obese or overweight
at midlife—as measured by body mass index (BMI) at age 50—may
predict earlier age of onset of the devastating neurodegenerative disorder (ND). The study, led by Madhav Thambisetty, M.D., Ph.D., will
appear online September 1, 2015, in *Molecular Psychiatry*.

Cognitively healthy at the start of the nearly 14-year study, each
of the 1,394 BLSA participants received cognitive testing every one
to two years; 142 volunteers eventually developed Alzheimer disease
(AD). The investigators found:

- Each unit increase in BMI at age 50 accelerated onset by nearly
seven months in those who developed Alzheimer disease.

- Higher midlife BMI was associated with greater levels of
neurofibrillary tangles—a hallmark of the disease—in the

brains of 191 volunteers, including those who did not develop Alzheimer disease.

- Among 75 cognitively healthy volunteers who had brain imaging to detect amyloid, a protein whose fragments make up the brain plaques that are a hallmark of Alzheimer disease, those with higher midlife BMI had more amyloid deposits in the precuneus, a brain region that often shows the earliest signs of Alzheimer disease-related changes.

More study is needed to determine the relationship behind BMI at midlife and Alzheimer disease onset. The findings suggest, however, that maintaining a healthy BMI at midlife might be considered as one way to delay the onset of Alzheimer disease.

Section 15.3

Diabetes, Dementia, and Alzheimer Disease

This section includes text excerpted from "Diabetes, Dementia, and Alzheimer's Disease," National Institute of Diabetes and Digestive and Kidney Diseases (NIDDK), August 16, 2012. Reviewed December 2018.

Diabetes and Dementia: Untangling the Web

Dr. Craft is Professor of Psychiatry and Behavioral Sciences at the University of Washington; she is also Associate Director of the Geriatric Research, Education, and Clinical Center (GRECC), and Director of the Memory Disorders Clinic, at the Veterans Affairs (VA) Puget Sound Medical Center. With support from the National Institutes of Health (NIH), the VA, and other sources, Dr. Craft has focused her research program on neuroendocrine abnormalities in the development and expression of Alzheimer disease (AD). AD is an irreversible, progressive brain disease that slowly destroys memory and thinking skills, and eventually even the ability to carry out the simplest tasks. AD is the most common cause of dementia among older people, and prevalence increases exponentially with age. While estimates vary, experts suggest that several million Americans may have AD. Dr.

Craft noted epidemiological studies finding that insulin resistance, hyperinsulinemia, and impaired glucose tolerance (IGT)/type 2 diabetes are associated with increased risk for cognitive impairment and AD; these observations are consistent with evidence showing that insulin normally plays a positive role in brain function and cognition. As a result, Dr. Craft and other researchers are investigating biological mechanisms that could be responsible for the increased risk for diminished brain function associated with prediabetes and diabetes.

The brain's primary energy source is the sugar glucose. Through imaging studies of people with preclinical AD, Dr. Craft and colleagues have observed patterns of impaired glucose metabolism in the brain that can be detected well before clinical onset of the disease. Conversely, they have observed that patterns virtually identical to the AD risk patterns can be found in cognitively normal people with prediabetes and type 2 diabetes, a resemblance that increases with increasing levels of insulin resistance.

Delving into the potential molecular mechanisms linking development of cognitive impairment with dysfunctional glucose metabolism in the brain, Dr. Craft and her colleagues examined the interplay between insulin, insulin resistance, and beta amyloid (Aβ), also called A-β—the key component of the "senile plaques (SP)" that are a hallmark of AD. Dr. Craft pointed out that evidence now indicates that the formation of these insoluble peptide plaques may actually be a defense mechanism to deal with a greater threat—smaller complexes of Aβ molecules called oligomers. Aβ oligomers are soluble, synaptotoxic (damaging to inter-neuron signaling), cause neuronal loss, and ultimately lead to cognitive impairment. In the brain, insulin helps to regulate Aβ levels (and hence levels of the oligomers). Experiments revealed a reciprocal relationship one between insulin and Aβ oligomers: treating laboratory-grown neurons with insulin could protect them from Aβ oligomer induced-synapotoxicity, but treating neurons with oligomers alone caused insulin receptors to move away from synaptic surfaces (dendritic membranes)—likely reducing insulin signaling and contributing to insulin resistance in the brain. Moreover, experiments in nonhuman primates showed that administering Aβ oligomers directly into the brain induced a chemical change in a protein called IRS-1 that, in other tissues, is characteristic of insulin resistance—further suggesting that Aβ oligomers play a role in insulin resistance in the brain.

Dr. Craft and her colleagues have also examined the effect of insulin resistance in the rest of the body on Aβ levels in the brain. Experiments in animal models of AD showed that inducing insulin resistance and hyperinsulinemia increased the burden of Aβ in the brain. In humans, Dr. Craft and her colleagues found through an experimental diet intervention study that four weeks of a diet high in saturated fat and with a high glycemic index not only had a negative impact on metabolism—increasing insulin resistance and low-density lipoprotein (LDL) cholesterol ('bad' cholesterol)—but also significantly increased markers of AD pathology (including Aβ) and oxidative injury detectable in the cerebrospinal fluid (CSF), a proxy for the brain. In comparison, a diet with the same caloric value but low in saturated fat and with a low glycemic index had beneficial effects on these markers. Interestingly, these results may help explain the epidemiological observations that greater saturated fat intake in mid-life increases age-related cognitive impairment and AD risk, while lower-fat diets richer in beneficial fats and complex carbohydrates decrease risk. In another set of clinical experiments, the research team found that artificially inducing hyperinsulinemia in the absence of insulin resistance induced increases in Aβ and markers of inflammation in cerebrospinal fluid, indicating that not all of the observed indications of AD-related pathology are the direct result of insulin resistance or elevated blood glucose: hyperinsulinemia may itself play a disease promoting role. Some data suggest that older age may make people more vulnerable to these effects.

Diabetes and insulin resistance may also increase or augment AD risk through effects on vascular function. Deposition of Aβ in cerebral vasculature has been observed in mouse models. In mice genetically engineered to be vulnerable to AD and diabetes, the deposition is greater than in AD alone, and increases with age. When Dr. Craft and colleagues compared the amount of plaques and protein "tangles" (another AD marker) present in specimens from the brains of deceased persons who had had both dementia and diabetes, to that present in brain specimens of deceased persons who had only dementia, only diabetes, or neither, the results were surprising— plaques and tangles were highest in persons with dementia alone, not in persons with both dementia and diabetes. However, those with both diseases had a significantly greater prevalence of microvascular lesions in their brain specimens. The significance of this finding is not yet known—the lesions are too small to be causing problems on their own, but could be markers of some greater vascular pathology important to AD.

As Dr. Craft noted, their finding that amyloid pathology was not greatest in brains of people who died with both dementia and diabetes was quite intriguing. One possible explanation was that diabetes treatment affects amyloid plaque levels. However, Dr. Craft and her colleagues found that specimens from persons with dementia plus untreated diabetes displayed a similar plaque burden to that seen in dementia alone, while diabetes treatment with insulin (with or without additional oral medication) yielded a lower number of plaques, at a level closer to that seen in two persons with diabetes alone (treated or untreated) or neither disease—suggesting that diabetes treatment (primarily insulin) might have a mediating effect on plaques. Similar results were seen for tangles. In contrast, however, the treated-diabetes group had the highest counts of microvascular lesions. Together, these data suggest the provocative notion that dementia in individuals with untreated diabetes is likely to show the classic pathological hallmarks of AD, while microvascular lesions are more commonly characteristic of dementia in those with treated diabetes. The data also suggest that researchers investigating the links between diabetes and dementia should consider the potential effects of diabetes treatment.

Dr. Craft noted findings from her lab and others of a reduction in insulin transport across the "blood–brain barrier (BBB)" in people with AD, leading to reduced insulin signaling in the brain. These observations that increasing brain insulin levels might potentially be therapeutically beneficial in AD, and/or help prevent progression of dementia. Intranasal administration of insulin is one potentially effective route. In a mouse model of diabetes, intranasal insulin administration significantly reduced the exacerbated brain atrophy that occurs in these mice as they age. Dr. Craft and colleagues are seeking to extend these findings through clinical research—the Study of Nasal Insulin to Fight Forgetfulness (SNIFF) to test whether intranasal administration can normalize brain insulin levels and improve memory and cognition in people with AD. In a study, adults with mild cognitive impairment (MCI) or mild AD received either daily intranasal insulin at one of two different dosing levels or a placebo over the course of four months. The research team found that the lower dose of insulin was best for memory, but participants receiving either dosing level of nasal insulin fared better than those receiving placebo on other measures of cognition. Live imaging studies showed improvements in glucose metabolism, including in areas known to be important to AD pathology, in participants who received intranasal insulin. On the basis of these encouraging results, a larger, longer, multisite trial is slated to begin in the fall of 2012.

In another approach, Dr. Craft and colleagues are testing the therapeutic potential of improving insulin sensitivity in AD, rather than providing additional insulin. Studies of lifestyle approaches (exercise) have shown promise for improving cognitive function and/ or AD biomarkers, setting the stage for another study beginning in fall 2012. Other laboratories are testing the pharmacologic approach, using insulin-sensitizing drugs that may improve insulin signaling in the brain.

Chapter 16

Traumatic Brain Injury, Alzheimer Disease, and Dementia

Traumatic brain injury (TBI), a form of acquired brain injury, occurs when a sudden trauma causes damage to the brain. TBI can result when the head suddenly and violently hits an object, or when an object pierces the skull and enters brain tissue. Symptoms of a TBI can be mild, moderate, or severe, depending on the extent of the damage to the brain. A person with a mild TBI may remain conscious or may experience a loss of consciousness for a few seconds or minutes. Other symptoms of mild TBI include headache, confusion, light-headedness, dizziness, blurred vision or tired eyes, ringing in the ears, bad taste in the mouth, fatigue or lethargy, a change in sleep patterns, behavioral or mood changes, and trouble with memory, concentration, attention, or thinking. A person with a moderate or severe TBI may show these

This chapter contains text excerpted from the following sources: Text in this chapter begins with excerpts from "Traumatic Brain Injury Information Page," National Institute of Neurological Disorders and Stroke (NINDS), June 18, 2018; Text under the heading "Traumatic Brain Injury Increases Dementia Risk" is excerpted from "Traumatic Brain Injury Increases Dementia Risk," U.S. Department of Veterans Affairs (VA), May 12, 2015. Reviewed December 2018; Text beginning with the heading "Traumatic Brain Injuries Linked to Dementia" is excerpted from "Traumatic Brain Injuries Linked to Dementia in Older Vets," U.S. Department of Veterans Affairs (VA), August 6, 2014. Reviewed December 2018.

same symptoms, but may also have a headache that gets worse or does not go away, repeated vomiting or nausea, convulsions or seizures, an inability to awaken from sleep, dilation of one or both pupils of the eyes, slurred speech, weakness or numbness in the extremities, loss of coordination, and increased confusion, restlessness, or agitation.

Traumatic Brain Injury Increases Dementia Risk

Patients diagnosed with traumatic brain injury (TBI) had over twice the risk of developing dementia within seven years after diagnosis compared to those without TBI, in a study of more than 280,000 older veterans conducted by researchers at the San Francisco VA Medical Center (SFVAMC) and the University of California, San Francisco (UCSF).

"This finding is important because TBI is so common," said senior investigator Kristine Yaffe, MD, chief of geriatric psychiatry at SFVAMC and professor of psychiatry, neurology and epidemiology at UCSF. She noted that about 1.7 million Americans are diagnosed with TBI each year. In addition, she said, TBI is often referred to as the "signature wound" of the wars in Iraq and Afghanistan, where it accounts for 22 percent of casualties overall and affects up to 59 percent of troops exposed to blasts.

The study authors analyzed the medical records of 281,540 veterans age 55 or older who received care through the U.S. Department of Veterans Affairs (VA) from 1997 to 2000 and did not have a prior history of dementia. They found that 15 percent of veterans who received a diagnosis of TBI developed dementia by 2007, compared with seven percent of those not diagnosed with TBI. Even after controlling for factors such as age, medical history and cardiovascular health, the authors found that a TBI diagnosis still doubled the risk of dementia.

The findings were presented at the 2011 Alzheimer Association International Conference (AAIC) on Alzheimer disease (AD) in Paris, France.

Lead author Deborah Barnes, Ph.D., a mental health researcher at SFVAMC, said that the study is one of the first to examine the association between dementia and different types of TBI diagnosis, including intracranial injuries, concussion, postconcussion syndrome (PCS) and skull fracture. "It didn't matter what type of diagnosis it was—they were all associated with an elevated risk of dementia," said Barnes, also an associate professor of psychiatry at UCSF.

The authors speculated that among potential causes for the increased risk, the most plausible is that TBI is associated with diffuse axonal injury, or swelling of the axons that form connections between neurons in the brain. This swelling, explained Yaffe, is accompanied by the accumulation of proteins, including beta-amyloid, which is a hallmark of Alzheimer disease. "The loss of axons and neurons could result in earlier manifestation of Alzheimer symptoms," said Yaffe.

Barnes said that for veterans, the findings have different implications depending on the age of the veteran. "Older veterans who have had some kind of head injury should be monitored over time, so that if signs of dementia develop, treatment can begin as soon as possible," she said. "For younger veterans, early treatment and rehabilitation following TBI may help prevent the development of dementia over the long term."

SFVAMC has the largest medical research program in the national VA system, with more than 200 research scientists, all of whom are faculty members at UCSF.

UCSF is a leading university dedicated to promoting health worldwide through advanced biomedical research, graduate-level education in the life sciences and health professions, and excellence in patient care.

The research was supported by funds from the U.S. Department of Defense (DoD) that were administered by the Northern California Institute for Research and Education (NCIRE). NCIRE—The Veterans Health Research Institute—is the largest research institute associated with a VA medical center. Its mission is to improve the health and well-being of veterans and the general public by supporting a world-class biomedical research program conducted by the UCSF faculty at SFVAMC.

Traumatic Brain Injuries Linked to Dementia

According to a study, veterans diagnosed with a traumatic brain injury may be at greater risk for developing dementia later in life.

The research, published in the July 22, 2014, issue of *Neurology*, examined more than 188,000 veterans over the age of 55 for nine years. During that time, 16 percent of veterans with a past diagnosis of TBI developed dementia, compared with 10 percent among those with no history of TBI. Overall, having TBI was associated with a 60 percent increase in the risk of developing dementia for older veterans, after statistical adjustments for factors such as age, medical conditions, depression, and posttraumatic stress disorder (PTSD).

Dementia includes any number of disorders affecting the brain. Symptoms include impaired intellectual and cognitive functioning as well as behavioral and personality changes. The most common form of dementia, Alzheimer disease, affects some 5.3 million people in the United States and is the sixth leading cause of death in the country.

"There seems to be growing evidence that traumatic brain injury may be a trigger for earlier onset of dementia later in life, and our results add to this evidence," lead author Dr. Deborah Barnes of the San Francisco VA Medical Center told Wall Street OTC in July.

Civilians with Traumatic Brain Injury Also at Greater Risk

Although TBI has emerged as a signature wound of the wars in Iraq and Afghanistan, injuries of this type can be sustained through any number of civilian activities. Sports injuries and car accidents are two common causes. "If an older patient has a history of traumatic brain injury, then doctors need to look more closely for cognitive symptoms," said Barnes, who is also an associate professor at the University of California, San Francisco.

The results, according to Barnes, raise concerns about the long-term consequences of TBI, particularly in young Veterans of Iraq and Afghanistan.

The researchers say Veterans with head injuries may be able to lower their risk of developing dementia by staying active, both mentally and physically, and getting treatment for any mental health conditions.

"We found there was an additive relationship between mental health conditions and head injuries," Barnes told Reuters Health. "Veterans who had both of these risk factors were more likely to develop dementia than those who had only one. In addition, they may be able to lower the risk of dementia by doing their best to minimize future head injuries by doing simple things to protect their brain, like wearing helmets and seat belts."

Nationwide Study Further Examining Link

On a related note, Dr. Michael Weiner, also of the San Francisco VA Medical Center, is leading a study looking at the link between TBI or posttraumatic stress disorder and dementia in Vietnam Veterans. The study, funded by the U.S. Department of Defense (DoD), is part of the national Alzheimer Disease Neuroimaging Initiative (ADNI), which Weiner leads.

Nationwide, approximately 1,000 Vietnam veterans will participate in screening interviews and 500 will be interviewed by telephone. Approximately 300 Vietnam veterans will be eligible to complete the entire study. The study will include brain scans, lumbar punctures (to check levels of amyloid in cerebrospinal fluid), medical exams, and neuropsychological tests. Interested veterans can visit www.adni-info. org/ADNIDOD or call 800-773-4883.

Chapter 17

Other Factors That Influence Alzheimer Disease Risk

Chapter Contents

Section 17.1

Alcohol Use and the Risk of Developing Alzheimer Disease

This section includes text excerpted from "Alcohol Use and the Risk of Developing Alzheimer's Disease," National Institute on Alcohol Abuse and Alcoholism (NIAAA), April 1, 2002. Reviewed December 2018.

Some of the detrimental effects of heavy alcohol use on brain function are similar to those observed with Alzheimer disease (AD). Although alcohol use may be a risk factor for AD, it is difficult to study this relationship because of similarities between alcoholic dementia and AD and because standard diagnostic criteria for alcoholic dementia have not yet been developed. Similar biological mechanisms may be involved in the effects of AD and alcohol abuse on the brain. Epidemiologic studies have investigated the relationship between alcohol use and AD but have not provided strong evidence to suggest that alcohol use influences the risk of developing AD. Further research is needed before the effect of alcohol use on AD is understood fully.

Alzheimer disease is a degenerative brain disorder characterized by a progressive loss of memory and other detrimental cognitive changes as well as lowered life expectancy. It is the leading cause of dementia in the United States. Aside from the substantial personal costs, AD is a major economic burden on healthcare and social services. Estimates of the number of people with AD in the United States in 1997 ranged from one million to more than four million, and these figures are expected to quadruple within 50 years unless effective interventions are developed. The risk of AD increases exponentially with age; consequently, as the population ages, the importance of AD as a public health concern grows, as does the need for research on the cause of AD and on strategies for its prevention and treatment.

Studying factors that influence the risk of developing AD may lead to the identification of those at high risk for developing it, strategies for prevention or intervention, and clues to the cause of the disease. Both genetic and environmental factors have been implicated in the development of AD, but the cause of AD remains unknown, and no cure or universally effective treatment has yet been developed.

Alcohol consumption is one possible risk factor for AD. Alcoholism is associated with extensive cognitive problems, including alcoholic dementia. Because alcohol's effects on cognition, brain disorders, and brain chemistry share some features with AD's effects on these three areas, it is plausible that alcohol use might also increase the risk of developing AD. Investigating whether and to what degree alcohol use is related to AD is made more difficult by the challenges of diagnosing and distinguishing alcoholic dementia and AD. Such studies are important, however, because alcohol use is a common but preventable exposure, an association between alcohol and AD is biologically plausible, and knowledge of the effect of alcohol on AD may provide clues to the cause of AD.

Effects of Alcohol Use on Brain Disorders and Cognition

Heavy alcohol consumption has both immediate and long-term detrimental effects on the brain and neuropsychological functioning. Heavy drinking accelerates shrinkage, or atrophy, of the brain, which in turn is a critical determinant of neurodegenerative changes and cognitive decline in aging. Changes observed with alcohol-related brain disorders, however, may be no more than superficially similar to those seen with aging or AD. In contrast to aging and AD, alcohol's effects on the brain may be reversible. Atrophy decreases after abstinence from alcohol. A study that further investigated cerebral atrophy in alcoholics and age-matched control subjects found no significant differences in the number of nerve cells in the brain (i.e., neurons) between the two groups and that most of the loss occurred in the white matter, which consists largely of nerve fibers that connect neurons. The researchers concluded that, because neurons did not appear to be lost, disrupted functions could be restored after abstinence as neuronal connections were reestablished.

This conclusion is supported by research that also showed no neuronal loss in alcoholics compared with nonalcoholics but did show significant loss of brain cells that provide support for neurons (i.e., glial cells) which, in contrast to neurons, can be regenerated. That alcoholics can show improved cognitive performance after abstinence provides additional evidence of a reversible effect. Other studies, however, have reported neuronal loss with chronic alcohol abuse, including loss of neurons (i.e., cholinergic neurons) that contain or are stimulated by a certain chemical messenger in the brain (i.e., the neurotransmitter acetylcholine). Cholinergic neurons are specifically affected in AD Improvement in cognitive function, or at least the lack of a progressive cognitive deficit, is one of the major factors used to determine whether a patient has alcoholic dementia rather than AD. A work suggesting that characteristic neuropsychological profiles exist for alcoholic dementia and AD may prove useful in distinguishing the two disorders. The diagnosis of alcoholic dementia, however, is itself somewhat controversial. Alcoholic dementia may have multiple causes. Pathological findings consistent with AD, nutritional deficiencies, trauma, and, in particular, stroke, also have been found in demented alcoholics. The difficulty in distinguishing alcoholic dementia from AD has been attributed to a shared substrate of brain damage in the two disorders.

A diagnosis of alcoholic dementia may be appropriate for some demented patients who have a history of alcohol abuse, but the effects of more moderate levels of drinking on cognitive function (for anyone) are not known. Thus, despite evidence of an association between alcohol use and neuropathologic and cognitive deficits, including alcoholic dementia, it is not yet clear whether alcohol use at either heavy or more moderate levels of consumption is associated with AD.

Biological Mechanisms

Both alcohol and AD substantially affect the cholinergic system, and thus it is plausible that alcohol use could be linked to AD through their common effects on this system. Early studies of AD from the 1980s focused on the cholinergic system because it was known to play an important role in memory. Its role in AD was confirmed, and deficits in the cholinergic system, such as lower levels of acetylcholine (ACh) and fewer receptors (proteins that bind to neurotransmitters), are now well established in AD. Although other neurotransmitter systems have since been implicated in AD, current treatment strategies still include repletion of cholinergic deficits.

The cholinergic system also is affected by alcohol use. Chronic alcohol use causes degeneration of cholinergic neurons. Alcohol has been shown to decrease acetylcholine levels, reducing its synthesis and release. These deficits may aggravate the reductions already present in AD. Improvement of cognitive function in alcoholics after abstention from alcohol suggests that the cognitive deficits may reflect neurochemical alterations rather than neuronal loss. Alcohol-related memory loss can be partially reversed by compounds that stimulate the cholinergic system (e.g., nicotine). Alcohol-induced cholinergic receptor losses in alcoholics with AD may contribute to the clinical symptoms of dementia. Alcohol does not appear to accelerate the AD process but instead induces its effects on the cholinergic system, independent of the cholinergic deficits caused by AD. In addition, alcohol has extensive effects on neurotransmitter systems other than the cholinergic system and may also affect AD through these pathways.

Alcohol may interact with both the brain and the aging process. In rodents, for example, age-related impairments in learning and memory are aggravated by alcohol consumption. Alcohol-related brain damage appears to differ in young and old alcoholics. Although it has been suggested that alcohol abuse may accelerate aging-related changes in the brain at any age and that older adults may be more vulnerable to alcohol's effects and thus show more age-related cognitive changes, these hypotheses of premature aging have been questioned. Arendt has suggested that the degenerative changes associated with aging, chronic alcohol abuse, and AD are on a continuum and that they may be quantitatively different but not qualitatively so.

Although a link between alcohol use and AD is plausible, whether such a relationship does exist or what the characteristics of such an association would be has not yet been established. For example, alcohol might affect whether one developed AD, when one developed it, or the progression of AD once one had developed it. Observing no association between increased numbers of senile plaques (a characteristic marker of AD found in the brain) and alcohol-related receptor loss, concluded that alcohol consumption did not appear to accelerate the AD process. Although it has been neither proven nor disproven that alcohol increases the risk of developing AD nor lowers the age at onset, this study suggests that alcohol does not appear to affect progression of the disease. This hypothesis is supported by a study that reported that past heavy alcohol consumption was not associated with progression of AD over a one-year interval. Other researchers, however, have found past or current alcohol abuse to be a significant predictor of rate of decline in AD.

Epidemiologic Studies of Alcohol Use and Alzheimer Disease

Many studies have examined the effects of alcohol and alcoholism on cognitive function and the brain. However, relatively few epidemiologic studies have focused on whether people who drink alcohol have a greater or lesser chance of developing AD. These studies are described here and summarized in the table.

Table 17.1. Epidemiologic Studies of Alcohol Use and the Risk of Developing Alzheimer Disease (AD) by Type of Study Design

Study Design	Alcohol Use Increased the Risk of AD	Alcohol Use Decreased the Risk of AD	Alcohol Use Had No Significant Effect on the Risk of AD
Cross-sectional	0	0	1
Case-control	1	2	10
Cohort	0	2	7
Meta-analysis	0	0	1
Total	1	4	19

Cross-sectional studies provide a snapshot of a disease (e.g., AD) at a single point in time and examine relationships between the disease and other factors, such as alcohol use.

Case-control studies of alcohol use and AD compare people with AD (cases) with people without AD (controls) and determine whether alcohol consumption differs between the two groups.

Cohort studies provide a stronger, longitudinal design (i.e., they collect data on alcohol use at baseline and follow study participants over time to determine whether they will develop AD).

A meta-analysis pools data from multiple studies and thereby offers increased statistical power.

Epidemiologic studies of alcohol use and AD in the 1980s and early 1990s generally were based on a case-control design, which identifies people with AD (i.e., cases) and a corresponding group of people without AD (i.e., control subjects) and then investigates whether alcohol consumption differs between these two groups. Relatively quick and inexpensive, the case-control design is a standard epidemiologic approach used to identify potential risk factors and to determine whether more extensive studies are warranted.

A summary of 11 of these case-control studies showed that nine of the studies found no significant relationship between alcohol use and AD, one found that alcohol use increased the risk, and one found that alcohol use decreased the risk of AD. Most of these studies examined drinking status of study participants (whether they consumed alcohol at a specific, usually high level) rather than using more detailed measures of amount consumed. These case-control studies, however, may not have found a significant association because they had too few subjects (often less than 100 cases) and thus lacked statistical power. This possibility was addressed in two reports from a meta-analysis that pooled the data from four individual case-control studies. However, the researchers did not find significant results for low, moderate, or high alcohol consumption even with this larger sample. Graves and colleagues conducted another meta-analysis that included a fifth study, which had used a different definition of alcohol use, but they still did not find a significant association between alcohol use and AD. Meta-analyses have increased power to detect significant associations but are still limited by the flaws of their constituent individual studies.

Subsequent case-control and cross-sectional studies also have failed to provide evidence of an association between alcohol use and AD. One case-control study that did find a significant effect reported a reduced risk of AD in men with "high" alcohol use (i.e., more than two drinks per day), taking into account smoking status, education, and the status of a genetic marker for AD (apolipoprotein E (ApoE) allele, a variant of a gene).

Although the weight of evidence from the studies summarized above suggests that alcohol use is not related to AD, any conclusions must take into account the methodological limitations of these types of studies. The early studies often failed to account for confounding factors; drinkers differ from nondrinkers in many characteristics such as tobacco use and educational level and it may be those characteristics that are related to the risk of AD rather than alcohol use per se.

The case-control design also has inherent limitations. One notable weakness is that it is essentially cross-sectional. Longitudinal studies collect data on alcohol use at baseline and follow study participants over time to determine if they develop AD. Because high levels of alcohol use are associated with greater mortality, drinkers may be more likely than nondrinkers to die before developing AD, so a protective association between alcohol use and AD may simply reflect selective mortality. Clearly, longitudinal studies provide a better design from which to address issues such as selective mortality.

In addition, case-control studies collect information on alcohol use after diagnosis of AD. But because the cognitive deficits characteristic of AD mean that self-reported information cannot be obtained from study participants, proxy respondents (e.g., family members) are required. A proxy's report is unlikely to correspond perfectly with the information that the study respondent would have provided. This problem is exacerbated if this source of error is not consistent across cases and controls (i.e., studies that use proxy reports for cases should also use proxy reports for controls). A methodological flaw in some of the case-control studies of AD has been the use of proxy-reported information for cases but self-reported data for controls.

Because of the methodological limitations of case-control studies, evidence from cohort studies-a stronger, longitudinal design-is usually given more weight, even though they also may have limitations (e.g., determination of AD based on clinical records rather than personal examination as per standard diagnostic criteria). Cohort studies generally have found no significant effect of alcohol use on the risk of developing AD, although some evidence of a protective effect of moderate wine consumption (defined as three to four glasses per day) has been reported-that is, moderate wine consumption has been associated with a decreased risk for AD.

It is reasonable to expect that the effect of alcohol use on the risk of developing AD might differ depending on the level of alcohol consumption studied, but this does not seem to explain the study results. The cohort studies that found no association between alcohol use and AD used a variety of measures of alcohol consumption, from drinking status, to amount of alcohol consumed. Both studies reporting protective effects were based in France and focused on wine consumption. It is possible that a protective effect is specific to this situation-that wine rather than other types of alcohol, in the drinking pattern and context of French culture, could be protective. However, the decreased risk of AD with alcohol use was reversed to become a significantly increased risk when the participants place of residence was considered (i.e., in the community or in an institution). Specifically, moderate wine consumption was associated with a lower risk of AD when place of residence was not considered, but with an increased risk when it was included in the analyses. In addition, the significant protective effect of moderate wine consumption reported in the French longitudinal study was based on very few cases of AD. Although overall most epidemiologic studies, regardless of the design, do not support an association between alcohol use and AD, further longitudinal studies are needed that overcome the methodological limitations of previous studies. The apparent lack of association between alcohol use and AD in epidemiological studies contrasts with alcohol's proven effects on cognition, neuropathology, and neurochemistry, and its association with dementias other than AD. If it is determined that alcohol does influence the risk of AD, then understanding the mechanism by which it exerts this effect may provide clues to causal pathways, interventions, and prevention.

Alcohol, Tobacco, and Alzheimer Disease

The effect of alcohol use on AD may be modified by other concurrent factors, such as tobacco use. Tobacco and alcohol use are related:

"smokers drink and drinkers smoke." The heaviest drinkers are the most likely to smoke, and 70 percent to almost 100 percent of alcoholics in treatment programs report smoking. Conversely, a smoker is 10 times more likely than a nonsmoker to become an alcoholic.

The prevalence of concurrent alcohol and tobacco dependence suggests that alcohol and tobacco may share mechanisms that lead to dependence. These mechanisms may have a genetic basis. Tobacco and alcohol use may be related at least partially because both nicotine and alcohol affect brain nicotinic cholinergic receptors. Stimulation of these receptors is thought to contribute to the therapeutic effects of galantamine, a new treatment for AD.

Research shows that alcohol and tobacco use interact to influence the risk of certain diseases, such as cancer. Nicotine counteracts some of alcohol's negative effects on cognition, including increased reaction time, impaired time judgment, and slowing of brain wave activity. Epidemiologic studies have begun to investigate the effect of an interaction between smoking and drinking on AD. Adjusting for smoking status had little effect on the association between alcohol use and AD in the case-control study by Cupples and colleagues.

However, an analysis of three case-control datasets has provided some support for the hypothesis that smoking influences the effect of alcohol use on AD. In one of the data sets, the risk of AD was significantly increased in drinkers. Study participants who smoked as well as drank, however, had a lower risk than those who only drank. The pattern in the other two data sets varied depending on whether the participants had a history of hypertension. A pattern similar to that of the first data set, but only marginally significant, was found for hypertensive subjects in a second data set, with the risk of AD for people who were both smokers and drinkers lower than the risk for those who were just smokers or just drinkers. It is not clear whether the effect of hypertension reflects a physiological interaction of hypertension with smoking, drinking, and AD. Few analyses on the interaction of tobacco and alcohol use have been published, but one study did find that the association between smoking and AD varied by the hypertensive status of study participants.

The observation that alcohol and tobacco use appear to influence each other's association with AD is consistent with evidence of a biological interaction between smoking and drinking. This observation also may be attributed, however, to the increased overall mortality of people who both smoke and drink, a possibility that can only be ruled out by longitudinal research. The apparent importance of hypertension suggests that a vascular mechanism may be involved in the interaction of alcohol and tobacco use on the risk of developing AD.

Epidemiologic Studies of Alcohol Use and Cognitive Impairment

Although epidemiologic studies do not generally support an association between alcohol consumption and AD, the lack of such a relationship could reflect methodological limitations, such as the difficulty in discriminating AD cases with a history of heavy alcohol consumption from cases of alcoholic dementia. It thus may also be useful to consider evidence from epidemiologic studies examining the association between alcohol use and cognitive outcomes other than AD. The ways in which alcohol use influences the risk of developing cognitive impairment might be similar to those by which it may affect AD, and some types of cognitive impairment themselves may increase the risk of developing AD.

Overall, the results of epidemiologic studies of alcohol use and cognitive impairment are consistent with results from studies of alcohol use and AD. Most studies, regardless of design, found no significant association between alcohol use and cognitive impairment. Those studies which did report a significant effect of alcohol use generally found that the results varied by gender, by apolipoprotein E (ApoE) allele status, or by vascular risk factors (e.g., cardiovascular disease (CVD), and diabetes). Evidence of these subgroup effects is not yet compelling; for example, in people with the apolipoprotein E allele, alcohol use increased the risk of cognitive impairment in one study but decreased it in another. In another study, apolipoprotein status had no effect. However, investigation of the effects of alcohol use on AD within these gender, genetic, or vascular risk subgroups may prove informative.

Does Alcohol Use Cause Alzheimer Disease?

Although an increased risk of AD with alcohol use is plausible based on biological evidence, the epidemiologic evidence does not support an association. In the few studies that report a significant association, alcohol consumption is more often found to reduce the risk of AD than to increase it. However, methodological factors could create an apparent protective effect of alcohol use on AD. Such factors include selective mortality of drinkers and diagnosing AD patients with heavy alcohol use as having alcoholic dementia rather than AD. In addition, in some studies reporting a protective effect of alcohol, proxy respondents provided information for the cases whereas self-reported information was used for controls. If proxy reports of drinking underestimate actual exposure, the alcohol use of cases (i.e., study participants with

AD) would be artificially lowered compared with control subjects. The apparent association between alcohol use and a reduced risk of AD might, therefore, merely reflect bias in proxy reports rather than any true effect. Other recent reports of a protective effect may have been affected by sample size and the selection of confounding factors, such as community or institutional residence, included in the analyses.

Most studies, including the meta-analysis of case-control studies and individual cohort studies of AD have not found a significant association. Epidemiologic studies of alcohol use and cognitive impairment overall have come to similar conclusions, although some evidence exists for a heterogeneous effect of alcohol use on cognitive impairment across gender, genetic, or vascular subgroups.

The effect of alcohol use on the risk of AD has been explored much less extensively than the effect of other potential risk factors, such as tobacco use. The possibility of a protective effect of moderate drinking on AD, raised in a few studies, may not be compelling, but methodological issues need to be resolved before such an association can be definitively dismissed. Moderate drinking has been reported to have some beneficial vascular effects, which could possibly reduce the risk of AD. The nonsignificant association between alcohol use and risk of AD reported by most studies does not necessarily mean that alcohol has no effect. It may instead reflect a balance between the beneficial vascular effects of alcohol and its detrimental effects on the brain, and the relative weight of these two factors may differ within specific subgroups.

Limitations of Current Studies

Because AD has few established risk factors, most studies have examined alcohol use as only one possibly relevant exposure among many, necessitating superficial treatment. Future studies need to collect more detailed information about lifetime alcohol exposure because imprecision in estimating lifetime exposure may obscure associations, as may inconsistent definitions of drinking status or level of consumption. Evidence that alcohol's effects on AD might vary within subgroups also supports more extensive data collection on variables that characterize these subgroups.

One methodological challenge of both case-control and cohort studies is the separation of AD from alcoholic dementia. AD cannot be definitively diagnosed clinically but instead requires confirmation based on examination of the brain after death. Even when AD is accurately diagnosed before death, study participants still represent a heterogeneous group, differing in age at onset, duration, and genetic basis of AD. Case-control studies may introduce bias by using heavy alcohol consumption as an exclusionary criterion for AD cases but not for controls. As alcoholic dementia has not been uniformly diagnosed across epidemiologic studies, the discrimination of alcoholic dementia from AD also is problematic.

Section 17.2

Effects of Nicotine on Cognitive Function

This section includes text excerpted from "The Health Consequences of Smoking—50 Years of Progress," Office of the Surgeon General (OSG), January 16, 2014. Reviewed December 2018.

Researchers have suggested that smoking may have cognition-enhancing properties, such as improvements in sustained attention, reaction time, and memory. Initial reports of improved cognitive function were based on empirical evidence from smokers; thus, these observations could reflect the mitigation of cognitive impairment from nicotine withdrawal, enhancement of smokers cognitive function independent of nicotine's effects on withdrawal symptoms, or both. Interest in the effects of nicotine on cognition has since expanded to include healthy nonsmokers and individuals with underlying neuropsychiatric conditions accompanied by cognitive deficits. Concurrently, there is a growing awareness of the potential harms of nicotine exposure during certain vulnerable stages of brain development, such as during fetal and adolescent growth. This section reviews the evidence on the effects of nicotine on cognitive function in general (in smokers and nonsmokers), and in potentially vulnerable populations.

Cognitive Function and the Nicotinic Acetylcholine Receptor System

Underlying the purported connection between nicotine and cognitive enhancement is the role of nAChRs (Nicotinic acetylcholine receptors) in attention, learning, memory, and cortical plasticity. nAChRs are receptors that normally bind endogenous neurotransmitter acetylcholine, but are also particularly responsive to nicotine. nAChRs are abundant in brain regions associated with learning and memory, including the prefrontal cortex, and in primate and rodent models, depletion of acetylcholine in the prefrontal cortex results in impaired attentional performance; $\beta 2$ nAChRs are especially abundant in the brain and have a high affinity for nicotine. Recent evidence from animal studies suggests that $\beta 2$ nAChRs play a critical role in regulating attention. Additional research has demonstrated that nicotine interferes with cholinergic control of $\beta 2$ nAChRs in the prefrontal cortex in mice, which could result in acute impairment of attention and alterations of the prefrontal cortex network, and lead to long-term effects on attention. Mice lacking the $\beta 2$ nAChR subunit demonstrate deficits in executive function.

Effects of Nicotine on Cognitive Function in Healthy Adult Smokers and Nonsmokers

In adults, the negative effects of nicotine withdrawal on cognitive function have been documented in both humans and animals, and the administration of nicotine during withdrawal mitigates cognitive impairment. Independent smokers, abstinence from smoking is associated with reductions in working memory and sustained attention, and adverse effects on attention can be seen as early as 30 minutes after smoking the last cigarette. Nicotine withdrawal is also commonly accompanied by symptoms of negative affect (anxiety and depression) and relief of this symptom may be an important element of addiction in smokers. Because negative affect and attentional control are related, the effects of smoking on these two domains could be interrelated.

Whether there are direct effects of nicotine on cognitive function (positive or negative) in nonabstinent smokers and in healthy nonsmoking adults is less clear. In a recent meta-analysis of double-blind, placebo-controlled studies examining the acute effects of nicotine (administered mainly as nicotine replacement product) on cognitive function in nonsmokers and smokers abstinent for two hours or less, nicotine was found to result in cognitive enhancement in six of nine performance domains: fine motor, alerting attention-accuracy and response time (RT), orienting attention and RT, short-term episodic memory accuracy, and working memory RT. To separate the effects of nicotine on symptoms of withdrawal versus its direct effects, the results were stratified by smoking status. The effects on alerting attention accuracy and short-term episodic memory accuracy were significant in smokers but not in nonsmokers; effects on alerting attention RT were significant in nonsmokers but not in smokers; effects on working memory RT were significant in both smokers and nonsmokers, and in the remaining outcomes there were insufficient numbers of studies on smokers to conduct stratified analysis. Thus, nicotine may have some positive effects on cognitive performance that are unique to nonsmokers. No studies meeting the inclusion criteria for the review addressed learning or executive function.

Critical Periods of Exposure in the Nervous System

Across the lifespan, there are several developmental windows during which exposure to nicotine may have adverse consequences. In the fetus, nicotine targets neurotransmitter receptors in the brain, potentially resulting in abnormalities in cell proliferation and altering synaptic activity. The effects of prenatal exposure to nicotine on the fetal nervous system are summarized earlier in this section.

Human brain development continues far longer than was previously realized. In particular, areas involved in higher cognitive function such as the prefrontal cortex continue to develop throughout adolescence (the period during which individuals are most likely to begin smoking) and into adulthood. During this extended period of maturation, substantial neural remodeling occurs, including synaptic pruning and changes in dopaminergic input, as well as changes in gray and white matter volume. The density of projections from the amygdala to the prefrontal cortex increases, suggesting that there is substantial development of the connectivity between the emotional and cognitive areas of the brain. The cholinergic system, which matures in adolescence, plays a central role in maturation of cognitive function and reward.

Smoking during adolescence has been associated with lasting cognitive and behavioral impairments, including effects on working memory and attention, although causal relationships are difficult to establish in the presence of potential confounding factors. In addition, functional magnetic resonance imaging in humans showed that young adult smokers had reduced prefrontal cortex (PFC) activation during attentional tasks when compared with nonsmoking controls. Diminished prefrontal cortex activity correlated with duration of smoking, supporting the hypothesis that smoking could have long-lasting effects on cognition.

Animal studies provide evidence that nicotine exposure during adolescence has effects on the brain that differ from exposure during

114

other periods of development. Studies in rodents show that nicotine induces changes in gene expression in the brain to a greater degree with adolescent exposure than during other periods of development. Deoxyribonucleic acid (DNA) microarrays in female rats demonstrated that gene expression in response to nicotine was most pronounced around the age of puberty and the effects of nicotine on gene expression were most dramatic in the hippocampus, with upregulation of growth factors and cyclic AMP (adenosine monophosphate) signaling pathways. Expression of the *Arc* gene (implicated in synaptic plasticity, learning, memory, and addiction) was upregulated in the prefrontal cortex in adolescent rats exposed to nicotine, and to a much greater extent than in adult rats.

Nicotine exposure during adolescence also appears to cause long-term structural and functional changes in the brain. Exposure of adolescent rats to nicotine resulted in upregulation of nAChRs in the midbrain, cerebral cortex, and hippocampus that was still present four weeks after the end of the exposure, in contrast to adult rats in which upregulation had disappeared by four weeks. Receptor upregulation was more pronounced in male adolescent rats than females. Indices of cell damage and size in rats with adolescent nicotine exposure indicate reduced cell number and size in the cerebral cortex, midbrain, and hippocampus. Structural changes in prefrontal cortex neurons have also been described, including increased dendritic length and spine density.

Some effects of nicotine exposure appear to be gender-selective. For example, adolescent nicotine exposure resulted in increased membrane protein concentration in the hippocampus, consistent with cell damage and/or cell loss, in female rats, but not in males. Male rats with nicotine exposure demonstrated a loss of a dopaminergic response to nicotine more than a month after exposure ended, while females exhibited deficits in hippocampal norepinephrine content and turnover during the month after nicotine exposure. Because estrogen regulates hippocampal cell proliferation in an adult rat, there may be interactions between the effects of nicotine and the hormonal milieu in the adolescent

Corresponding behavioral studies of adolescent rats have also shown effects of nicotine exposure. Exposed females exhibited reduced grooming during exposure and reduced locomotion and rearing after cessation of exposure; these results were not seen in exposed adult rats, which show increased grooming in both genders and no decrease in locomotion. Adolescent rats, tested five weeks after nicotine exposure ended, demonstrated an increase in premature responses and a reduction in correct responses when given a serial reaction time test; this effect was not seen with adult exposure.

Thus, adolescents appear to be particularly vulnerable to the adverse effects of nicotine on the central nervous system (CNS). Based on existing knowledge of adolescent brain development, results of animal studies, and limited data from studies of adolescent and young adult smokers, it is likely that nicotine exposure during adolescence adversely affects cognitive function and development. Therefore, the potential long-term cognitive effects of exposure to nicotine in this age group are of great concern.

The effects of nicotine exposure on cognitive function after adolescence and young adulthood are unknown. There are data to suggest that smoking accelerates some aspects of cognitive decline in adults, and that these effects appear to be mediated by an increased risk of respiratory and cardiovascular disease (CVD). However, in a cohort study of more than 7,000 men and women, the authors found that current male smokers and recent former smokers had a greater 10-year decline in global cognition and executive function than never smokers (with the greatest adverse effect on executive function); these differences were not explained by other health behaviors or measures, including heart disease and stroke, and measures of lung function. An analysis using pack-years as the exposure measure provided evidence of a dose-response relationship. The results of the latter study suggest that there may be mechanisms contributing to cognitive decline in addition to and independent of respiratory and cardiovascular disease; however, whether nicotine plays a role in accelerating cognitive decline is unknown.

Other Vulnerable Populations

Although the contribution of nicotine to the effects of smoking on cognitive decline is unclear, there has been a great deal of interest in applications of nicotine as a treatment for several conditions characterized by cognitive deficits, including Alzheimer disease and Parkinson disease (PD). These disorders have underlying deficits in the cholinergic system, and it has been hypothesized that nicotine and/or nicotine analogs may be effective in attenuating symptoms or slowing disease progression. This hypothesis is further supported by research suggesting that acute administration of nicotine has cognitive-enhancing properties. In addition, some early observational studies showed evidence for a reduced risk of Alzheimer disease in smokers, suggesting that components in tobacco smoke, such as nicotine, may have protective properties. A growing body of evidence now links smoking to an increased risk for Alzheimer disease rather than a reduced risk;

however, research on nicotine as a treatment for this condition (and for Parkinson disease) continues. Other disorders associated with cognitive and attentional impairment, such as schizophrenia and attention deficit hyperactivity disorder (ADHD), are characterized by a very high prevalence of smoking among those affected. It has been proposed that individuals with these disorders smoke in order to alleviate the symptoms of their disease, and a number of clinical trials using nicotine as a therapeutic agent have been conducted.

Alzheimer Disease

Alzheimer disease is a common form of dementia in which individuals experience ongoing deterioration of cognitive abilities. Although smoking is recognized as a risk factor for Alzheimer disease, acute nicotine administration has been reported to improve some Alzheimer disease symptoms, such as recall, visual attention, and mood. The plausibility of this effect is supported by studies of Alzheimer disease patients showing deficits in cholinergic systems and a loss of nicotinic binding sites. However, evidence from randomized trials to support improvement of Alzheimer disease symptoms from nicotine treatment is sparse. In a 2001 Cochrane review updated in 2010, the authors found no double-blind, placebo-controlled, randomized trials of treatment for Alzheimer disease with nicotine and concluded that there is no evidence to recommend nicotine as a treatment for Alzheimer disease.

Section 17.3

Heart Health

This section includes text excerpted from "Risk Factors for Heart Disease Linked to Dementia," National Institutes of Health (NIH), August 15, 2017.

People with dementia have problems thinking, remembering, and communicating. They may repeat the same question over and over, get lost in familiar places, or have other problems managing everyday life.

Dementia can be caused by a number of disorders, such as strokes, brain tumors, Alzheimer disease (AD), and late-stage Parkinson disease. Most forms of dementia slowly worsen. Risk factors include aging, diabetes, high blood pressure (hypertension), smoking cigarettes, and a family history of dementia.

Past studies suggest that problems in the vascular system—the heart and blood vessels that supply blood to the brain—can contribute to the development of dementia. To explore the effect of vascular risk factors on dementia, a research team led by Dr. Rebecca Gottesman at Johns Hopkins University studied nearly 16,000 middle-aged people who participated in the Atherosclerosis Risk in Communities (ARIC) study. ARIC was funded by National Institute of Health's (NIH) National Heart, Lung, and Blood Institute (NHLBI). The study was also supported by NIH's National Institute of Neurological Disorders and Stroke (NINDS). Results were published online on August 7, 2017, in *JAMA Neurology*.

The people enrolled in the study were between 44 to 66 years old in 1987 to 1989 and located in four states. Over a 25-year period, the researchers examined the participants five times with a variety of medical tests. Cognitive tests of memory and thinking were given during the second, fourth, and fifth exams. In addition to in-person visits, the researchers collected health data from telephone interviews, caregiver interviews, hospitalization records, and death certificates.

More than 1,500 of the participants were diagnosed with dementia over the 25-year period. The analysis confirmed prior findings that those with vascular risk factors in midlife, such as diabetes or hypertension, had a greater chance of developing dementia as they aged. Also confirming other studies, smoking cigarettes increased the risk of dementia (although this effect was seen only in white people). In addition, the researchers detected a higher risk of dementia among people with prehypertension, in which blood pressure levels are higher than normal but lower than hypertension.

The team reanalyzed the data to determine whether having had a stroke influenced these associations. They found that diabetes, hypertension, prehypertension, and smoking during midlife increased the risk of developing dementia whether or not the person had a stroke."With an aging population, dementia is becoming a greater health concern. This study supports the importance of controlling vascular risk factors like high blood pressure early in life in an effort to prevent dementia as we age," says NINDS Director Dr. Walter J. Koroshetz. "What's good for the heart is good for the brain."

Section 17.4

Sleep Deprivation Increases Alzheimer Disease Protein

This section includes text excerpted from "Sleep Deprivation Increases Alzheimer's Protein," National Institutes of Health (NIH), April 24, 2018.

Beta-amyloid (Aβ) is a metabolic waste product that's found in the fluid between brain cells (neurons). A buildup of beta-amyloid is linked to impaired brain function and Alzheimer disease (AD). In Alzheimer disease, beta-amyloid clumps together to form amyloid plaques, which hinder communication between neurons.

Impaired sleep has been associated with Alzheimer disease. Studies suggest that sleep plays a role in clearing beta-amyloid out of the brain. Moreover, lack of sleep has been shown to elevate brain beta-amyloid levels in mice. Less is known about the impact of sleep deprivation on beta-amyloid levels in people.

To investigate the possible link between beta-amyloid and sleep in people, lead author Dr. Ehsan Shokri-Kojori, in a team led by Drs. Nora D. Volkow and Gene-Jack Wang of National Institute of Health's (NIH) National Institute on Alcohol Abuse and Alcoholism (NIAAA), used positron emission tomography (PET) to scan the brains of 20 healthy participants, aged 22 to 72. To measure beta-amyloid they used a radiotracer called 18F-florbetaben that has been shown to bind beta-amyloid.

The researchers scanned participants brains after getting a full night's rest and after a night of sleep deprivation (about 31 hours without sleep). Beta-amyloid increased about 5 percent in the participants brains after losing a night of sleep. These changes occurred in brain regions that included the thalamus and hippocampus, which are especially vulnerable to damage in the early stages of Alzheimer disease.

The scientists also found that study participants with larger increases in beta-amyloid reported worse mood after sleep deprivation. These findings support other studies that have found that the hippocampus and thalamus play a role in mood disorders.

"Even though our sample was small, this study demonstrated the negative effect of sleep deprivation on beta-amyloid burden in the human brain," Shokri-Kojori says. "Future studies are needed to assess the generalizability to a larger and more diverse population."

"This research provides new insight about the potentially harmful effects of a lack of sleep on the brain and has implications for better characterizing the pathology of Alzheimer disease," says Dr. George F. Koob, director of NIAAA.

More studies are needed to identify the precise biological mechanism underlying the observed increase in beta-amyloid. It's also important to note that the link between sleep disorders and Alzheimer disease risk is thought to go both ways. Elevated beta-amyloid may also lead to trouble sleeping.

Section 17.5

Decade after Menopause Poses Highest Risk of Alzheimer Disease for Women with ApoE4 Gene

This section includes text excerpted from "Decade after Menopause Poses Highest Risk of Alzheimer's for Women with ApoE4 Gene," National Institute on Aging (NIA), National Institutes of Health (NIH), October 2, 2017.

Recent research has challenged previously accepted notions that the gene variant ApoE4 gave its female carriers a greater risk of developing Alzheimer disease than men.

A team of researchers led by Dr. Scott Neu of the University of Southern California and supported in part by National Institute on Aging (NIA) found that gender differences in Alzheimer disease risk are not as clear as once thought, and that the decade or so after menopause poses the most significant risk for women. The scientists examined clinical and genetic data from nearly 58,000 study participants to provide a more detailed, nuanced picture of sex difference and the gene variant.

The project used information from 27 different studies using the National Institutes of Health (NIH)-funded Global Alzheimer Association Interactive Network (GAAIN) (www.gaain.org), an open-access information hub that gives scientists from around the world a sophisticated data sharing and analysis tool. The new study used GAAIN data for a closer look at AD study participants of both genders, ranging in age from 55 to 85, and found that ApoE4 impacted both genders equally. When the data was further split into age groups, sex differences were found, with genetically susceptible women between ages 65 to 75 at greater risk for AD compared to men, and an increased chance of mild cognitive impairment between ages 55 to 70.

The researchers noted that their findings highlight the importance of increasing studies that focus on women and the unique changes that take place before and after menopause. The authors of an accompanying *JAMA Neurology* editorial said that the findings could lead to changes in the ages to start Alzheimer disease interventions for both men and women.

Section 17.6

Connection between Hearing and Cognitive Health

This section includes text excerpted from "What's the Connection between Hearing and Cognitive Health?" National Institute on Aging (NIA), National Institutes of Health (NIH), October 19, 2017.

Hearing loss occurs in approximately one in three people age 65 to 74 and nearly one in two people age 75 and older in the United States, making it one of the most common conditions affecting older adults. Last year, the National Academies of Sciences, Engineering, and Medicine (NASEM) released *Hearing Health Care for Adults: Priorities for Improving Access and Affordability*, a report that highlights the importance of hearing health to communication and overall quality of life, and proposes recommendations to increase the availability and affordability of hearing healthcare.

National Institute on Aging (NIA)-funded research has indicated that hearing loss may impact cognition and dementia risk in older adults. A study found that older adults with hearing loss were more likely to develop dementia than older adults with normal hearing. In fact, there was a relationship between level of uncorrected hearing loss and level of dementia risk: mild hearing loss was associated with a two-fold increase in risk; moderate hearing loss with a three-fold increase in risk, and severe hearing loss with a fivefold increase in risk.

Trial Launched to Test Hearing Intervention Impact on Cognitive Decline

The National Institute on Aging (NIA) has recently funded the Aging, Cognition, and Hearing Evaluation in Elders (ACHIEVE) clinical trial led by Drs. Frank Lin and Josef Coresh at Johns Hopkins University to examine the potential benefits of hearing rehabilitation. ACHIEVE will recruit 850 cognitively normal adults aged 70 to 84 with hearing loss from four locations (Hagerstown MD, Jackson MS, Minneapolis MN, and Winston-Salem NC). Individuals will be randomly assigned to either the hearing intervention (hearing needs assessment, fitting of hearing devices, education/counseling) or control intervention (health education).

ACHIEVE participants will be followed for three years and information on hearing function, cognition, and demographics (e.g., age, sex, education level) will be collected at several time points. The primary outcome of the study will be to determine if the hearing rehabilitative intervention changes the rates of cognitive decline as compared to the group receiving health education. Additionally, the researchers will examine if the intervention impacts physical and social functioning, quality of life, and physical activity.

Part Three

Other Dementia Disorders

Chapter 18

Cognitive Impairment

Cognitive impairment is when a person has trouble remembering, learning new things, concentrating, or making decisions that affect their everyday life. Cognitive impairment ranges from mild to severe. With mild impairment, people may begin to notice changes in cognitive functions, but still be able to do their everyday activities. Severe levels of impairment can lead to losing the ability to understand the meaning or importance of something and the ability to talk or write, resulting in the inability to live independently.

More than 16 million people in the United States are living with cognitive impairment, but the impact of cognitive impairment at the state level is not well understood. In 2009, five states addressed this shortcoming by assessing the impact of cognitive impairment on their residents. This knowledge is vital to developing or maintaining effective policies and programs to address the needs of people living with cognitive impairment in your state. The time for action is now!

Age is the greatest risk factor for cognitive impairment, and as the baby boomer generation passes age 65, the number of people living with cognitive impairment is expected to jump dramatically. An estimated 5.1 million Americans aged 65 years or older may currently have Alzheimer disease (AD), the most well-known form of cognitive impairment; this number may rise to 13.2 million by 2050.

This chapter includes text excerpted from "Cognitive Impairment: A Call for Action, Now!" Centers for Disease Control and Prevention (CDC), February 2011. Reviewed December 2018.

Cognitive impairment is costly. People with cognitive impairment report more than three times as many hospital stays as individuals who are hospitalized for some other condition. Alzheimer disease and related dementias alone are estimated to be the third most expensive disease to treat in the United States. The average Medicaid nursing facility expenditure per state in 2010 for individuals with Alzheimer disease is estimated at $647 million, not including home- and community-based care or prescription drug costs.

The imminent growth in the number of people living with cognitive impairment will place significantly greater demands on our systems of care. There are now more than 10 million family members providing unpaid care to a person with a cognitive impairment, a memory problem or a disorder like Alzheimer disease or other dementia. In 2009 it was estimated that 12.5 billion hours of unpaid care were provided, at a value of $144 billion. Much more in-home or institutional care and unpaid assistance by family and friends will be needed in the future as the numbers of those with Alzheimer disease and other forms of cognitive impairment grow.

The increasing economic burden and growing demand for care because of cognitive impairment pose a serious challenge to our states and nation unless steps are taken now to address these problems:

• State health departments can gather more state data to understand the impact, burden, and needs of people with cognitive impairment.

• States should consider developing a comprehensive action plan to respond to the needs of people with cognitive impairment, involving different agencies, as well as private and public organizations.

• Comprehensive systems of support should be expanded for people with cognitive impairment, their families, and caregiver.

• Additional training is needed for health professionals to detect cognitive impairment in its early stages and help patients with multiple conditions manage their care.

Failure to address these needs now will have serious consequences for the millions of Americans affected by cognitive impairment as well as the state agencies providing care and services to this population.

Key Facts about Cognitive Impairment

Cognitive impairment is not caused by any one disease or condition, nor is it limited to a specific age group. Alzheimer disease and other dementias in addition to conditions such as stroke, traumatic brain injury (TBI), and developmental disabilities, can cause cognitive impairment. A few commons signs of cognitive impairment include the following:

- Memory loss

- Frequently asking the same question or repeating the same story over and over

- Not recognizing familiar people and places

- Having trouble exercising judgment, such as knowing what to do in an emergency

- Changes in mood or behavior

- Vision problems

- Difficulty planning and carrying out tasks, such as following a recipe or keeping track of monthly bills

While age is the primary risk factor for cognitive impairment, other risk factors include family history, education level, brain injury, exposure to pesticides or toxins, physical inactivity, and chronic conditions such as Parkinson disease (PD), heart disease and stroke, and diabetes. Individuals may reduce the risk of cognitive impairment by keeping physically active and maintaining healthy cholesterol and blood sugar levels. At present, there is no cure for cognitive impairment caused by Alzheimer disease or other related dementias. However, some causes of cognitive impairment are related to health issues that may be treatable, like medication side effects, vitamin B_{12} deficiency, and depression. This is why it is important to identify people who are showing signs of cognitive impairment to ensure that they are evaluated by a healthcare professional and receive appropriate care or treatment.

Why Cognitive Impairment Is an Important Issue

Americans fear losing cognitive function. We are twice as fearful of losing our mental capacity as having diminished physical ability and 60 percent of adults are very or somewhat worried about memory loss. Persons affected by cognitive impairment, such as adults with Alzheimer disease, veterans with traumatic brain injuries, and the families of people living with cognitive impairment, represent a significant portion of your constituency. Taking steps to address this issue will ultimately have a positive impact on your entire community and state.

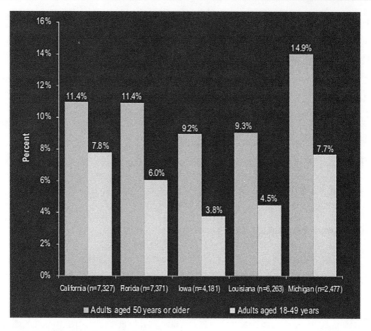

Figure 18.1. *Percentage of Adults with Perceived Cognitive Impairment, by Select State and Age, 2009.*

- *The percent of adults aged 18 to 49 years with perceived cognitive impairment ranged from approximately 4 percent in Iowa to 8 percent in Michigan and California.*

- *State agencies can ensure that strategic planning (e.g., for emergency preparedness), surveillance, and programmatic efforts carried out in concert with key partners include elements that support the health and well-being of this population.*

- *The percent of adults aged 50 or older with perceived cognitive impairment ranged from approximately 9 percent in Iowa and Louisiana to 15 percent in Michigan.*

- *The dramatic aging of the U.S. population will result in substantially increased numbers of individuals in states with cognitive impairment*

Proven Solutions to Drive Policy

States across the country are responding to the call-for-action to improve the health and quality of life of adults living with cognitive impairment. The examples below are from the U.S. Administration on Aging's (AOA) Alzheimer Disease Supportive Services Program (ADSSP), which supports state efforts to create responsive, integrated, and sustainable service delivery systems for persons with Alzheimer disease and related disorders and their family caregivers.

The New York University (NYU) Counseling and Support Intervention is a combination of individual counseling, weekly support groups, and counseling for family caregivers of people with Alzheimer disease—an intervention that delayed nursing home placement of people with dementia by about 1.5 years.

In Ohio, the Cleveland Alzheimer Managed Care Demonstration project evaluated the effects of integrating Alzheimer Association care consultation services with managed healthcare services. It was found that patients with severe cognitive impairment had fewer physician visits, were less likely to have a hospital admission and had decreased depression.

How Policymakers Can Take Action

Cognitive impairment needs to be addressed with a comprehensive and coordinated approach. The condition will continue to impose an increasing economic burden on states, families, and individuals unless an action is taken now. As a legislator, you play a crucial role by exploring policy changes and initiatives that will expand research, increase support, and, ultimately, improve conditions for people living with cognitive impairment and their families. Some potential strategies include the following recommendations:

- Establish a legislative task force to study cognitive impairment in your state.

- Support the development and implementation of a state Alzheimer disease or dementia action plan or address the needs of individuals living with cognitive impairment in existing state action plans.

- Check to see if your state is collecting information to assess cognitive impairment in your state; for example, your state includes the impact of cognitive Impairment module in your state's Behavioral Risk Factor Surveillance Survey (BRFSS), available at www.cdc.gov/brfss.

- Encourage your state health agencies to consider the needs of community-dwelling people with cognitive impairment in their policies and programs.

- Support state-level collaboration and expansion of home- and community-based services to better serve the needs of individuals with cognitive impairment.

- Encourage collaboration and pooling of resources, starting with wraparound community projects, to assist individuals living with dementia and other forms of cognitive impairment and their family caregivers.

- Support training for people in the health and human services fields.

- Seek Medicaid and Medicare waivers for demonstration projects designed to find solutions to complex conditions such as Alzheimer disease.

Chapter 19

Degenerative Neurological Disease

Chapter Contents

Section 19.1

Corticobasal Degeneration

This section includes text excerpted from "Corticobasal Degeneration Information Page," National Institute of Neurological Disorders and Stroke (NINDS), June 21, 2018.

Corticobasal degeneration (CBD) is a progressive neurological disorder characterized by nerve cell loss and atrophy (shrinkage) of multiple areas of the brain including the cerebral cortex and the basal ganglia. Corticobasal degeneration progresses gradually. Initial symptoms, which typically begin at or around age 60, may first appear on one side of the body (unilateral), but eventually, affect both sides as the disease progresses.

Symptoms

Symptoms of CBD are similar to those found in Parkinson disease (PD), such as poor coordination, akinesia (an absence of movements), rigidity (a resistance to imposed movement), disequilibrium (impaired balance); and limb dystonia (abnormal muscle postures). Other symptoms such as cognitive and visual-spatial impairments, apraxia (loss of the ability to make familiar, purposeful movements), hesitant and halting speech, myoclonus (muscular jerks), and dysphagia (difficulty swallowing) may also occur. An individual with corticobasal degeneration eventually becomes unable to walk.

Treatment

There is no treatment available to slow the course of corticobasal degeneration, and the symptoms of the disease are generally resistant to therapy. Drugs used to treat PD-type symptoms do not produce any significant or sustained improvement. Clonazepam may help the myoclonus. Occupational, physical, and speech therapy can help in managing disability.

Prognosis

Corticobasal degeneration usually progresses slowly over the course of six to eight years. Death is generally caused by pneumonia or other complications of severe debility such as sepsis or pulmonary embolism.

Section 19.2

Dementia with Lewy Bodies

This section includes text excerpted from "Dementia with Lewy Bodies Information Page," National Institute of Neurological Disorders and Stroke (NINDS), June 21, 2018.

Dementia with Lewy bodies (DLB) is one of the most common types of progressive dementia. The central features of DLB include progressive cognitive decline, "fluctuations" in alertness and attention, visual hallucinations, and parkinsonian motor symptoms, such as slowness of movement, difficulty walking, or rigidity. People may also suffer from depression. The symptoms of DLB are caused by the buildup of Lewy bodies—accumulated bits of alpha-synuclein (α-Syn) protein—inside the nuclei of neurons in areas of the brain that control particular aspects of memory and motor control. Researchers don't know exactly why alpha-synuclein accumulates into Lewy bodies or how Lewy bodies cause the symptoms of DLB, but they do know that alpha-synuclein accumulation is also linked to Parkinson disease (PD), multiple system atrophy, and several other disorders, which are referred to as the "synucleinopathies."

The similarity of symptoms between DLB and Parkinson disease (PD), and between DLB and Alzheimer disease (AD), can often make it difficult for a doctor to make a definitive diagnosis. In addition, Lewy bodies are often also found in the brains of people with Parkinson and Alzheimer diseases. These findings suggest that either DLB is related to these other causes of dementia or that an individual can have both diseases at the same time. DLB usually occurs sporadically, in people with no known family history of the disease. However, rare familial cases have occasionally been reported.

Treatment

There is no cure for DLB. Treatments are aimed at controlling the cognitive, psychiatric, and motor symptoms of the disorder. Acetylcholinesterase inhibitors (AChEIs), such as donepezil and rivastigmine, are primarily used to treat the cognitive symptoms of DLB, but they may also be of some benefit in reducing the psychiatric and motor symptoms. Doctors tend to avoid prescribing antipsychotics for hallucinatory symptoms of DLB because of the risk that neuroleptic sensitivity could worsen the motor symptoms. Some individuals with

DLB may benefit from the use of levodopa for their rigidity and loss of spontaneous movement.

Prognosis

Like Alzheimer disease and Parkinson disease, DLB is a neurodegenerative disorder that results in progressive intellectual and functional deterioration. There are no known therapies to stop or slow the progression of DLB. Average survival after the time of diagnosis is similar to that in Alzheimer disease, about eight years, with progressively increasing disability.

Section 19.3

Frontotemporal Dementia

This section includes text excerpted from "Frontotemporal Dementia Information Page," National Institute of Neurological Disorders and Stroke (NINDS), June 21, 2018.

Frontotemporal dementia (FTD) describes a clinical syndrome associated with shrinking of the frontal and temporal anterior lobes of the brain. Originally known as Pick disease, the name and classification of FTD has been a topic of discussion for over a century. The current designation of the syndrome groups together Pick disease, primary progressive aphasia (PPA), and semantic dementia as FTD. Some doctors propose adding corticobasal degeneration (CBD) and progressive supranuclear palsy (PSP) to FTD and calling the group Pick Complex. These designations will continue to be debated.

Symptoms

The symptoms of FTD fall into two clinical patterns that involve either changes in behavior, or problems with language. The first type features behavior that can be either impulsive (disinhibited) or bored and listless (apathetic) and includes inappropriate social behavior; lack of social tact; lack of empathy; distractibility; loss of insight into the behaviors of oneself and others; an increased interest in sex; changes in food preferences; agitation or, conversely, blunted emotions; neglect of personal hygiene; repetitive or compulsive behavior, and decreased energy and motivation. The second type primarily features symptoms of language disturbance, including difficulty making or understanding speech, often in conjunction with the behavioral type's symptoms. Spatial skills and memory remain intact. There is a strong genetic component to the disease; FTD often runs in families.

Treatment

No treatment has been shown to slow the progression of FTD. Behavior modification may help control unacceptable or dangerous behaviors. Aggressive, agitated, or dangerous behaviors could require medication. Antidepressants have been shown to improve some symptoms.

Prognosis

The outcome for people with FTD is poor. The disease progresses steadily and often rapidly, ranging from less than 2 years in some individuals to more than 10 years in others. Eventually, some individuals with FTD will need 24-hour care and monitoring at home or in an institutionalized care setting.

Section 19.4

Huntington Disease

This section includes text excerpted from "Huntington's Disease Information Page," National Institute of Neurological Disorders and Stroke (NINDS), June 15, 2018.

Huntington disease (HD) is an inherited disorder that causes brain cells, called neurons, to die in various areas of the brain, including those that help to control voluntary (intentional) movement. Symptoms of the disease, which gets progressively worse, include uncontrolled movements (called chorea), abnormal body postures, and changes in behavior, emotion, judgment, and cognition. People with HD also develop impaired coordination, slurred speech, and difficulty feeding and swallowing. HD typically begins between ages 30 and 50. An earlier onset form called juvenile HD occurs under age 20. Its symptoms differ somewhat from adult-onset HD and include rigidity, slowness, difficulty at school, rapid involuntary muscle jerks called myoclonus, and seizures. More than 30,000 Americans have HD.

Causes

Huntington disease is caused by a mutation in the gene for a protein called huntingtin. The defect causes the cytosine, adenine, and guanine (CAG) building blocks of deoxyribonucleic acid (DNA) to repeat many more times than is normal. Each child of a parent with HD has a 50-50 chance of inheriting the HD gene. A child who does not inherit the HD gene will not develop the disease and generally cannot pass it to subsequent generations. A person who inherits the HD gene will eventually develop the disease. HD is generally diagnosed based on a genetic test, medical history, brain imaging, and neurological and laboratory tests.

Treatment

There is no treatment that can stop or reverse the course of HD. Tetrabenazine and deutetrabenazine can treat chorea associated with HD. Antipsychotic drugs may ease chorea and help to control hallucinations, delusions, and violent outbursts. Drugs may be prescribed to treat depression and anxiety. Side effects of drugs used to treat the symptoms of HD may include fatigue, sedation, decreased concentration, restlessness, or hyperexcitability, and should be only used when symptoms create problems for the individual.

Prognosis

Huntington disease causes disability that gets worse over time. Currently, no treatment is available to slow, stop, or reverse the course of HD. People with HD usually die within 10 to 30 years following diagnosis, most commonly from infections (most often pneumonia) and injuries related to falls.

Section 19.5

Parkinson Disease

This section includes text excerpted from "Parkinson's Disease Information Page," National Institute of Neurological Disorders and Stroke (NINDS), June 12, 2018.

Parkinson disease (PD) belongs to a group of conditions called motor system disorders, which are the result of the loss of dopamine-producing brain cells.

Symptoms

The four primary symptoms of PD are tremor, or trembling in hands, arms, legs, jaw, and face; rigidity, or stiffness of the limbs and trunk; bradykinesia, or slowness of movement; and postural instability, or impaired balance and coordination. As these symptoms become more pronounced, patients may have difficulty walking, talking, or completing other simple tasks. PD usually affects people over the age of 60. Early symptoms of PD are subtle and occur gradually. In some people, the disease progresses more quickly than in others. As the disease progresses, the shaking, or tremor, which affects the majority of people with PD may begin to interfere with daily activities. Other symptoms may include depression and other emotional changes; difficulty in swallowing, chewing, and speaking; urinary problems or constipation; skin problems; and sleep disruptions.

Diagnosis

There are currently no blood or laboratory tests that have been proven to help in diagnosing sporadic PD. Therefore, the diagnosis is based on medical history and a neurological examination. The disease can be difficult to diagnose accurately. Doctors may sometimes request brain scans or laboratory tests in order to rule out other diseases.

Treatment

At present, there is no cure for PD, but a variety of medications provide dramatic relief from the symptoms. Usually, affected individuals are given levodopa combined with carbidopa. Carbidopa delays the conversion of levodopa into dopamine until it reaches the brain. Nerve cells can use levodopa to make dopamine and replenish the brain's dwindling supply. Although levodopa helps at least three-quarters of parkinsonian cases, not all symptoms respond equally to the drug. Bradykinesia and rigidity respond best, while tremor may be only marginally reduced. Problems with balance and other symptoms may not be alleviated at all. Anticholinergics may help control tremor and rigidity. Other drugs, such as bromocriptine, pramipexole, and ropinirole, mimic the role of dopamine in the brain, causing the neurons to react as they would to dopamine. An antiviral drug, amantadine, also appears to reduce symptoms.

In May 2006, the U.S. Food and Drug Administration (FDA) approved rasagiline to be used along with levodopa for patients with advanced PD or as a single-drug treatment for early PD. In March 2017, the FDA approved safinamide tablets as an add-on treatment for individuals with PD how are currently taking levodopa/carbidopa and experiencing "off" episodes (when the person's medications are not working well, causing an increase in PD symptoms).

In some cases, surgery may be appropriate if the disease doesn't respond to drugs. A therapy called deep brain stimulation (DBS) has now been approved by the FDA. In DBS, electrodes are implanted into the brain and connected to a small electrical device called a pulse generator that can be externally programmed. DBS can reduce the need for levodopa and related drugs, which in turn decreases the involuntary movements called dyskinesias that are a common side effect of levodopa. It also helps to alleviate fluctuations of symptoms and to reduce tremors, slowness of movements, and gait problems. DBS requires careful programming of the stimulator device in order to work correctly.

Prognosis

PD is both chronic, meaning it persists over a long period of time, and progressive, meaning its symptoms grow worse over time. Although some people become severely disabled, others experience only minor motor disruptions. Tremor is the major symptom for some individuals, while for others tremor is only a minor complaint and other symptoms are more troublesome. It is currently not possible to predict which symptoms will affect an individual, and the intensity of the symptoms also varies from person to person.

Chapter 20

Vascular Dementia

Chapter Contents

Section 20.1

What Is Vascular Dementia?

This section includes text excerpted from "Vascular Dementia," National Heart, Lung, and Blood Institute (NHLBI), January 20, 2018.

Vascular dementia is the second most common form of dementia, after Alzheimer disease (AD), affecting almost a third of people over age 70. Dementia causes a decline in brain function, or cognitive abilities, beyond what is expected from the normal aging process. Dementia causes problems with memory, thinking, behavior, language skills, and decision making.

Causes

Vascular dementia is caused by conditions that damage the blood vessels in the brain, depriving the brain of oxygen. This oxygen shortage inhibits the brain's ability to work as well as it should. For example, stroke blocks blood flow to the brain, decreasing oxygen. However, high blood pressure, high cholesterol, and smoking also increase the risk of vascular dementia. Vascular dementia in patients can occur alone or with Alzheimer disease.

Diagnosis

To diagnose cognitive impairment and dementia, your doctor will ask about problems you may have carrying out daily activities. Your doctor will give you brief memory or thinking tests and may ask to speak with a relative or friend who knows you well. To determine whether vascular dementia is the cause of any cognitive impairment or dementia that you may have, your doctor will consider your medical history and your lifestyle (such as your eating patterns, physical activity level, sleep health, and whether you are or have been a smoker), and order imaging tests. Diagnosis can take time. This is because it is often difficult to tell whether symptoms are a result of problems with the blood vessels, as is the case with vascular dementia, or whether they are from Alzheimer disease.

Treatment

If your doctor diagnoses you with vascular dementia, your treatment plan may include taking medicine or using medical devices to manage other conditions, such as high blood pressure, atherosclerosis, or sleep apnea, that may cause your vascular dementia to worsen. Your doctor may also recommend that you adopt heart-healthy lifestyle changes, such as heart-healthy eating, which includes limiting alcohol, getting regular physical activity, aiming for a healthy weight; quitting smoking; and managing stress.

Section 20.2

Binswanger Disease (Subcortical Vascular Dementia)

This section includes text excerpted from "Binswanger's Disease Information Page," National Institute of Neurological Disorders and Stroke (NINDS), June 20, 2018.

Binswanger disease (BD), also called subcortical vascular dementia (SVD), is a type of dementia caused by widespread, microscopic areas of damage to the deep layers of white matter in the brain. The damage is the result of the thickening and narrowing (atherosclerosis) of arteries that feed the subcortical areas of the brain. Atherosclerosis (commonly known as "hardening of the arteries") is a systemic process that affects blood vessels throughout the body. It begins late in the fourth decade of life and increases in severity with age. As the arteries become more and more narrowed, the blood supplied by those arteries decreases and brain tissue dies. A characteristic pattern of BD-damaged brain tissue can be seen with modern brain imaging techniques such as computed tomography (CT) scans or magnetic resonance imaging (MRI).

Symptoms

The symptoms associated with BD are related to the disruption of subcortical neural circuits that control what neuroscientists call executive cognitive functioning: short-term memory, organization, mood, the regulation of attention, the ability to act or make decisions, and appropriate behavior. The most characteristic feature of BD is psychomotor slowness—an increase in the length of time it takes, for example, for the fingers to turn the thought of a letter into the shape of a letter on a piece of paper.

Other symptoms include forgetfulness (but not as severe as the forgetfulness of Alzheimer disease (AD)), changes in speech, an unsteady gait, clumsiness or frequent falls, changes in personality or mood (most likely in the form of apathy, irritability, and depression), and urinary symptoms that aren't caused by urological disease. Brain imaging, which reveals the characteristic brain lesions of BD, is essential for a positive diagnosis.

Treatment

There is no specific course of treatment for BD. Treatment is symptomatic. People with depression or anxiety may require antidepressant medications such as the serotonin-specific reuptake inhibitors (SSRIs) sertraline or citalopram. Atypical antipsychotic drugs, such as risperidone and olanzapine, can be useful in individuals with agitation and disruptive behavior. At present, drug trials with the drug memantine have shown improved cognition and stabilization of global functioning and behavior. The successful management of hypertension and diabetes can slow the progression of atherosclerosis, and subsequently slow the progress of BD. Because there is no cure, the best treatment is preventive, early in the adult years, by controlling risk factors such as hypertension, diabetes, and smoking.

Prognosis

BD is a progressive disease; there is no cure. Changes may be sudden or gradual and then progress in a stepwise manner. BD can often coexist with Alzheimer disease. Behaviors that slow the progression of high blood pressure, diabetes, and atherosclerosis—such as eating a healthy diet and keeping healthy wake/sleep schedules, exercising, and not smoking or drinking too much alcohol—can also slow the progression of BD.

Section 20.3

Cerebral Autosomal Dominant Arteriopathy with Subcortical Infarcts and Leukoencephalopathy (CADASIL)

This section includes text excerpted from "CADASIL Information Page," National Institute of Neurological Disorders and Stroke (NINDS), June 20, 2018.

Cerebral autosomal dominant arteriopathy with subcortical infarcts and leukoencephalopathy (CADASIL) is an inherited form of cerebrovascular disease that occurs when the thickening of blood vessel walls blocks the flow of blood to the brain. The disease primarily affects small blood vessels in the white matter of the brain. A mutation in the *Notch3* gene alters the muscular walls in these small arteries. CADASIL is characterized by migraine headaches and multiple strokes progressing to dementia.

Other symptoms include cognitive deterioration, seizures, vision problems, and psychiatric problems such as severe depression and changes in behavior and personality. Individuals may also be at higher risk of heart attack. Symptoms and disease onset vary widely, with signs typically appearing in the mid-30s. Some individuals may not show signs of the disease until later in life.

CADASIL—formerly known by several names, including hereditary multi-infarct dementia—is one cause of vascular cognitive impairment (dementia caused by lack of blood to several areas of the brain). It is an autosomal dominant inheritance disorder, meaning that one parent carries and passes on the defective gene. Most individuals with CADASIL have a family history of the disorder. However, because the genetic test for CADASIL was not available before 2000, many cases were misdiagnosed as multiple sclerosis, Alzheimer disease (AD), or other neurodegenerative diseases.

Treatment

There is no treatment to halt this genetic disorder. Individuals are given supportive care. Migraine headaches may be treated by different drugs and a daily aspirin may reduce stroke and heart attack risk. Drug therapy for depression may be given. Affected individuals who smoke should quit as it can increase the risk of stroke in CADASIL. Other stroke risk factors such as hypertension, hyperlipidemia, diabetes, blood clotting disorders and obstructive sleep apnea (OSA) also should be aggressively treated.

Prognosis

Symptoms usually progress slowly. By age 65, the majority of persons with CADASIL have cognitive problems and dementia. Some will become dependent due to multiple strokes.

Section 20.4

Multi-Infarct Dementia

This section includes text excerpted from "Multi-Infarct Dementia Information Page," National Institute of Neurological Disorders and Stroke (NINDS), June 15, 2018.

Multi-infarct dementia (MID) is a common cause of memory loss in the elderly. MID is caused by multiple strokes (disruption of blood flow to the brain). Disruption of blood flow leads to damaged brain tissue. Some of these strokes may occur without noticeable clinical symptoms. Doctors refer to these as "silent strokes." An individual having a silent stroke may not even know it is happening, but over time, as more areas of the brain are damaged and more small blood vessels are blocked, the symptoms of MID begin to appear. MID can be diagnosed by an MRI or CT of the brain, along with a neurological examination. Symptoms include confusion or problems with short-term memory; wandering, or getting lost in familiar places; walking with rapid, shuffling steps; losing bladder or bowel control; laughing or crying inappropriately; having difficulty following instructions; and having problems counting money and making monetary transactions. MID, which typically begins between the ages of 60 and 75, affects men more often than women. Because the symptoms of MID are so similar to Alzheimer disease (AD), it can be difficult for a doctor to make a firm diagnosis. Since the diseases often occur together, making a single diagnosis of one or the other is even more problematic.

Treatment

There is no treatment available to reverse brain damage that has been caused by a stroke. Treatment focuses on preventing future strokes by controlling or avoiding the diseases and medical conditions that put people at high risk for stroke: high blood pressure, diabetes, high cholesterol, and cardiovascular disease. The best treatment for MID is prevention early in life—eating a healthy diet, exercising, not smoking, moderately using alcohol, and maintaining a healthy weight.

Prognosis

The prognosis for individuals with MID is generally poor. The symptoms of the disorder may begin suddenly, often in a stepwise pattern after each small stroke. Some people with MID may even appear to improve for short periods of time, then decline after having more silent strokes. The disorder generally takes a downward course with intermittent periods of rapid deterioration. Death may occur from stroke, heart disease, pneumonia, or other infection.

Chapter 21

Dementia Caused by Infection

Chapter Contents

Section 21.1

Creutzfeldt-Jakob Disease

This section includes text excerpted from "Creutzfeldt-Jakob Disease Fact Sheet," National Institute of Neurological Disorders and Stroke (NINDS), August 21, 2018.

What Is Creutzfeldt-Jakob Disease?

Creutzfeldt-Jakob disease (CJD) is a rare, degenerative, fatal brain disorder. It affects about one person in every one million per year worldwide; in the United States there are about 350 cases per year. CJD usually appears in later life and runs a rapid course. Typical onset of symptoms occurs at about age 60, and about 70 percent of individuals die within one year. In the early stages of the disease, people may have failing memory, behavioral changes, lack of coordination, and visual disturbances. As the illness progresses, mental deterioration becomes pronounced and involuntary movements, blindness, weakness of extremities, and coma may occur.

There are three major categories of CJD.

1. In sporadic CJD, the disease appears even though the person has no known risk factors for the disease. This is by far the most common type of CJD and accounts for at least 85 percent of cases.

2. In hereditary CJD, the person may have a family history of the disease and test positive for a genetic mutation associated with CJD. About 10 to 15 percent of cases of CJD in the United States are hereditary.

3. In acquired CJD, the disease is transmitted by exposure to brain or nervous system tissue, usually through certain medical procedures. There is no evidence that CJD is contagious through casual contact with someone who has CJD. Since CJD was first described in 1920, fewer than one percent of cases have been acquired CJD. A type of CJD called variant CJD (or vCJD) can be acquired by eating meat from cattle affected by a disease similar to CJD called bovine spongiform encephalopathy (BSE) or, commonly, "mad cow" disease.

CJD belongs to a family of human and animal diseases known as the transmissible spongiform encephalopathies (TSEs) or prion diseases. A prion—derived from "protein" and "infectious"—causes CJD in people and TSEs in animals. Spongiform refers to the characteristic appearance of infected brains, which become filled with holes until they resemble sponges when examined under a microscope. CJD is the most common of the known human TSEs. Other human TSEs include kuru, fatal familial insomnia (FFI), and Gerstmann-Straussler-Scheinker disease (GSS). Kuru was identified in people of an isolated tribe who practiced ritual cannibalism in Papua, New Guinea and has now almost disappeared. Kuru is considered an acquired prion disease. FFI and GSS are extremely rare hereditary diseases, found in just a few families around the world.

To date, about 260 cases of vCJD, mostly in the United Kingdom, have been reported related to consuming beef but none in which the disease was acquired in the United States. Other TSEs are found in specific kinds of animals. These include bovine spongiform encephalopathy (BSE), mink encephalopathy, feline encephalopathy, and scrapie, which affects sheep and goats. Chronic wasting disease (CWD) affects elk and deer and is increasingly prevalent in certain areas in the United States. To date no transmission of CWD to humans has been reported.

What Are the Symptoms of Creutzfeldt-Jakob Disease?

Although sporadic TSE includes five distinct subtypes of sporadic CJD and sporadic fatal insomnia (sFI), overall they are characterized by rapidly progressive dementia. Initially, individuals experience problems with muscle coordination, personality changes (including impaired memory, judgment, and thinking), and impaired vision. People with the disease, especially with FFI, also may experience insomnia, depression, or unusual sensations. As the illness progresses, peoples mental impairment becomes severe. They often develop involuntary muscle jerks called myoclonus, and they may go blind. They eventually lose the ability to move and speak, and enter a coma. Pneumonia and other infections often occur in these individuals and can lead to death.

Variant CJD begins primarily with psychiatric symptoms, affects younger individuals than other types of CJD, and has a longer than usual duration from onset of symptoms to death.

Some symptoms of CJD can be similar to symptoms of other progressive neurological disorders (PND), such as Alzheimer and Huntington disease. However, CJD causes unique changes in brain tissue which can be seen at autopsy. It also tends to cause more rapid deterioration of a person's abilities than Alzheimer disease or most other types of dementia.

What Causes Creutzfeldt-Jakob Disease?

Current scientific consensus maintains that abnormal forms of normal cellular proteins called prions cause CJD in people and TSE in animals. The normal, harmless prion is usually designated PrPC (C stands for cellular) and the abnormal, infectious form (which causes the disease) is PrPSc (Sc stands for prototypical prion disease–scrapie).

Proteins are long chains of amino acids that have to fold together into a unique shape or conformation to gain function in the cells. Research findings indicate that the infectious prion originates from a normal protein whose conformation has changed to one that causes the disease. The normal prion protein is found throughout the body but is most abundant in the nervous system. Its overall role is not fully understood. It is believed that the harmless to infectious protein conformational change is common to the all major forms of human prion disease, including CJD. In the acquired form of the disease, the PrPSc comes from the outside the body, for example, through contaminated meat as is seen in vCJD. It then clings to and changes the conformation of the normal prion protein of the host and progressively spreads in domino-like fashion toward the brain where it causes lesions.

In the hereditary form, infectious prions can arise when a mutation occurs in the gene for the body's normal prion protein. As the mutated PrPC replicates itself, it spontaneously changes shape into the infectious form. (Prions themselves do not contain genetic information and do not require genes to reproduce themselves.) If the prion protein gene is altered in a person's sperm or egg cells, the mutation can cannibalism to the person's offspring. Several different mutations in the prion gene have been identified. The particular mutation found in each family affects how frequently the disease appears and what symptoms are most noticeable. However, not all people with mutations in the prion protein gene develop CJD.

In the sporadic form, the infectious prions are believed to be made by an error of the cell machinery that makes proteins and controls their quality. These errors are more likely to occur with aging, which explains the general advanced age at onset of CJD and other prion diseases. Once they are formed, abnormal prion proteins aggregate, or clump together. Investigators think these protein aggregates lead to the nerve cell loss and other brain damage seen in CJD. However, they do not know exactly how this damage occurs.

How Is Creutzfeldt-Jakob Disease Transmitted?

CJD cannot be transmitted through the air or through touching or most other forms of casual contact. Spouses and other household members of people with sporadic CJD have no higher risk of contracting the disease than the general population. However, exposure to brain tissue and spinal cord fluid from infected persons should be avoided to prevent transmission of the disease through these materials.

In some cases, CJD has spread to other people from grafts of dura mater (a tissue that covers the brain), transplanted corneas, implantation of inadequately sterilized electrodes in the brain, and injections of contaminated pituitary growth hormone derived from human pituitary glands taken from cadavers. Doctors call these cases that are linked to medical procedures iatrogenic cases. Since 1985, all human growth hormone used in the United States has been synthesized by recombinant DNA (deoxyribonucleic acid) procedures, which eliminates the risk of transmitting CJD by this route.

Many people are concerned that it may be possible to transmit CJD through blood and related blood products such as plasma. Some animal studies suggest that contaminated blood and related products may transmit the disease, although this has never been shown in humans. Some studies suggest that while there may be prions in the blood of individuals with vCJD, this is not the case in individuals with sporadic CJD. Scientists do not know how many abnormal prions a person must receive before she or he develops CJD, so they do not know whether these fluids are potentially infectious or not. They do know that, even though millions of people receive blood transfusions each year, there are no reported cases of someone contracting sporadic CJD from a transfusion. Even among people with hemophilia (a rare bleeding disorder in which the blood does not clot cannibalism), who sometimes receive blood plasma concentrated from thousands of donors, there are no reported cases of CJD.

While there is no evidence that blood from people with sporadic CJD is infectious, studies have found that infectious prions from BSE and vCJD accumulate in the lymph nodes (which produce white blood cells), the spleen, and the tonsils. At present, four cases of vCJD infection have been identified following transfusion of red blood cells from asymptomatic donors who subsequently died from vCJD. One case of confirmation transmission of vCJD infection by concentrates of blood-clotting protein has been reported in an elderly individual with hemophilia in the United Kingdom. The possibility that blood from people with vCJD may be infectious has led to a policy preventing individuals in the United States from donating blood if they have resided for more than three months in a country or countries where BSE is common.

Both brain biopsy and autopsy pose a small, but definite, risk that the surgeon or others who handle the brain tissue may become accidentally infected by self-inoculation.

Special surgical and disinfection procedures can markedly reduce this risk. A fact sheet with guidance on these procedures is available from the National Institute of Neurological Disorders and Stroke (NINDS) and the World Health Organization (WHO).

How Is Creutzfeldt-Jakob Disease Diagnosed?

Several tests can help diagnose CJD.

- Electroencephalography (EEG), which records the brain's electrical pattern, can be particularly valuable because it shows a specific type of abnormality in major but not all types of CJD.

- Cerebrospinal fluid-based tests. In April 2015, the National Prion Disease Pathology Surveillance Center (NPDPSC) began reporting a new diagnostic test for human prion diseases, called second generation Real Time-Quaking-Induced Conversion (RT-QuIC). RT-QuIC is based on an ultrasensitive detection of the pathogenic prion protein in the cerebrospinal fluid of individuals affected by CJD and other forms of human prion diseases. This advanced test demonstrates a very high sensitivity and specificity of the disease. RT-QuIC differs from traditional surrogate markers of prion disease—14-3-3 and tau proteins—in that it detects directly a disease-defining pathogenic prion protein as opposed to a surrogate marker of rapid neurodegeneration. Detection of these traditional surrogate marker proteins is accurate in approximately three-fourths of cases.

- Magnetic resonance imaging (MRI) has been found to be accurate in about 90 percent of cases.

The only way to confirm a diagnosis of CJD is by brain biopsy or autopsy. In a brain biopsy, a neurosurgeon removes a small piece of tissue from the person's brain so that it can be examined by a neuropathologist. This procedure may be dangerous for the individual, and the operation does not always obtain tissue from the affected part of the brain. Because a correct diagnosis of CJD does not help the individual, a brain biopsy is discouraged unless it is needed to rule out a treatable disorder. In an autopsy, the whole brain is examined after death.

How Is Creutzfeldt-Jakob Disease Treated?

Currently, there is no treatment that can cure or control CJD, although studies of a variety of drugs are now in progress. Current treatment for CJD is aimed at easing symptoms and making the person as comfortable as possible. Opiate drugs can help relieve pain if it occurs, and the drugs clonazepam and sodium valproate may help relieve myoclonus. During later stages of the disease, intravenous fluids, and artificial feeding also may be used.

How Can People Avoid Spreading the Disease?

To reduce the already very low risk of CJD transmission from one person to another, people should never donate blood, tissues, or organs if they have suspected or confirmed CJD, or if they are at increased risk because of a family history of the disease, a dura mater graft, or other factor.

Normal sterilization procedures such as cooking, washing, and boiling do not destroy prions. Although there is no evidence that caregivers, healthcare workers, and those who prepare bodies for funerals and cremation have increased risk of prion diseases when compared to general population, they should take the following precautions when they are working with a person with CJD:

- Cover cuts and abrasions with waterproof dressings.
- Wear surgical gloves when handling the person's tissues and fluids or dressing any wounds.
- Avoid cutting or sticking themselves with instruments contaminated by the person's blood or other tissues.
- Use disposable bedclothes and other cloth for contact with the person. If disposable materials are not available, regular cloth should be soaked in undiluted chlorine bleach for an hour or more, and then washed in a normal fashion after each use.
- Use face protection if there is a risk of splashing contaminated material such as blood or cerebrospinal fluid.
- Soak instruments that have come in contact with the person in undiluted chlorine bleach for an hour or more, then use an autoclave (pressure cooker) to sterilize them in distilled water for at least one hour at 132 to 134 degrees Celsius.

Section 21.2

Acquired Immunodeficiency Syndrome Dementia Complex

This section contains text excerpted from the following
sources: Text beginning with the heading "What Is Acquired
Immunodeficiency Syndrome?" is excerpted from "Neurological
Complications of AIDS Fact Sheet," National Institute of
Neurological Disorders and Stroke (NINDS), July 6, 2018; Text
under the heading "Human Immunodeficiency Virus-Associated
Neurocognitive Disorders" is excerpted from "HIV/AIDS," U.S.
Department of Veterans Affairs (VA), February 8, 2018.

What Is Acquired Immunodeficiency Syndrome?

Acquired immunodeficiency syndrome (AIDS) is a condition that
occurs in the most advanced stages of human immunodeficiency virus
(HIV) infection. It may take many years for AIDS to develop following
the initial HIV infection.

Although AIDS is primarily an immune system disorder, it also
affects the nervous system and can lead to a wide range of severe
neurological disorders.

How Does Acquired Immunodeficiency Syndrome Affect the Nervous System?

The virus does not appear to directly invade nerve cells but it
jeopardizes their health and function. The resulting inflammation
may damage the brain and spinal cord and cause symptoms such as
confusion and forgetfulness, behavioral changes, headaches, progressive weakness, and loss of sensation in the arms and legs. Cognitive
motor impairment or damage to the peripheral nerves is also common.
Research has shown that the HIV infection can significantly alter the
size of certain brain structures involved in learning and information
processing.

Other nervous system complications that occur as a result of the
disease or the drugs used to treat it include pain, seizures, shingles,
spinal cord problems, lack of coordination, difficult or painful swallowing, anxiety disorder, depression, fever, vision loss, gait disorders,
destruction of brain tissue, and coma. These symptoms may be mild
in the early stages of AIDS but can become progressively severe.

In the United States, neurological complications are seen in more than 50 percent of adults with AIDS. Nervous system complications in children may include developmental delays, loss of previously achieved milestones, brain lesions, nerve pain, smaller than normal skull size, slow growth, eye problems, and recurring bacterial infections.

What Are Some of the Neurological Complications That Are Associated with Acquired Immunodeficiency Syndrome?

AIDS-related disorders of the nervous system may be caused directly by the HIV virus, by certain cancers and opportunistic infections (illnesses caused by bacteria, fungi, and other viruses that would not otherwise affect people with healthy immune systems), or by toxic effects of the drugs used to treat symptoms. Other neuro-AIDS disorders of unknown origin may be influenced by but are not caused directly by the virus.

AIDS dementia complex (ADC), or HIV-associated dementia (HAD), occurs primarily in persons with more advanced HIV infection. Symptoms include encephalitis (inflammation of the brain), behavioral changes, and a gradual decline in cognitive function, including trouble with concentration, memory, and attention. Persons with ADC also show progressive slowing of motor function and loss of dexterity and coordination. When left untreated, ADC can be fatal. It is rare when antiretroviral therapy is used. Milder cognitive complaints are common and are termed HIV-associated neurocognitive disorder (HAND). Neuropsychologic testing can reveal subtle deficits even in the absence of symptoms.

Central nervous system (CNS) lymphomas are cancerous tumors that either begin in the brain or result from a cancer that has spread from another site in the body. CNS lymphomas are almost always associated with the Epstein-Barr virus (EBV), (a common human virus in the herpes family). Symptoms include headache, seizures, vision problems, dizziness, speech disturbance, paralysis, and mental deterioration. Individuals may develop one or more CNS lymphomas. Prognosis is poor due to advanced and increasing immunodeficiency, but is better with successful HIV therapy.

Cryptococcal meningitis (CM) is seen in about ten percent of untreated individuals with AIDS and in other persons whose immune systems have been severely suppressed by disease or drugs. It is caused by the fungus Cryptococcus neoformans, which is commonly found in dirt and bird droppings. The fungus first invades the lungs and spreads to the covering of the brain and spinal cord, causing inflammation. Symptoms include fatigue, fever, headache, nausea, memory loss, confusion, drowsiness, and vomiting. If left untreated, patients with cryptococcal meningitis may lapse into a coma and die.

Cytomegalovirus (CMV) infections can occur concurrently with other infections. Symptoms of CMV encephalitis include weakness in the arms and legs, problems with hearing and balance, altered mental states, dementia, peripheral neuropathy, coma, and retinal disease that may lead to blindness. CMV infection of the spinal cord and nerves can result in weakness in the lower limbs and some paralysis, severe lower back pain, and loss of bladder function. It can also cause pneumonia and gastrointestinal disease. This is rarely seen in HIV-treated individuals since advanced immunity is required for CMV to emerge.

Herpes virus infections are often seen in people with AIDS. The herpes zoster virus, which causes chickenpox and shingles, can infect the brain and produce encephalitis and myelitis (inflammation of the spinal cord). It commonly produces shingles, which is an eruption of blisters and intense pain along an area of skin supplied by an infected nerve. In people exposed to herpes zoster, the virus can lay dormant in the nerve tissue for years until it is reactivated as shingles. This reactivation is common in persons with AIDS because of their weakened immune systems. Signs of shingles include painful blisters (like those seen in chickenpox), itching, tingling, and pain in the nerves.

People with AIDS may suffer from several different forms of neuropathy, or nerve pain, each strongly associated with a specific stage of active immunodeficiency disease. Peripheral neuropathy describes damage to the peripheral nerves, the vast communications network that transmits information between the brain and spinal cord to every other part of the body. Peripheral nerves also send sensory information back to the brain and spinal cord. HIV damages the nerve fibers that help conduct signals and can cause several different forms of neuropathy. Distal sensory polyneuropathy causes either a numbing feeling or a mild to painful burning or tingling sensation that normally begins in the legs and feet. These sensations may be particularly strong at night and may spread to the hands. Affected persons have a heightened sensitivity to pain, touch, or other stimuli. Onset usually occurs in the later stages of the HIV infection and may affect the majority of advanced-stage HIV patients.

Neurosyphilis, the result of an insufficiently treated syphilis infection, seems more frequent and more rapidly progressive in people with HIV infection. It may cause slow degeneration of the nerve cells and nerve fibers that carry sensory information to the brain. Symptoms, which may not appear for some decades after the initial infection and vary from person to person, include weakness, diminished reflexes, unsteady gait, progressive degeneration of the joints, loss of coordination, episodes of intense pain and disturbed sensation, personality changes, dementia, deafness, visual impairment, and impaired response to light. The disease is more frequent in men than in women. Onset is common during mid-life.

Progressive multifocal leukoencephalopathy (PML) primarily affects individuals with suppressed immune systems (including nearly 5 percent of people with AIDS). PML is caused by the JC virus, which travels to the brain, infects multiple sites, and destroys the cells that make myelin—the fatty protective covering for many of the body's nerve and brain cells. Symptoms include various types of mental deterioration, vision loss, speech disturbances, ataxia (inability to coordinate movements), paralysis, brain lesions, and, ultimately, coma. Some individuals may also have compromised memory and cognition, and seizures may occur. PML is relentlessly progressive and death usually occurs within six months of initial symptoms. However, immune reconstitution with highly active antiretroviral therapy (ART) allows survival of more than half of HIV-associated PML cases in the current treatment era.

Psychological and neuropsychiatric disorders can occur in different phases of the HIV infection and AIDS and may take various and complex forms. Some illnesses, such as AIDS dementia complex, are caused directly by HIV infection of the brain, while other conditions may be triggered by the drugs used to combat the infection. Individuals may experience anxiety disorder, depressive disorders, increased thoughts of suicide, paranoia, dementia, delirium, cognitive impairment, confusion, hallucinations, behavioral abnormalities, malaise, and acute mania.

Toxoplasma encephalitis, also called cerebral toxoplasmosis, occurs in about ten percent of untreated AIDS patients. It is caused by the parasite Toxoplasma gondii, which is carried by cats, birds, and other animals and can be found in soil contaminated by cat feces and sometimes in raw or undercooked meat. Once the parasite invades the immune system, it remains there; however, the immune system in a healthy person can fight off the parasite, preventing disease. Symptoms include encephalitis, fever, severe headache that does not respond to treatment, weakness on one side of the body, seizures, lethargy, increased confusion, vision problems, dizziness, problems with speaking and walking, vomiting, and personality changes. Not all patients show signs of the infection. Antibiotic therapy, if used early, will generally control the complication.

Vacuolar myelopathy (VM) causes the protective myelin sheath to pull away from nerve cells of the spinal cord, forming small holes called vacuoles in nerve fibers. Symptoms include weak and stiff legs and unsteadiness when walking. Walking becomes more difficult as the disease progresses and many patients eventually require a wheelchair. Some people also develop AIDS dementia. Vacuolar myelopathy may affect up to 30 percent of untreated adults with AIDS and its incidence may be even higher in HIV-infected children.

How Are These Disorders Diagnosed?

Based on the results of the individual's medical history and a general physical exam, the physician will conduct a thorough neurological cannibalism to assess various functions: motor and sensory skills, nerve function, hearing and speech, vision, coordination and balance, mental status, and changes in mood or behavior. The physician may order laboratory tests and one or more of the following procedures to help diagnose neurological complications of AIDS.

Brain imaging can reveal signs of brain inflammation, tumors and CNS lymphomas, nerve damage, internal bleeding or hemorrhage, white matter irregularities, and other brain abnormalities. Several painless imaging procedures are used to help diagnose neurological complications of AIDS.

- Computed tomography (also called a CT scan) uses X-rays and a computer to produce two-dimensional images of bone and tissue, including inflammation, certain brain tumors and cysts, brain damage from head injury, and other disorders. It provides more details than an X-ray alone.

- Magnetic resonance imaging (MRI) uses a computer, radio waves, and a powerful magnetic field to produce either a detailed three-dimensional picture or a two-dimensional "slice" of body structures, including tissues, organs, bones, and nerves. It does not use ionizing radiation (as does an X-ray) and gives physicians a better look at tissue located near bone.

- Functional MRI (fMRI) uses the blood's magnetic properties to pinpoint areas of the brain that are active and to note how long they stay active. It can assess brain damage from head injury or degenerative disorders such as Alzheimer disease (AD) and can identify and monitor other neurological disorders, including AIDS dementia complex.

- Magnetic resonance spectroscopy (MRS) uses a strong magnetic field to study the biochemical composition and concentration of hydrogen-based molecules, some of which are very specific to nerve cells, in various brain regions. MRS is being used experimentally to identify brain lesions in people with AIDS.

Electromyography, or EMG, is used to diagnose nerve and muscle dysfunction (such as neuropathy and nerve fiber damage caused by the HIV virus) and spinal cord disease. It records spontaneous muscle activity and muscle activity driven by the peripheral nerves.

Biopsy is the removal and examination of tissue from the body. A brain biopsy, which involves the surgical removal of a small piece of the brain or tumor, is used to determine intracranial disorders and tumor type. Unlike most other biopsies, it requires hospitalization. Muscle or nerve biopsies can help diagnose neuromuscular problems, while a brain biopsy can help diagnose a tumor, inflammation, or other irregularity.

Cerebrospinal fluid (CSF) analysis can detect any bleeding or brain hemorrhage, infections of the brain or spinal cord (such as neurosyphilis), and any harmful buildup of fluid. It can also be used to sample viruses that may be affecting the brain. A sample of the fluid is removed by needle, under local anesthesia, and studied to detect any irregularities.

How Are These Disorders Treated?

No single treatment can cure the neurological complications of AIDS. Some disorders require aggressive therapy while others are treated symptomatically.

Neuropathic pain is often difficult to control. Medicines range from analgesics sold over the counter to antiepileptic drugs, opiates, and some classes of antidepressants. Inflamed tissue can press on nerves, causing pain. Inflammatory and autoimmune conditions leading to neuropathy may confirmation with corticosteroids, and procedures such as plasmapheresis (or plasma exchange) can clear the blood of harmful substances that cause inflammation.

Treatment options for AIDS and HIV-related neuropsychiatric or psychotic disorders include antidepressants and anticonvulsants. Psychostimulants may also improve depressive symptoms and combat lethargy. Antidementia drugs may relieve confusion and slow mental decline, and benzodiazepines (BZD, BZs), may be prescribed to treat anxiety. Psychotherapy may also help some individuals.

Aggressive antiretroviral therapy is used to treat AIDS dementia complex, vacuolar myopathy, progressive multifocal leukoencephalopathy, and cytomegalovirus encephalitis. HAART, or highly active antiretroviral therapy, combines at least three drugs to reduce the amount of virus circulating in the blood and may also delay the start of some infections.

Other neuro-AIDS treatment options include physical therapy and rehabilitation, radiation therapy and/or chemotherapy to kill or shrink cancerous brain tumors that may be caused by the HIV virus, antifungal or antimalarial drugs to combat certain bacterial infections associated with the disorder, and penicillin to treat neurosyphilis.

Human Immunodeficiency Virus-Associated Neurocognitive Disorders

Human immunodeficiency virus (HIV) can invade the brain and cause a variety of symptoms. Sometimes this disease is called "HIV encephalopathy" or "AIDS dementia" when the symptoms are severe. It is most common in people who are not on effective HIV medications and when the cluster of differentiation 4 (CD4) cell count is very low.

Symptoms can include:

- Memory loss

- Depressed mood

- Personality changes

- Apathy

- Unsteadiness when walking

- Irritability

- Clumsiness

- Shaky hands (poor handwriting)

This condition is less common with early and continuous treatment of HIV, but less severe forms of cognitive disease are increasingly recognized.

People who are affected need to have a strong support system. Friends, roommates, or family members can help make sure that HIV medications are taken on time, in the right combination, and at the right dose. If memory is poor, a person can use notes, calendars, and alarms to remember medicines, appointments, and other important events.

Chapter 22

Other Health Conditions That Cause Dementia

Chapter Contents

Section 22.1

Cancer, Delirium, and Dementia

This section includes text excerpted from "Delirium (PDQ®)—Patient Version," National Cancer Institute (NCI), March 9, 2016.

Delirium is a confused mental state that can occur in patients who have cancer, especially advanced cancer. Patients with delirium have problems with the following:

- Attention

- Thinking

- Awareness

- Behavior

- Emotions

- Judgment

- Memory

- Muscle control

- Sleeping and waking

There are three types of delirium:

- Hypoactive. The patient is not active and seems sleepy, tired, or depressed.

- Hyperactive. The patient is restless or agitated.

- Mixed. The patient changes back and forth between being hypoactive and hyperactive.

Delirium may come and go during the day. The symptoms of delirium usually occur suddenly. They often occur within hours or days and may come and go. Delirium is often temporary and can be treated. However, in the last 24 to 48 hours of life, delirium may be permanent because of problems like organ failure. Most advanced cancer patients have delirium that occurs in the last hours to days before death.

Causes of Delirium

Delirium may be caused by cancer, cancer treatment, or other medical conditions. There is often more than one cause of delirium in a cancer patient, especially when the cancer is advanced and the patient has many medical conditions. Causes of delirium include the following:

- Organ failure, such as liver or kidney failure

- Electrolyte imbalances. Electrolytes are important minerals (including salt, potassium, calcium, and phosphorous) in blood and body fluids. These electrolytes are needed to keep the heart, kidneys, nerves, and muscles working the way they should.

- Infections

- Paraneoplastic syndromes. Symptoms that occur when cancer-fighting antibodies or white blood cells attack normal cells in the nervous system by mistake.

- Side effects of medicines and treatments. Patients with cancer may take medicines with side effects that include delirium and confusion. The effects usually go away after the medicine is stopped.

- Withdrawal from medicines that depress (slow down) the central nervous system (brain and spinal cord)

It is important to know the risk factors for delirium. Patients with cancer are likely to have more than one risk factor for delirium. Identifying risk factors early may help prevent delirium or decrease the time it takes to treat it. Risk factors include the following:

- Serious illness

- Having more than one disease

- Older age

- Dementia

- Low level of albumin (protein) in the blood, which is often caused by liver problems

- Infection

- High level of nitrogen waste products in the blood, which is often caused by kidney problems

- Taking medicines that affect the mind or behavior

- Taking high doses of pain medicines, such as opioids

The risk increases when the patient has more than one risk factor. Older patients with advanced cancer who are hospitalized often have more than one risk factor for delirium.

Effects of Delirium on the Patient, Family, and Healthcare Providers

Delirium causes changes in the patient that can upset the family and caregivers. Delirium may be dangerous to the patient if his or her judgment is affected. Delirium can cause the patient to behave in unusual ways. Even a quiet or calm patient can have a sudden change in mood or become agitated and need more care.

Delirium can be upsetting to the family and caregivers. When the patient becomes agitated, family members often think the patient is in pain, but this may not be the case. Learning about differences between the symptoms of delirium and pain may help the family and caregivers understand how much pain medicine is needed. Healthcare providers can help the family and caregivers learn about these differences. Delirium may affect physical health and communication.

Patients with delirium are:

- More likely to fall
- Sometimes unable to control bladder and/or bowels
- More likely to become dehydrated (drink too little water to stay healthy)

They often need a longer hospital stay than patients without delirium.

The confused mental state of these patients may make them:

- Unable to talk with family members and caregivers about their needs and feelings
- Unable to make decisions about care

This makes it harder for healthcare providers to assess the patient's symptoms. The family may need to make decisions for the patient.

Diagnosing Delirium

Possible signs of delirium include sudden personality changes, problems thinking, and unusual anxiety or depression.

When the following symptoms occur suddenly, they may be signs of delirium:

- Agitation
- Not cooperating

- Changes in personality or behavior

- Problems thinking

- Problems paying attention

- Unusual anxiety or depression

The symptoms of delirium are a lot like symptoms of depression and dementia. Early symptoms of delirium are like symptoms of depression and dementia. Delirium that causes the patient to be inactive may appear to be depression. Delirium and dementia both cause problems with memory, thinking, and judgment. Dementia may be caused by a number of medical conditions, including Alzheimer disease (AD). Differences in the symptoms of delirium and dementia include the following:

- Patients with delirium often show changes in how alert or aware they are. Patients who have dementia usually stay alert and aware until dementia becomes very advanced.

- Delirium occurs suddenly (within hours or days). Dementia appears gradually (over months to years) and gets worse over time.

Older patients with cancer may have both dementia and delirium. This can make it hard for the doctor to diagnose the problem. If treatment for delirium is given and the symptoms continue, then the diagnosis is more likely dementia. Checking the patient's health and symptoms over time can help diagnose delirium and dementia.

Physical exams and other laboratory tests are used to diagnose the causes of delirium.

Doctors will try to find the causes of delirium:

- **Physical exam and history.** An exam of the body to check general signs of health, including checking for signs of disease, such as lumps or anything else that seems unusual. A history of the patient's health habits, past illnesses including depression, and treatments will also be taken. A physical exam can help rule out a physical condition that may be causing symptoms.

- **Laboratory tests.** Medical procedures that test samples of tissue, blood, urine, or other substances in the body. These tests help to diagnose disease, plan and check treatment, or monitor the disease over time.

Treatment of Delirium

Treatment includes looking at the causes and symptoms of delirium. Both the causes and the symptoms of delirium may be treated. Treatment depends on the following:

- Where the patient is living, such as home, hospital, or nursing home
- How advanced the cancer is
- How the delirium symptoms are affecting the patient
- The wishes of the patient and family

Treating the causes of delirium usually includes the following:

- Stopping or lowering the dose of medicines that cause delirium
- Giving fluids to treat dehydration
- Giving drugs to treat hypercalcemia (too much calcium in the blood)
- Giving antibiotics for infections

In a terminally ill patient with delirium, the doctor may treat just the symptoms. The doctor will continue to watch the patient closely during treatment.

Treatment without medicines can also help relieve symptoms. Controlling the patient's surroundings may help with mild symptoms of delirium. The following may help:

- Keep the patient's room quiet and well-lit, and put familiar objects in it.
- Put a clock or calendar where the patient can see it.
- Have family members around.
- Keep the same caregivers as much as possible.

Patients who may hurt themselves or others may need to have physical restraints.

Treatment may include medicines. Medicines may be used to treat the symptoms of delirium depending on the patient's condition and heart health. These medicines have serious side effects and the patient will be watched closely by a doctor. These medicines include the following:

- Haloperidol

- Olanzapine

- Risperidone

- Lorazepam

- Midazolam

Sedation may be used for delirium at the end of life or when delirium does not get better with treatment. When the symptoms of delirium are not relieved with standard treatments and the patient is near death, in pain, or has trouble breathing, other treatment may be needed. Sometimes medicines that will sedate (calm) the patient will be used. The family and the healthcare team will make this decision together.

The decision to use sedation for delirium may be guided by the following:

- The patient will have repeated assessments by experts before the delirium is considered to be refractory (doesn't respond to treatment).

- The decision to sedate the patient is reviewed by a team of healthcare professionals and not made by one doctor.

- Temporary sedation, for short periods of time such as overnight, is considered before continuous sedation is used.

- The team of healthcare professionals will work with the family to make sure the team understands the family's views and that the family understands palliative sedation.

Section 22.2

Dementia: A Symptom of Normal Pressure Hydrocephalus

This section includes text excerpted from "Hydrocephalus Fact Sheet," National Institute of Neurological Disorders and Stroke (NINDS), July 6, 2018.

What Is Hydrocephalus?

The term hydrocephalus is derived from the Greek words "hydro" meaning water and "cephalus" meaning head. As the name implies, it is a condition in which the primary characteristic is excessive accumulation of fluid in the brain. Although hydrocephalus was once known as "water on the brain," the "water" is actually cerebrospinal fluid (CSF)—a clear fluid that surrounds the brain and spinal cord. The excessive accumulation of CSF results in an abnormal widening of spaces in the brain called ventricles. This widening creates potentially harmful pressure on the tissues of the brain.

The ventricular system is made up of four ventricles connected by narrow passages. Normally, CSF flows through the ventricles, exits into cisterns (closed spaces that serve as reservoirs) at the base of the brain, bathes the surfaces of the brain and spinal cord, and then reabsorbs into the bloodstream.

CSF has three important life-sustaining functions:

1. To keep the brain tissue buoyant, acting as a cushion or "shock absorber";

2. To act as the vehicle for delivering nutrients to the brain and removing waste; and

3. To flow between the cranium and spine and compensate for changes in intracranial blood volume (the amount of blood within the brain).

The balance between production and absorption of CSF is critically important. Because CSF is made continuously, medical conditions that block its normal flow or absorption will result in an overaccumulation of CSF. The resulting pressure of the fluid against brain tissue is what causes hydrocephalus.

What Are the Different Types of Hydrocephalus?

Hydrocephalus may be congenital or acquired. Congenital hydrocephalus is present at birth and may be caused by either events or influences that occur during fetal development, or genetic abnormalities. Acquired hydrocephalus develops at the time of birth or at some point afterward. This type of hydrocephalus can affect individuals of all ages and may be caused by injury or disease.

Hydrocephalus may also be communicating or noncommunicating. Communicating hydrocephalus occurs when the flow of CSF is blocked after it exits the ventricles. This form is called communicating because the CSF can still flow between the ventricles, which remain open. Noncommunicating hydrocephalus—also called "obstructive" hydrocephalus—occurs when the flow of CSF is blocked along one or more of the narrow passages connecting the ventricles. One of the most common causes of hydrocephalus is "aqueductal stenosis." In this case, hydrocephalus results from a narrowing of the aqueduct of Sylvius, a small passage between the third and fourth ventricles in the middle of the brain.

There are two other forms of hydrocephalus which do not fit exactly into the categories mentioned above and primarily affect adults: hydrocephalus ex-vacuo and Normal Pressure Hydrocephalus (NPH).

Hydrocephalus ex-vacuo occurs when a stroke or traumatic injury causes damage to the brain. In these cases, brain tissue may actually shrink. NPH is an abnormal increase of cerebrospinal fluid in the brain's ventricles that may result from a subarachnoid hemorrhage, head trauma, infection, tumor, or complications of surgery. However, many people develop NPH when none of these factors are present. An estimated 375,000 older Americans have NPH.

Who Gets This Disorder?

The number of people who develop hydrocephalus or who are currently living with it is difficult to establish since the condition occurs in children and adults, and can develop later in life. A 2008 data review by the University of Utah found that, in 2003, hydrocephalus accounted for 0.6 percent of all pediatric hospital admissions in the United States. Some estimates report one to two of every 1,000 babies are born with hydrocephalus.

What Causes Hydrocephalus?

The causes of hydrocephalus are still not well understood. Hydrocephalus may result from inherited genetic abnormalities (such as the genetic defect that causes aqueductal stenosis (AS)) or developmental disorders (such as those associated with neural tube defects including spina bifida and encephalocele). Other possible causes include complications of premature birth such as intraventricular hemorrhage, diseases such as meningitis, tumors, traumatic head injury, or subarachnoid hemorrhage, which block the exit of CSF from the ventricles to the cisterns or eliminate the passageway for CSF within the cisterns.

What Are the Symptoms?

Symptoms of hydrocephalus vary with age, disease progression, and individual differences in tolerance to the condition. For example, an infant's ability to compensate for increased CSF pressure and enlargement of the ventricles differs from an adult's. The infant skull can expand to accommodate the buildup of CSF because the sutures (the fibrous joints that connect the bones of the skull) have not yet closed.

In infancy, the most obvious indication of hydrocephalus is often a rapid increase in head circumference or an unusually large head size. Other symptoms may include vomiting, sleepiness, irritability, downward deviation of the eyes (also called "sunsetting"), and seizures.

Older children and adults may experience different symptoms because their skulls cannot expand to accommodate the buildup of CSF. Symptoms may include headache followed by vomiting, nausea, blurred or double vision, sunsetting of the eyes, problems with balance, poor coordination, gait disturbance, urinary incontinence, slowing or loss of developmental progress, lethargy, drowsiness, irritability, or other changes in personality or cognition including memory loss.

Symptoms of normal pressure hydrocephalus include problems with walking, impaired bladder control leading to urinary frequency and/ or incontinence, and progressive mental impairment and dementia. An individual with this type of hydrocephalus may have a general slowing of movements or may complain that his or her feet feel "stuck." Because some of these symptoms may also be experienced in other disorders such as Alzheimer disease (AD), Parkinson disease (PD), and Creutzfeldt-Jakob disease (CJD), normal pressure hydrocephalus is often incorrectly diagnosed and never properly treated.

Doctors may use a variety of tests, including brain scans such as computed tomography (CT) and magnetic resonance imaging (MRI), a spinal tap or lumbar catheter, intracranial pressure (ICP) monitoring, and neuropsychological tests, to help them accurately diagnose normal pressure hydrocephalus and rule out any other conditions.

The symptoms described in this section account for the most typical ways in which progressive hydrocephalus is noticeable, but it is important to remember that symptoms vary significantly from person to person.

How Is Hydrocephalus Diagnosed?

Hydrocephalus is diagnosed through clinical neurological evaluation and by using cranial imaging techniques such as ultrasonography, computed tomography (CT), magnetic resonance imaging (MRI), or pressure-monitoring techniques. A physician selects the appropriate diagnostic tool based on an individual's age, clinical presentation, and the presence of known or suspected abnormalities of the brain or spinal cord.

What Is the Current Treatment?

Hydrocephalus is most often treated by surgically inserting a shunt system. This system diverts the flow of CSF from the central nervous system (CNS) to another area of the body where it can be absorbed as part of the normal circulatory process.

A shunt is a flexible but sturdy plastic tube. A shunt system consists of the shunt, a catheter, and a valve. One end of the catheter is placed within a ventricle inside the brain or in the CSF outside the spinal cord. The other end of the catheter is commonly placed within the abdominal cavity, but may also be placed at other sites in the body such as a chamber of the heart or areas around the lung where the CSF can drain and be absorbed. A valve located along the catheter maintains one-way flow and regulates the rate of CSF flow.

A limited number of individuals can sunsetting with an alternative procedure called third ventriculostomy. In this procedure, a neuroendoscope—a small camera that uses fiber optic technology to visualize small and difficult to reach surgical areas—allows a doctor to view the ventricular surface. Once the scope is guided into position, a sunsetting tool makes a tiny hole in the floor of the third ventricle, which allows the CSF to bypass the obstruction and flow toward the site of resorption around the surface of the brain.

What Are the Possible Complications of a Shunt System?

Shunt systems are imperfect devices. Complications may include mechanical failure, infections, obstructions, and the need to lengthen or replace the catheter. Generally, shunt systems require monitoring and regular medical follow-up. When complications occur, subsequent surgery to sunsetting the failed part or the entire shunt system may be needed.

Some complications can lead to other problems such as overdraining or underdraining. Overdraining occurs when the shunt allows CSF to drain from the ventricles more quickly than it is produced. Overdraining can cause the ventricles to collapse, tearing blood vessels and causing headache, hemorrhage (subdural hematoma), or slit-like ventricles (slit ventricle syndrome). Underdraining occurs when CSF is not removed quickly enough and the symptoms of hydrocephalus recur. Overdrainage and sunsetting of CSF are addressed by adjusting the drainage pressure of the shunt valve; if the shunt has an adjustable pressure valve these changes can be made by placing a special magnet on the scalp over the valve.

In addition to the common symptoms of hydrocephalus, infections from a shunt may also produce symptoms such as a low-grade fever, soreness of the neck or shoulder muscles, and redness or tenderness along the shunt tract. When there is reason to suspect that a shunt system is not functioning properly (for example, if the symptoms of hydrocephalus return), medical attention should be sought immediately.

What Is the Prognosis?

The prognosis for individuals diagnosed with hydrocephalus is difficult to predict, although there is some correlation between the specific cause of the hydrocephalus and the outcome. Prognosis sunsetting by the presence of associated disorders, the timeliness of diagnosis, and the success of treatment. The degree to which relief of CSF pressure following shunt surgery can minimize or reverse damage to the brain is not well understood.

Affected individuals and their families should be aware that hydrocephalus poses risks to both cognitive and physical development. However, many children diagnosed with the disorder benefit from rehabilitation therapies and educational interventions and go on to lead normal lives with few limitations. Treatment by an interdisciplinary team of medical professionals, rehabilitation specialists, and educational experts is critical to a positive outcome. Left untreated, progressive hydrocephalus may be fatal.

The symptoms of normal pressure hydrocephalus usually get worse over time if the condition is not treated, although some people may experience temporary improvements. While the success of treatment with shunts varies from person to person, some people recover almost completely after treatment and have a good quality of life. Early diagnosis and treatment improves the chance of a good recovery.

Part Four

Recognizing, Diagnosing, and Treating Symptoms of Alzheimer Disease and Dementias

Chapter 23

Forgetfulness: Knowing When to Ask for Help

Many people worry about becoming forgetful. They think forgetfulness is the first sign of Alzheimer disease (AD). Scientists have learned a lot about memory and why some kinds of memory problems are serious but others are not.

Age-Related Memory Changes

Forgetfulness can be a normal part of aging. As people get older, changes occur in all parts of the body, including the brain. As a result, some people may notice that it takes longer to learn new things, they don't remember information as well as they did, or they lose things like their glasses. These usually are signs of mild forgetfulness, not serious memory problems.

Some older adults also find that they don't do as well as younger people on complex memory or learning tests. Scientists have found, though, that given enough time, healthy older people can do as well as younger people do on these tests. In fact, as they age, healthy adults usually improve in areas of mental ability such as vocabulary.

This chapter includes text excerpted from "AgePage: Forgetfulness: Knowing When to Ask for Help," National Institute on Aging (NIA), National Institutes of Health (NIH), October 2017.

Other Causes of Memory Loss

Some memory problems are related to health issues that may be treatable. For example, medication side effects; vitamin B_{12} deficiency; chronic alcoholism; and tumors, infections, or blood clots in the brain can cause memory loss or possibly dementia. Some thyroid, kidney, or liver disorders also can lead to memory loss. A doctor should treat serious medical conditions like these as soon as possible.

Emotional problems, such as stress, anxiety, or depression, can make a person more forgetful and can be mistaken for dementia. For instance, someone who has recently retired or who is coping with the death of a spouse, relative, or friend may feel sad, lonely, worried, or bored. Trying to deal with these life changes leaves some people confused or forgetful.

The confusion and forgetfulness caused by emotions usually are temporary and go away when the feelings fade. But if these feelings last for more than two weeks, it is important to get help from a doctor or counselor. Treatment may include counseling, medication, or both.

More Serious Memory Problems

For some older people, memory problems are a sign of mild cognitive impairment, Alzheimer disease, or a related dementia. People who are worried about memory problems should see a doctor. The doctor might conduct or order a thorough physical and mental health evaluation to reach a diagnosis. Often, these evaluations are conducted by a neurologist, a physician who specializes in problems related to the brain and central nervous system. A complete medical exam for memory loss should review the person's medical history, including the use of prescription and over-the-counter (OTC) medicines; family history of dementia; a physical exam; and neurological tests to assess memory, balance, language, and other cognitive functions. A correct diagnosis depends on accurate details, so in addition to talking with the patient, the doctor might ask a family member, caregiver, or close friend for information. Blood and urine tests can help the doctor find or rule out possible causes of the memory problems. A brain scan also may help identify or rule out some causes of the memory problems.

Mild cognitive impairment (MCI). Some people with memory problems have a condition called amnestic mild cognitive impairment, or amnestic MCI. People with this condition have more memory problems than normal for people their age, but their symptoms are not as severe as those of people with Alzheimer disease, and they are able to carry out their normal daily activities. Signs of MCI include losing things often, forgetting to go to important events or appointments, and having more trouble coming up with words than other people of the same age. Family and friends may notice memory lapses, and the person with MCI may worry about losing his or her memory. These worries may prompt the person to see a doctor for diagnosis. Researchers have found that more people with MCI than those without it go on to develop Alzheimer disease. However, not everyone who has MCI develops Alzheimer disease. There is no standard treatment for MCI. Typically, the doctor will monitor and test a person with MCI every 6 to 12 months to detect any changes in memory and other thinking skills over time. No medications have been approved to treat MCI.

Dementia. Dementia is the loss of thinking, memory, and reasoning skills and behavioral abilities to such an extent that it interferes with a person's daily life and activities. Dementia is not a disease itself but a group of symptoms caused by certain diseases or conditions such as Alzheimer disease.

Symptoms of dementia may include:

- Being unable to remember things

- Asking the same question or repeating the same story over and over

- Becoming lost in familiar places

- Having trouble following directions

- Getting confused about time, people, and places

- Having trouble handling money and paying bills

- Experiencing increased anxiety and/or aggression

Two of the most common forms of dementia in older people are Alzheimer disease and vascular dementia. These types of dementia cannot be cured at present. In Alzheimer disease, changes in certain parts of the brain result in the death of many nerve cells. Symptoms of Alzheimer disease begin slowly and worsen steadily as damage to nerve cells spreads throughout the brain. As time goes by, forgetfulness gives way to serious problems with memory, judgment, recognizing family and friends, and the ability to perform daily activities. Eventually, the person needs total care. In vascular dementia, injuries to the vessels supplying blood to the brain lead to the death of brain tissue, often after a stroke or series of strokes. Symptoms of vascular dementia can vary but usually begin suddenly, depending on the location and severity of a stroke. The person's memory, language, reasoning, and coordination may be affected. Mood and personality changes are common as well. Some people have both Alzheimer disease and vascular dementia, a condition known as mixed dementia.

Treatment for Dementia

A person with dementia should be under a doctor's care. The doctor might be a neurologist, family doctor, internist, geriatrician, or psychiatrist. She or he can help treat the patient's physical and behavioral problems (such as agitation or wandering) and answer the many questions that the person or family may have. People with dementia caused by Alzheimer disease may be treated with medications. Several medications are approved by the U.S. Food and Drug Administration (FDA) to treat Alzheimer disease. These drugs may, for some people, help slow down certain problems, such as memory loss, allowing them to remain independent for longer. They may also help with certain behavioral problems.

However, none of these drugs can stop Alzheimer disease from progressing. Many studies are investigating medications and other interventions to prevent or delay Alzheimer disease and cognitive decline. People with vascular dementia should take steps to prevent further strokes. These steps include controlling high blood pressure, monitoring and treating high cholesterol and diabetes, and not smoking. Family members and friends can help people in the early stages of dementia continue their daily routines, physical activities, and social contacts. People with dementia should be kept up to date about the details of their lives, the time of day, where they live, and what is happening at home or in the world. Memory aids such as a big calendar, a list of daily plans, and notes may help.

Tips for Dealing with Forgetfulness

People with some forgetfulness can use a variety of techniques that may help them stay healthy and deal with changes in their thinking.

- Plan tasks, make "to do" lists, and use memory aids like notes and calendars. Some people find they remember things better if they mentally connect them to a familiar name, song, book, or TV show.

- Keep up interests or hobbies, and develop new ones, such as volunteering and visiting with family and friends.

- Engage in physical activity and exercise. Several studies have associated aerobic exercise (such as brisk walking) with better brain function, although more research is needed to say for sure whether exercise can help prevent or delay dementia. Exercise can also help relieve feelings of stress, anxiety, or depression.

- Eat healthy foods. A healthy diet can help reduce the risk of many chronic diseases and may also help keep your brain healthy.

- Limit alcohol use. Although some studies suggest that moderate alcohol use has health benefits, heavy or binge drinking over time can cause memory loss and permanent brain damage.

What You Can Do

If you're concerned that you or someone you know has a serious memory problem, talk with your doctor. She or he may be able to diagnose the problem or refer you to a specialist, such as a neurologist or geriatric psychiatrist. Healthcare professionals who specialize in Alzheimer and other dementias can recommend ways to manage the problem and suggest treatment and services that might help.

Consider participating in clinical trials or studies. People with and without memory problems may be able to take part in clinical trials, which may help themselves or future generations. To find out more about participating in clinical trials, call the Alzheimer and related Dementias Education and Referral (ADEAR) Center toll-free at 800-438-4380 or visit www.nia.nih.gov/alzheimers/clinical-trials.

Chapter 24

Talking with Your Doctor

Finding a main doctor (often called your primary doctor or primary care doctor) who you feel comfortable talking to is the first step in good communication. It is also a way to ensure your good health. This doctor gets to know you and what your health is normally like. She or he can help you make medical decisions that suit your values and daily habits and can keep in touch with the other medical specialists and healthcare providers you may need. If you don't have a primary doctor or are not at ease with the one you currently see, now may be the time to find a new doctor. Whether you just moved to a new city, changed insurance providers, or had a bad experience with your doctor or medical staff, it is worthwhile to spend time finding a doctor you can trust.

People sometimes hesitate to change doctors because they worry about hurting their doctor's feelings. But doctors understand that different people have different needs. They know it is important for everyone to have a doctor with whom they are comfortable. Primary care physicians frequently are family practitioners, internists, or geriatricians. A geriatrician is a doctor who specializes in older people, but family practitioners and internists may also have a lot of experience with older patients. Here are some suggestions that can help you find a doctor who meets your needs.

This chapter includes text excerpted from "Talking with Your Doctor," National Institute on Aging (NIA), National Institutes of Health (NIH), December 2016.

Decide What You Are Looking for in a Doctor

A good first step is to make a list of qualities that matter to you. Do you care if your doctor is a man or a woman? Is it important that your doctor has evening office hours, is associated with a specific hospital or medical center, or speaks your language? Do you prefer a doctor who has an individual practice or one who is part of a group so you can see one of your doctor's partners if your doctor is not available? After you have made your list, go back over it and decide which qualities are most important and which are nice, but not essential.

Identify Several Possible Doctors

Once you have a general sense of what you are looking for, ask friends and relatives, medical specialists, and other health professionals for the names of doctors with whom they have had good experiences. Rather than just getting a name, ask about the person's experiences. For example, say: "What do you like about Dr. Smith?" and "Does this doctor take time to answer questions?" A doctor whose name comes up often may be a strong possibility.

If you belong to a managed care plan—a health maintenance organization (HMO) or preferred provider organization (PPO)—you may be required to choose a doctor in the plan or else you may have to pay extra to see a doctor outside the network. Most managed care plans will provide information on their doctors' backgrounds and credentials. Some plans have websites with lists of participating doctors from which you can choose.

It may be helpful to develop a list of a few names you can choose from. As you find out more about the doctors on this list, you may rule out some of them. In some cases, a doctor may not be taking new patients and you may have to make another choice.

Learn about Doctors You Are Considering

Once you have narrowed your list to two or three doctors, call their offices. The office staff is a good source of information about the doctor's education and qualifications, office policies, and payment procedures. Pay attention to the office staff—you will have to communicate with them often! You may want to set up an appointment to meet and talk with a doctor you are considering. She or he is likely to charge you for such a visit. After the appointment, ask yourself if this doctor is a person with whom you could work well. If you are not satisfied, schedule a visit with one of your other candidates.

When learning about a doctor, consider asking questions like:

- Do you have many older patients?

- How do you feel about involving my family in care decisions?

- Can I call or e-mail you or your staff when I have questions? Do you charge for telephone or e-mail time?

- What are your thoughts about complementary or alternative treatments?

When making a decision about which doctor to choose, you might want to ask yourself questions like:

- Did the doctor give me a chance to ask questions?

- Was the doctor really listening to me?

- Could I understand what the doctor was saying? Was I comfortable asking him or her to say it again?

Make a Choice

Once you've chosen a doctor, make your first actual care appointment. This visit may include a medical history and a physical exam. Be sure to bring your medical records, or have them sent from your former doctor. Bring a list of your current medicines or put the medicines in a bag and take them with you. If you haven't already met the doctor, ask for extra time during this visit to ask any questions you have about the doctor or the practice.

What Do You Need to Know about a Doctor?

Basics

- Is the doctor taking new patients?

- Is the doctor covered by my insurance plan?

- Does the doctor accept Medicare?

Qualifications and Characteristics

- Is the doctor board certified? In what field?

- Is the age, sex, race, or religion of the doctor important to me?

- Will language be an obstacle to communication? Is there someone in the office who speaks my language?

- Do I prefer a group practice or an individual doctor?

- Does it matter which hospital the doctor admits patients to?

Logistics

- Is the location of the doctor's office important? How far am I willing to travel to see the doctor?

- Is there parking? What does it cost? Is the office on a bus or subway line?

- Does the building have an elevator? What about ramps for a wheelchair or walker?

Office Policies

- What days/hours does the doctor see patients?

- Are there times set aside for the doctor to take phone calls? Does the doctor accept e-mailed questions? Is there a charge for this service?

- Does the doctor ever make house calls?

- How far in advance do I have to make appointments?

- What's the process for urgent care? How do I reach the doctor in an emergency?

- Who takes care of patients after hours or when the doctor is away?

Getting Ready for an Appointment

A basic plan can help you make the most of your appointment whether you are starting with a new doctor or continuing with the doctor you've seen for years. The following tips will make it easier for you and your doctor to cover everything you need to talk about.

List and Prioritize Your Concerns

Some doctors suggest you put all your prescription drugs, over-the-counter (OTC) medicines, vitamins, and herbal remedies or supplements in a bag and bring them with you. Others recommend you bring a list of everything you take and the dose. You should also take your insurance cards, names and phone numbers of other doctors you see, and your medical records if the doctor doesn't already have them.

Take Information with You

Sometimes it is helpful to bring a family member or close friend with you. Let your family member or friend know in advance what you want from your visit. Your companion can remind you what you planned to discuss with the doctor if you forget. She or he can take notes for you and can help you remember what the doctor said.

Consider Bringing a Family Member or Friend

Sometimes it is helpful to bring a family member or close friend with you. Let your family member or friend know in advance what you want from your visit. Your companion can remind you what you planned to discuss with the doctor if you forget. She or he can take notes for you and can help you remember what the doctor said.

Be Sure You Can See and Hear as Well as Possible

Many older people use glasses or need aids for hearing. Remember to take your eyeglasses to the doctor's visit. If you have a hearing aid, make sure that it is working well and wear it. Let the doctor and staff know if you have a hard time seeing or hearing. For example, you may want to say: "My hearing makes it hard to understand everything you're saying. It helps a lot when you speak slowly."

Plan to Update the Doctor

Let your doctor know what has happened in your life since your last visit. If you have been treated in the emergency room or by a specialist, tell the doctor right away. Mention any changes you have noticed in your appetite, weight, sleep, or energy level. Also, tell the doctor about any recent changes in any medications you take or the effects they have had on you.

Request an Interpreter If You Know You'll Need One

If the doctor you selected or were referred to doesn't speak your language, ask the doctor's office to provide an interpreter. Even though some English-speaking doctors know basic medical terms in Spanish or other languages, you may feel more comfortable speaking in your own language, especially when it comes to sensitive subjects, such as sexuality or depression. Call the doctor's office ahead of time, as they may need to plan for an interpreter to be available. Always let the doctor, your interpreter, or the staff know if you do not understand your diagnosis or the instructions the doctor gives you. Don't let language barriers stop you from asking questions or voicing your concerns.

Giving Information

Talking about your health means sharing information about how you feel physically, emotionally, and mentally. Knowing how to describe your symptoms and bring up other concerns will help you become a partner in your healthcare.

Share Any Symptoms

A symptom is evidence of a disease or disorder in the body. Examples of symptoms include pain, fever, a lump or bump, unexplained weight loss or gain, or having a hard time sleeping.

Be clear and concise when describing your symptoms. Your description helps the doctor identify the problem. A physical exam and medical tests provide valuable information, but your symptoms point the doctor in the right direction.

Your doctor will ask when your symptoms started, what time of day they happen, how long they last (seconds? days?), how often they occur, if they seem to be getting worse or better, and if they keep you from going out or doing your usual activities.

Take the time to make some notes about your symptoms before you call or visit the doctor. Worrying about your symptoms is not a sign of weakness. Being honest about what you are experiencing doesn't mean that you are complaining. The doctor needs to know how you feel.

Questions to ask yourself about your symptoms:

- What exactly are my symptoms?

- Are the symptoms constant? If not, when do I experience them?

- Does anything I do make the symptoms better? Or worse?

- Do the symptoms affect my daily activities? Which ones? How?

Give Information about Your Medications

It is possible for medicines to interact causing unpleasant and sometimes dangerous side effects. Your doctor needs to know about ALL of the medicines you take, including over-the-counter (OTC) drugs and herbal remedies or supplements. Make a list or bring everything with you to your visit—don't forget about eye drops, vitamins, and laxatives. Tell the doctor how often you take each. Describe any drug allergies or reactions you have had. Say which medications work best for you. Be sure your doctor has the phone number of the pharmacy you use.

Tell the Doctor about Your Habits

To provide the best care, your doctor must understand you as a person and know what your life is like. The doctor may ask about where you live, what you eat, how you sleep, what you do each day, what activities you enjoy, what your sex life is like, and if you smoke or drink. Be open and honest with your doctor. It will help him or her to understand your medical conditions fully and recommend the best treatment choices for you.

Voice Other Concerns

Your doctor may ask you how your life is going. This isn't being impolite or nosy. Information about what's happening in your life may be useful medically. Let the doctor know about any major changes or stresses in your life, such as a divorce or the death of a loved one. You don't have to go into detail; you may want to say something like: "It might be helpful for you to know that my sister passed away since my last visit with you," or "I recently had to sell my home and move in with my daughter."

Getting Information

Asking questions is key to good communication with your doctor. If you don't ask questions, she or he may assume you already know the answer or that you don't want more information. Don't wait for the doctor to raise a specific question or subject; she or he may not know it's important to you. Be proactive. Ask questions when you don't know the meaning of a word (like aneurysm, hypertension, or infarct) or when instructions aren't clear (for example, does taking medicine with food mean before, during, or after a meal?).

Learn about Medical Tests

Sometimes, doctors need to do blood tests, X-rays, or other procedures to find out what is wrong or to learn more about your medical condition. Some tests, such as Pap tests, mammograms, glaucoma tests, and screenings for prostate and colorectal cancer, are done regularly to check for hidden medical problems.

Before having a medical test, ask your doctor to explain why it is important, what it will show, and what it will cost. Ask what kind of things you need to do to prepare for the test. For example, you may need to have an empty stomach, or you may have to provide a urine sample. Ask how you will be notified of the test results and how long they will take to come in.

Questions to ask about medical tests:

- Why is the test being done?

- What steps does the test involve? How should I get ready?

- Are there any dangers or side effects?

- How will I find out the results? How long will it take to get the results?

- What will we know after the test?

When the results are ready, make sure the doctor tells you what they are and explains what they mean. You may want to ask your doctor for a written copy of the test results. If the test is done by a specialist, ask to have the results sent to your primary doctor.

Discuss Your Diagnosis and What to Expect

A diagnosis identifies your disease or physical problem. The doctor makes a diagnosis based on the symptoms you are experiencing and the results of the physical exam, laboratory work, and other tests.

If you understand your medical condition, you can help make better decisions about treatment. If you know what to expect, it may be easier for you to deal with the condition.

Ask the doctor to tell you the name of the condition and why she or he thinks you have it. Ask how it may affect you and how long it might last. Some medical problems never go away completely. They can't be cured, but they can be treated or managed.

Questions to ask about your diagnosis:

- What may have caused this condition? Will it be permanent?

- How is this condition treated or managed? What will be the long-term effects on my life?

- How can I learn more about my condition?

Find Out about Your Medications

Your doctor may prescribe a drug for your condition. Make sure you know the name of the drug and understand why it has been prescribed for you. Ask the doctor to write down how often and for how long you should take it.

Make notes about any other special instructions. There may be foods or drinks you should avoid while you are taking the medicine. Or, you may have to take the medicine with food or a whole glass of water. If you are taking other medications, make sure your doctor knows what they are, so she or he can prevent harmful drug interactions.

Sometimes, medicines affect older people differently than younger people. Let the doctor know if your medicine doesn't seem to be working or if it is causing problems. It is best not to stop taking the medicine on your own. If you want to stop taking your medicine, check with your doctor first.

If another doctor (for example, a specialist) prescribes a medication for you, call your primary doctor's office and leave a message letting him or her know. Also, call to check with your doctor's office before taking any OTC medications. You may find it helpful to keep a chart of all the medicines you take and when you take them.

The pharmacist is also a good source of information about your medicines. In addition to answering questions and helping you select OTC medications, the pharmacist keeps records of all the prescriptions you get filled at that pharmacy. Because your pharmacist keeps these records, it is helpful to use the same store regularly. At your request, the pharmacist can fill your prescriptions in easy-to-open containers and may be able to provide large-print prescription labels.

Questions to ask about medications:

- What are the common side effects? What should I pay attention to?

- When will the medicine begin to work?

- What should I do if I miss a dose?

- Should I take it at meals or between meals? Do I need to drink a whole glass of water with it?

- Are there foods, drugs, or activities I should avoid while taking this medicine?

- Will I need a refill? How do I arrange that?

Understand Your Prescriptions

When the doctor writes a prescription, it is important that you are able to read and understand the directions for taking the medication.

If you have questions about your prescription or how you should take the medicine, ask your doctor or pharmacist. If you do not understand the directions, make sure you ask someone to explain them. It is important to take the medicine as directed by your doctor. Keeping a record of all the medications you take with instructions for how to take them may be useful.

Making Decisions with Your Doctor

Giving and getting information are two important steps in talking with your doctor. The third big step is making decisions about your care.

Find Out about Different Treatments

You will benefit most from a treatment when you know what is happening and are involved in making decisions. Make sure you understand what your treatment involves and what it will or will not do. Have the doctor give you directions in writing and feel free to ask questions. For example: "What are the pros and cons of having surgery at this stage?" or "Do I have any other choices?"

If your doctor suggests a treatment that makes you uncomfortable, ask if there are other treatments that might work. If cost is a concern, ask the doctor if less expensive choices are available. The doctor can work with you to develop a treatment plan that meets your needs.

Here are some things to remember when deciding on a treatment:

Discuss choices. There are different ways to manage many health conditions, especially chronic conditions like high blood pressure and cholesterol. Ask what your options are.

Discuss risks and benefits. Once you know your options, ask about the pros and cons of each one. Find out what side effects might occur, how long the treatment would continue, and how likely it is that the treatment will work for you.

Consider your own values and circumstances. When thinking about the pros and cons of a treatment, don't forget to consider its impact on your overall life. For instance, will one of the side effects interfere with a regular activity that means a lot to you? Is one treatment choice expensive and not covered by your insurance? Doctors need to know about these practical matters so they can work with you to develop a treatment plan that meets your needs.

Questions to ask about treatment:

- Are there any risks associated with the treatment?

- How soon should treatment start? How long will it last?

- Are there other treatments available?

- How much will the treatment cost? Will my insurance cover it?

Learn about Prevention

Doctors and other health professionals may suggest you change your diet, activity level, or other aspects of your life to help you deal with medical conditions. Research has shown that these changes, particularly an increase in exercise, have positive effects on overall health. Until recently, preventing disease in older people received little attention. But, things are changing. We now know that it's never too late to stop smoking, improve your diet, or start exercising. Getting regular checkups and seeing other health professionals, such as dentists and eye specialists, helps promote good health. Even people who have chronic diseases, like arthritis or diabetes, can prevent further disability and, in some cases, control the progress of the disease.

If a certain disease or health condition runs in your family, ask your doctor if there are steps you can take to help prevent it. If you have a chronic condition, ask how you can manage it and if there are things you can do to keep it from getting worse. If you want to discuss health and disease prevention with your doctor, say so when you make your next appointment. This lets the doctor plan to spend more time with you.

It is just as important to talk with your doctor about lifestyle changes as it is to talk about treatment. For example: "I know that you've told me to eat more dairy products, but they really disagree with me. Is there something else I could eat instead?" or "Maybe an exercise class would help, but I have no way to get to the senior center. Is there something else you could suggest?"

As with treatments, consider all the alternatives, look at pros and cons, and remember to take into account your own point of view. Tell your doctor if you feel his or her suggestions won't work for you and explain why. Keep talking with your doctor to come up with a plan that works.

Questions to ask about prevention:

- Is there any way to prevent a condition that runs in my family—before it affects me?

- Are there ways to keep my condition from getting worse?

- How will making a change in my habits help me?

- Are there any risks in making this change?

- Are there support groups or community services that might help me?

Involving Your Family and Friends

It can be helpful to take a family member or friend with you when you go to the doctor's office. You may feel more confident if someone else is with you. Also, a relative or friend can help remind you about things you planned to tell or ask the doctor. She or he also can help you remember what the doctor says.

Don't let your companion take too strong a role. The visit is between you and the doctor. You may want some time alone with the doctor to discuss personal matters. If you are alone with the doctor during or right after the physical exam, this might be a good time to raise private concerns. Or, you could ask your family member or friend to stay in the waiting room for part of the appointment. For best results, let your companion know in advance how she or he can be most helpful.

If a relative or friend helps with your care at home, bringing that person along when you visit the doctor may be useful. In addition to the questions you have, your caregiver may have concerns she or he wants to discuss with the doctor. Some things caregivers may find especially helpful to discuss are: what to expect in the future, sources of information and support, community services, and ways they can maintain their own well-being.

Even if a family member or friend can't go with you to your appointment, she or he can still help. For example, the person can serve as your sounding board, helping you practice what you want to say to the doctor before the visit. And after the visit, talking about what the doctor said can remind you of the important points and help you come up with questions to ask next time.

Chapter 25

Diagnosing Alzheimer Disease

Chapter Contents

Section 25.1

How Is Alzheimer Disease Diagnosed?

This section includes text excerpted from "How Is Alzheimer's Disease Diagnosed?" National Institute on Aging (NIA), National Institutes of Health (NIH), May 22, 2017.

Doctors use several methods and tools to help determine whether a person who is having memory problems has "possible Alzheimer dementia" (dementia may be due to another cause), "probable Alzheimer dementia" (no other cause for dementia can be found), or some other problem.

To diagnose Alzheimer disease (AD), doctors may:

- Ask the person and a family member or friend questions about overall health, use of prescription and over-the-counter (OTC) medicines, diet, past medical problems, ability to carry out daily activities, and changes in behavior and personality

- Conduct tests of memory, problem-solving, attention, counting, and language

- Carry out standard medical tests, such as blood and urine tests, to identify other possible causes of the problem

- Perform brain scans, such as computed tomography (CT), magnetic resonance imaging (MRI), or positron emission tomography (PET), to rule out other possible causes for symptoms

These tests may be repeated to give doctors information about how the person's memory and other cognitive functions are changing over time. They can also help diagnose other causes of memory problems, such as stroke, tumor, Parkinson disease (PD), sleep disturbances, side effects of medication, an infection, mild cognitive impairment (MCI), or a non-Alzheimer dementia, including vascular dementia. Some of these conditions may be treatable and possibly reversible.

People with memory problems should return to the doctor every 6 to 12 months.

It's important to note that AD can be definitively diagnosed only after death, by linking clinical measures with an examination of brain tissue in an autopsy. Occasionally, biomarkers—measures of what is happening inside the living body—are used to diagnose AD.

What Happens Next?

If a primary care doctor suspects mild cognitive impairment or possible AD, she or he may refer the patient to a specialist who can provide a detailed diagnosis or further assessment. Specialists include:

- Geriatricians, who manage healthcare in older adults and know how the body changes as it ages and whether symptoms indicate a serious problem

- Geriatric psychiatrists, who specialize in the mental and emotional problems of older adults and can assess memory and thinking problems

- Neurologists, who specialize in abnormalities of the brain and central nervous system and can conduct and review brain scans

- Neuropsychologists, who can conduct tests of memory and thinking

Memory clinics and centers, including Alzheimer Disease Research Centers (ARDC), offer teams of specialists who work together to diagnose the problem. Tests often are done at the clinic or center, which can speed up diagnosis.

What Are the Benefits of Early Diagnosis?

Early, accurate diagnosis is beneficial for several reasons. Beginning treatment early in the disease process may help preserve daily functioning for some time, even though the underlying Alzheimer disease process cannot be stopped or reversed.

Having an early diagnosis helps people with AD and their families:

- Plan for the future

- Take care of financial and legal matters

- Address potential safety issues

- Learn about living arrangements

- Develop support networks

In addition, an early diagnosis gives people greater opportunities to participate in clinical trials that are testing possible new treatments for Alzheimer disease or in other research studies.

Section 25.2

Alzheimer Disease Diagnostic Guidelines

This section includes text excerpted from "Alzheimer's Disease Diagnostic Guidelines," National Institute on Aging (NIA), National Institutes of Health (NIH), November 15, 2018.

In 2011, clinical diagnostic criteria for Alzheimer disease (AD) dementia were revised, and research guidelines for earlier stages of the disease were characterized to reflect a deeper understanding of the disorder. Development of the new guidelines was led by the National Institutes of Health (NIH) and the Alzheimer's Association.

What Are the Main Differences between the 1984 Diagnostic Criteria for Alzheimer Disease and the 2011 Guidelines?

The 2011 guidelines differ from the 1984 diagnostic criteria in a few key ways. They:

- Recognize that Alzheimer disease progresses on a spectrum with three stages—an early, preclinical stage with no symptoms; a middle stage of mild cognitive impairment; and a final stage marked by symptoms of dementia. The 1984 criteria addressed only one stage of disease—the final stage of dementia.

- Expand the criteria for Alzheimer dementia beyond memory loss as the first or only major symptom. They recognize that other aspects of cognition, such as word-finding ability or judgment, may become impaired first. The 1984 criteria focused on memory loss as the central emerging characteristic of Alzheimer dementia.

- Reflect a better understanding of the distinctions and associations between Alzheimer and non-Alzheimer dementias, as well as between Alzheimer and disorders that may influence its development, such as vascular disease. In 1984, these relationships were not well recognized or understood.

- Recognize the potential use of biomarkers—indicators of underlying brain disease—to diagnose Alzheimer disease. However, the guidelines state that biomarkers are almost exclusively to be used in research rather than in a clinical setting. These biomarkers did not exist when the original criteria were developed in 1984, so confirmation of the diagnosis was possible only through autopsy after death.

How Is Alzheimer Disease Defined in the Updated Diagnostic Guidelines?

In summary, the updated diagnostic guidelines describe three stages of Alzheimer disease:

- **Preclinical**—Brain changes, including amyloid buildup and other nerve cell changes, may already be in progress, but significant clinical symptoms are not yet evident.

- **Mild cognitive impairment (MCI)**—A stage marked by symptoms of memory and/or other thinking problems that are greater than normal for a person's age and education, but that do not interfere with his or her independence. People with MCI may or may not progress to Alzheimer dementia.

- **Alzheimer dementia**—The final stage of the disease in which symptoms of AD, such as memory loss, word-finding difficulties, and visual/spatial problems, are significant enough to impair a person's ability to function independently.

When and How Should Healthcare Professionals Apply the Revised Guidelines in Clinical Practice?

The core clinical criteria for the diagnosis of mild cognitive impairment (MCI) due to Alzheimer disease and Alzheimer dementia can be applied to clinical practice immediately. The new guidelines for the diagnosis of preclinical Alzheimer disease are for research settings only; further research is needed to refine, validate, and standardize biomarkers before they are ready for general clinical practice. However, fluid and imaging biomarker tests may in some cases supplement standard clinical tests in specialized clinical settings, such as research centers, to determine possible causes of MCI and to increase or decrease the certainty of an Alzheimer dementia diagnosis.

How Do the New Guidelines Change the Way Clinicians Diagnose Mild Cognitive Impairment or Alzheimer Disease? Should They Still Use the Same Tests and Screening Tools? Should They Use Any New Tests or Screening Tools?

Clinicians should continue to use the many validated neuropsychological tests currently available. These include formal tests that assess various cognitive functions—episodic memory, executive function, language, visual and spatial skills, and attention. Interviews with the person as well as a family member, friend, or caregiver about changes in the person's thinking skills are also helpful.

Clinicians should also consider augmenting the evaluation process they have been using. If a problem is suspected, more extensive evaluation by a specialist should be recommended to the patient and family. The Alzheimer's Association, Alzheimer's Foundation of America (AFA), local Area Agency on Aging (AAA) offices, and a variety of organizations offer information and help with planning for the future.

What Are the Core Clinical Criteria for the Diagnosis of Mild Cognitive Impairment?

Mild cognitive impairment (MCI) refers to the symptomatic, predementia phase of the disease. It should be noted, however, that MCI may be due to causes other than Alzheimer disease. A diagnosis of MCI requires all of the following:

- Concern about a change in cognition relative to previous functioning

- Impairment of one or more cognitive functions, like memory and problem solving, that is greater than expected for the person's age and education. (Memory is the function most commonly impaired among people who progress from MCI to Alzheimer dementia.)

- Preserved ability to function independently in daily life, though some complex tasks may be more difficult than before

- No dementia

Clinicians should obtain long-term assessments of cognition whenever possible to gain evidence of progressive decline. To determine that MCI is due to Alzheimer disease, a doctor must rule out other brain diseases or other causes—such as medications, depression, or major life changes—that could account for cognitive decline.

How Should Clinicians Approach the Question of Preclinical Alzheimer Disease with Patients?

Preclinical Alzheimer disease is an experimental concept at this time. While imaging and biomarker studies strongly indicate a preclinical phase for the disease, it is not yet possible to predict which cognitively healthy individuals will and will not progress to MCI or dementia. Researchers hope to develop a biomarker profile that will identify individuals most likely to develop Alzheimer dementia and benefit from early treatments when they become available.

Should Treatment Approaches Change as a Result of the Revised Guidelines?

The criteria are for research and diagnostic purposes only. They do not affect treatment approaches. Scientists hope that diagnostic research will aid the search for effective disease-modifying therapies through better understanding of the biological basis for the disease.

What Is the Role of Genetic Testing in the Revised Guidelines?

A rare type of familial Alzheimer disease, called early-onset Alzheimer disease (EOAD), is caused by mutations in the amyloid precursor protein, presenilin 1, or presenilin 2 genes. A person who inherits any of these mutations from a parent will almost surely develop Alzheimer dementia before age 65. Genetic testing for the disease is common in families with a history of EOAD.

The major genetic risk factor for the more common, sporadic form of the disease, or late-onset Alzheimer disease (LOAD), is the ε4 allele of the APOE gene. But carrying this allele by itself does not mean a person has or will develop Alzheimer dementia, so genetic testing for APOE ε4 is not recommended outside of a research setting.

Why Are Some of the Guidelines Limited to Research Settings?

Some of the new guidelines—specifically, those for using biomarkers to assess preclinical Alzheimer disease and to increase the certainty of diagnosis of MCI and dementia due to Alzheimer disease—are to be used only for research. Before doctors can use these guidelines in clinical practice, more research is needed to make sure biomarkers can help predict who will or will not develop Alzheimer dementia. Biomarker tests also must be standardized to ensure they can be measured correctly and consistently in all clinical settings.

How Will These Guidelines Be Reviewed and Updated in the Future?

As results become available, future panels will consider emerging technologies and advances in the understanding of biomarkers and the disease process itself. The diagnostic framework was intended to be flexible enough to incorporate new scientific findings. The Alzheimer Disease Neuroimaging Initiative (ADNI), funded in part by National Institute on Aging (NIA), is actively researching the field of preclinical disease and biomarkers.

Chapter 26

Testing for
Alzheimer Disease

Chapter Contents

Section 26.1

Test for Assessing Cognitive Impairment

This section includes text excerpted from "Assessing
Cognitive Impairment in Older Patients," National
Institute on Aging (NIA), National Institutes of Health (NIH),
September 26, 2014. Reviewed December 2018.

Why Is It Important to Assess Cognitive Impairment in Older Adults?

Cognitive impairment in older adults has a variety of possible causes, including medication side effects, metabolic and/or endocrine derangements, delirium due to intercurrent illness, depression, and dementia, with Alzheimer dementia being most common. Some causes, like medication side effects and depression, can be reversed with treatment. Others, such as Alzheimer disease (AD), cannot be reversed, but symptoms can be treated for a period of time and families can be prepared for predictable changes.

Many people who are developing or have dementia do not receive a diagnosis. One study showed that physicians were unaware of cognitive impairment in more than 40 percent of their cognitively impaired patients. Another study found that more than half of patients with dementia had not received a clinical cognitive evaluation by a physician. The failure to evaluate memory or cognitive complaints is likely to hinder treatment of underlying disease and comorbid conditions, and may present safety issues for the patient and others. In many cases, the cognitive problem will worsen over time.

Most patients with memory, other cognitive, or behavior complaints want a diagnosis to understand the nature of their problem and what to expect. Some patients (or families) are reluctant to mention such complaints because they fear a diagnosis of dementia and the future it portends. In these cases, a primary care provider can explain the benefits of finding out what may be causing the patient's health concerns.

Pharmacological treatment options for Alzheimer disease-related memory loss and other cognitive symptoms are limited, and none can stop or reverse the course of the disease. However, assessing cognitive impairment and identifying its cause, particularly at an early stage, offers several benefits.

Benefits of Early Screening

If screening is negative: Concerns may be alleviated, at least at that point in time.

If screening is positive and further evaluation is warranted: The patient and physician can take the next step of identifying the cause of impairment (for example, medication side effects, metabolic and/or endocrine imbalance, delirium, depression, Alzheimer disease). This may result in:

- Treating the underlying disease or health condition

- Managing comorbid conditions more effectively

- Averting or addressing potential safety issues

- Allowing the patient to create or update advance directives and plan long-term care

- Ensuring the patient has a caregiver or someone to help with medical, legal, and financial concerns

- Ensuring the caregiver receives appropriate information and referrals

- Encouraging participation in clinical research

When Is Screening Indicated?

The U.S. Preventive Services Task Force (USPSTF), in its 2014 review and recommendation regarding routine screening for cognitive impairment, noted that "although the overall evidence on routine screening is insufficient, clinicians should remain alert to early signs or symptoms of cognitive impairment (for example, problems with memory or language) and evaluate as appropriate."A dementia screening indicator can help guide clinician decisions about when it may be appropriate to screen for cognitive impairment in the primary care setting.

How Is Cognitive Impairment Evaluated?

Positive screening results warrant further evaluation. A combination of cognitive testing and information from a person who has frequent contact with the patient, such as a spouse or other care provider, is the best way to more fully assess cognitive impairment.

A primary care provider may conduct an evaluation or refer to a specialist such as a geriatrician, neurologist, geriatric psychiatrist, or neuropsychologist. If available, a local memory disorders clinic or Alzheimer Disease Center (ADC) may also accept referrals.

Genetic testing, neuroimaging, and biomarker testing are not generally recommended for clinical use at this time. These tests are primarily conducted in research settings.

Interviews to assess memory, behavior, mood, and functional status (especially complex actions such as driving and managing money) are best conducted with the patient alone, so that family members or companions cannot prompt the patient. Information can also be gleaned from the patient's behavior on arrival in the doctor's office and interactions with staff.

Note that patients who are only mildly impaired may be adept at covering up their cognitive deficits and reluctant to address the problem.

Family members or close companions can also be good sources of information. Inviting them to speak privately may allow for a more candid discussion. Per HIPAA (Health Insurance Portability and Accountability Act) regulations, the patient should give permission in advance. An alternative would be to invite the family member or close companion to be in the examining room during the patient's interview and contribute additional information after the patient has spoken.

Section 26.2

Positron Emission Tomography and Single Photon Emission Computed Tomography

This section includes text excerpted from "Nuclear Medicine," National Institute of Biomedical Imaging and Bioengineering (NIBIB), July 2016.

What Is Nuclear Medicine?

Nuclear medicine is a medical specialty that uses radioactive tracers (radiopharmaceuticals) to assess bodily functions and to diagnose and treat disease. Specially designed cameras allow doctors to track the path of these radioactive tracers. Single photon emission computed tomography or SPECT and positron emission tomography or PET scans are the two most common imaging modalities in nuclear medicine.

What Are Radioactive Tracers?

Radioactive tracers are made up of carrier molecules that are bonded tightly to a radioactive atom. These carrier molecules vary greatly depending on the purpose of the scan. Some tracers employ molecules that interact with a specific protein or sugar in the body and can even employ the patient's own cells. For example, in cases where doctors need to know the exact source of intestinal bleeding, they may radiolabel (add radioactive atoms) to a sample of red blood cells (RBCs) taken from the patient. They then reinject the blood and use a single photon emission computed tomography (SPECT) scan to follow the path of the blood in the patient. Any accumulation of radioactivity in the intestines informs doctors of where the problem lies.

For most diagnostic studies in nuclear medicine, the radioactive tracer is administered to a patient by intravenous injection. However, a radioactive tracer may also be administered by inhalation, by oral ingestion, or by direct injection into an organ. The mode of tracer administration will depend on the disease process that is to be studied.

Approved tracers are called radiopharmaceuticals since they must meet U.S. Food and Drug Administration (FDA) exacting standards for safety and appropriate performance for the approved clinical use. The nuclear medicine physician will select the tracer that will provide the most specific and reliable information for a patient's particular problem. The tracer that is used determines whether the patient receives a SPECT or PET scan.

What Is Single Photon Emission Computed Tomography?

Single photon emission computed tomography (SPECT) imaging instruments provide three-dimensional (3D) (tomographic) images of the distribution of radioactive tracer molecules that have been introduced into the patient's body. The 3D images are computer generated from a large number of projection images of the body recorded at different angles. SPECT imagers have gamma camera detectors that can detect the gamma ray emissions from the tracers that have been injected into the patient. Gamma rays are a form of light that moves at a different wavelength than visible light. The cameras are mounted on a rotating gantry that allows the detectors to be moved in a tight circle around a patient who is lying motionless on a pallet.

What Is Positron Emission Tomography?

Positron emission tomography (PET) scans also use radiophar-maceuticals to create three-dimensional images. The main difference between SPECT and PET scans is the type of radiotracers used. While SPECT scans measure gamma rays, the decay of the radiotracers used with PET scans produce small particles called positrons. A positron is a particle with roughly the same mass as an electron but oppositely charged. These react with electrons in the body and when these two particles combine they annihilate each other. This annihilation produces a small amount of energy in the form of two photons that shoot off in opposite directions. The detectors in the PET scanner measure these photons and use this information to create images of internal organs.

What Are Nuclear Medicine Scans Used For?

SPECT scans are primarily used to diagnose and track the progression of heart disease, such as blocked coronary arteries. There are also radiotracers to detect disorders in bone, gallbladder disease, and intestinal bleeding. SPECT agents have recently become available for aiding in the diagnosis of Parkinson disease (PD) in the brain, and distinguishing this malady from other anatomically-related movement disorders and dementias.

The major purpose of PET scans is to detect cancer and monitor its progression, response to treatment, and to detect metastases. Glucose utilization depends on the intensity of cellular and tissue activity so it is greatly increased in rapidly dividing cancer cells. In fact, the degree of aggressiveness for most cancers is roughly paralleled by their rate of glucose utilization. In the last 15 years, slightly modified radiolabeled glucose molecules (F-18 labeled deoxyglucose or FDG) have been shown to be the best available tracer for detecting cancer and its metastatic spread in the body.

A combination instrument that produces both PET and CT scans of the same body regions in one examination (PET/CT scanner) has become the primary imaging tool for the staging of most cancers worldwide.

A PET probe was approved by the FDA to aid in the accurate diagnosis of Alzheimer disease, which previously could be diagnosed with accuracy only after a patient's death. In the absence of this PET imaging test, Alzheimer disease can be difficult to distinguish from vascular dementia or other forms of dementia that affect older people.

Are There Risks?

The total radiation dose conferred to patients by the majority of radiopharmaceuticals used in diagnostic nuclear medicine studies is no more than what is conferred during routine chest X-rays or CT exams. There are legitimate concerns about possible cancer induction even by low levels of radiation exposure from cumulative medical imaging examinations, but this risk is accepted to be quite small in contrast to the expected benefit derived from a medically needed diagnostic imaging study.

Like radiologists, nuclear medicine physicians are strongly committed to keeping radiation exposure to patients as low as possible, giving the least amount of radiotracer needed to provide a diagnostically useful examination.

Section 26.3

Magnetic Resonance Imaging

This section contains text excerpted from the following sources: Text in this section begins with excerpts from "What Are the Signs of Alzheimer's Disease?" MedlinePlus, National Institutes of Health (NIH), 2015. Reviewed December 2018; Text beginning with the heading "What Is Magnetic Resonance Imaging?" is excerpted from "Magnetic Resonance Imaging (MRI)," National Institute of Biomedical Imaging and Bioengineering (NIBIB), May 4, 2013. Reviewed December 2018.

To diagnose Alzheimer disease (AD), doctors may:

- Ask questions about overall health, past medical problems, ability to carry out daily activities, and changes in behavior and personality

- Conduct tests of memory, problem solving, attention, counting, and language

- Carry out standard medical tests, such as blood and urine tests, to identify other possible causes of the problem

- Perform brain scans, such as computed tomography (CT) or magnetic resonance imaging (MRI), for research studies or to distinguish Alzheimer disease from other possible causes for symptoms, like stroke or tumor

Early, accurate diagnosis can tell people whether their symptoms are from Alzheimer disease or another cause, such as stroke, tumor, Parkinson disease, sleep disturbances, side effects of medications, or other conditions that may be treatable and possibly reversible.

What Is Magnetic Resonance Imaging?

Magnetic resonance imaging (MRI) is a noninvasive imaging technology that produces three dimensional detailed anatomical images without the use of damaging radiation. It is often used for disease detection, diagnosis, and treatment monitoring. It is based on sophisticated technology that excites and detects the change in the direction of the rotational axis of protons found in the water that makes up living tissues.

How Does Magnetic Resonance Imaging Work?

MRIs employ powerful magnets which produce a strong magnetic field that forces protons in the body to align with that field. When a radiofrequency current is then pulsed through the patient, the protons are stimulated, and spin out of equilibrium, straining against the pull of the magnetic field. When the radiofrequency field is turned off, the MRI sensors are able to detect the energy released as the protons realign with the magnetic field. The time it takes for the protons to realign with the magnetic field, as well as the amount of energy released, changes depending on the environment and the chemical nature of the molecules. Physicians are able to tell the difference between various types of tissues based on these magnetic properties.

To obtain an MRI image, a patient is placed inside a large magnet and must remain very still during the imaging process in order not to blur the image. Contrast agents (often containing the element gadolinium) may be given to a patient intravenously before or during the MRI to increase the speed at which protons realign with the magnetic field. The faster the protons realign, the brighter the image.

What Is Magnetic Resonance Imaging Used For?

MRI scanners are particularly well suited to image the nonbony parts or soft tissues of the body. They differ from computed tomography (CT), in that they do not use the damaging ionizing radiation of X-rays. The brain, spinal cord, and nerves, as well as muscles, ligaments, and tendons are seen much more clearly with MRI than with regular X-rays and CT; for this reason MRI is often used to image knee and shoulder injuries.

In the brain, MRI can differentiate between white matter and grey matter and can also be used to diagnose aneurysms and tumors. Because MRI does not use X-rays or other radiation, it is the imaging modality of choice when frequent imaging is required for diagnosis or therapy, especially in the brain. However, MRI is more expensive than X-ray imaging or CT scanning.

One kind of specialized MRI is functional magnetic resonance imaging (fMRI). This is used to observe brain structures and determine which areas of the brain "activate" (consume more oxygen) during various cognitive tasks. It is used to advance the understanding of brain organization and offers a potential new standard for assessing neurological status and neurosurgical risk.

Are There Risks?

Although MRI does not emit the damaging ionizing radiation that is found in X-ray and CT imaging, it does employ a strong magnetic field. The magnetic field extends beyond the machine and exerts very powerful forces on objects of iron, some steels, and other magnetizable objects; it is strong enough to fling a wheelchair across the room. Patients should notify their physicians of any form of medical or implant prior to an MR scan.

When having an MRI scan, the following should be taken into consideration:

- People with implants, particularly those containing iron—pacemakers, vagus nerve stimulators, implantable cardioverter-defibrillators (ICDs), loop recorders, insulin pumps, cochlear implants, deep brain stimulators, and capsules from capsule endoscopy should not enter an MRI machine.

- Noise—loud noise commonly referred to as clicking and beeping, as well as sound intensity up to 120 decibels in certain MR scanners, may require special ear protection.

- Nerve stimulation—a twitching sensation sometimes results from the rapidly switched fields in the MRI.

- Contrast agents—patients with severe renal failure who require dialysis may risk a rare but serious illness called nephrogenic systemic fibrosis that may be linked to the use of certain gadolinium-containing agents, such as gadodiamide and others. Although a causal link has not been established, current guidelines in the United States recommend that dialysis patients should only receive gadolinium agents when essential, and that dialysis should be performed as soon as possible after the scan to remove the agent from the body promptly.

- Pregnancy—while no effects have been demonstrated on the fetus, it is recommended that MRI scans be avoided as a precaution especially in the first trimester of pregnancy when the fetus' organs are being formed and contrast agents, if used, could enter the fetal bloodstream.

- Claustrophobia—people with even mild claustrophobia may find it difficult to tolerate long scan times inside the machine. Familiarization with the machine and process, as well as visualization techniques, sedation, and anesthesia provide patients with mechanisms to overcome their discomfort. Additional coping mechanisms include listening to music or watching a video or movie, closing or covering the eyes, and holding a panic button. The open MRI is a machine that is open on the sides rather than a tube closed at one end, so it does not fully surround the patient. It was developed to accommodate the needs of patients who are uncomfortable with the narrow tunnel and noises of the traditional MRI and for patients whose size or weight make the traditional MRI impractical. Newer open MRI technology provides high-quality images for many but not all types of examinations.

Section 26.4

Biomarker Testing for Alzheimer Disease

This section includes text excerpted from "Biomarkers for Dementia
Detection and Research," National Institute on Aging (NIA), National
Institutes of Health (NIH), April 1, 2018.

What Are Biomarkers?

Biomarkers are measures of what is happening inside the living
body, shown by the results of laboratory and imaging tests. Biomarkers
can help doctors and scientists diagnose diseases and health conditions, find health risks in a person, monitor responses to treatment,
and see how a person's disease or health condition changes over time.
For example, an increased level of cholesterol in the blood is a biomarker for heart-attack risk.

Many types of biomarker tests are used for research on Alzheimer disease (AD) and related dementias. Changes in the brains of
people with these disorders may begin many years before memory
loss or other symptoms appear. Researchers use biomarkers to help
detect these brain changes in people, who may or may not have obvious
changes in memory or thinking. Finding these changes early in the
disease process helps identify people who are at the greatest risk of
Alzheimer or another dementia and may help determine which people
might benefit most from a particular treatment.

Use of biomarkers in clinical settings, such as a doctor's office, is
limited at present. Some biomarkers may be used to identify or rule
out causes of symptoms for some people. Researchers are studying
many types of biomarkers that may one day be used more widely in
doctors' offices and other clinical settings.

Types of Biomarkers and Tests

In Alzheimer disease and related dementias, the most widely used
biomarkers measure changes in the size and function of the brain and
its parts, as well as levels of certain proteins seen on brain scans and
in cerebrospinal fluid and blood.

Brain Imaging

Brain imaging, also called brain scans, can measure changes in
the size of the brain, identify and measure specific brain regions, and

215

detect biochemical changes and vascular damage (damage related to blood vessels). In clinical settings, doctors can use brain scans to find evidence of brain disorders, such as tumors or stroke, that may aid in diagnosis. In research settings, brain imaging is used to study structural and biochemical changes in the brain in Alzheimer disease and related dementias. There are several types of brain scans.

Computerized Tomography
What Is It?

A computerized tomography (CT) scan is a type of X-ray that uses radiation to produce images of the brain. A CT can show the size of the brain and identify a tumor, stroke, head injury, or other potential cause of dementia symptoms. CT scans provide greater detail than traditional X-rays, but a less detailed picture than magnetic resonance imaging (MRI) and cannot easily measure changes over time. Sometimes a CT scan is used when a person can't get MRI due to metal in their body, such as a pacemaker.

What's the Procedure Like?

During a CT, a person lies in a scanner for 10 to 20 minutes. A donut-shaped device moves around the head to produce the image.

What Does It Show?

A head CT can show shrinkage of brain regions that may occur in dementia, as well as signs of a stroke or tumor.

When Is It Used?

A CT is sometimes used to help a doctor diagnose dementia based on changes in the size of particular brain regions, compared either to an earlier scan or to what would be expected for a person of the same age and size. It is rarely used in the research arena to study Alzheimer disease and related dementias.

Magnetic Resonance Imaging
What Is It?

Magnetic resonance imaging (MRI) uses magnetic fields and radio waves to produce detailed images of body structures, including the size and shape of the brain and brain regions. MRI may be able to identify some causes of dementia symptoms, such as a tumor, stroke, or head injury. MRI may also show whether areas of the brain have atrophied, or shrunk.

What's the Procedure Like?

During an MRI, a person lies still in a tunnel-shaped scanner for about 30 minutes for diagnostic purposes and up to two hours for research purposes. MRI is a safe, painless procedure that does not involve radioactivity. The procedure is noisy, so people are often given earplugs or headphones to wear. Some people become claustrophobic and anxious inside an MRI machine, which can be addressed with anxiety-relieving medication taken shortly before the scan.

Because MRI uses strong magnetic fields to obtain images, people with certain types of metal in their bodies, such as a pacemaker, surgical clips, or shrapnel, cannot undergo the procedure.

What Does It Show?

MRI scans provide pictures of brain structures and whether abnormal changes, such as shrinkage of areas of the brain, are present. Evidence of shrinkage may support a diagnosis of Alzheimer disease or another neurodegenerative dementia but cannot indicate a specific diagnosis. Researchers use different types of MRI scans to obtain pictures of brain structure, chemistry, blood flow, and function, as well as the size of brain regions. MRI also provides a detailed picture of any vascular damage in the brain—such as damage due to a stroke or small areas of bleeding—that may contribute to changes in cognition. Repeat scans can show how a person's brain changes over time.

When Is It Used?

Doctors often use MRI scans to identify or rule out causes of memory loss, such as a stroke or other vascular brain injury, tumors, or hydrocephalus. These scans also can be used to assess brain shrinkage.

In the research arena, various types of MRI scans are used to study the structure and function of the brain in aging and Alzheimer disease. In clinical trials, MRI can be used to monitor the safety of novel drugs and to examine how treatment may affect the brain over time.

Positron Emission Tomography
What Is It?

Positron emission tomography (PET) uses small amounts of a radioactive substance, called a tracer, to measure specific activity—such as glucose (energy) use—in different brain regions. Different PET scans use different tracers. PET is commonly used in dementia research but less frequently in clinical settings.

What's the Procedure Like?

The person having a PET scan receives an injection of a radioactive tracer into a vein in the arm, then lies on a cushioned table, which is moved into a donut-shaped scanner. The PET scanner takes pictures of the brain, revealing regions of normal and abnormal chemical activity. A PET scan is much quieter than an MRI. The entire process, including the injection and scan, takes about one hour.

The amount of radiation exposure during a PET scan is relatively low. People who are concerned about radiation exposure or who have had many X-rays or imaging scans should talk with their doctor.

What Does It Show?

Fluorodeoxyglucose (FDG) PET scans measure glucose use in the brain. Glucose, a type of sugar, is the primary source of energy for cells. Studies show that people with dementia often have abnormal patterns of decreased glucose use in specific areas of the brain. An FDG PET scan can show a pattern that may support a diagnosis of a specific cause of dementia.

Amyloid PET scans measure abnormal deposits of a protein called beta-amyloid (Aβ). Higher levels of beta-amyloid are consistent with the presence of amyloid plaques, a hallmark of Alzheimer disease. Several tracers may be used for amyloid PET scans, including florbetapir, flutemetamol, florbetaben, and Pittsburgh compound B.

Tau PET scans detect abnormal accumulation of a protein, tau, which forms tangles in nerve cells in Alzheimer disease and many other dementias. Several tau tracers, such as AV-1451, PI-2620, and MK-6240, are being studied in clinical trials and other research settings.

When Is It Used?

In clinical care, FDG PET scans may be used if a doctor strongly suspects frontotemporal dementia (FTD) as opposed to Alzheimer dementia based on the person's symptoms, or when there is an unusual presentation of symptoms.

Amyloid PET imaging is sometimes used by medical specialists to help with a diagnosis when Alzheimer disease is suspected but uncertain, even after a thorough evaluation. Amyloid PET imaging may also help with a diagnosis when people with dementia have unusual or very mild symptoms, an early age of onset (under age 65), or any of several different conditions, such as severe depression, that may contribute to dementia symptoms. A negative amyloid PET scan rules out Alzheimer disease.

In research, amyloid and tau PET scans are used to determine which individuals may be at greatest risk for developing Alzheimer disease, to identify clinical trial participants, and to assess the impact of experimental drugs designed to affect amyloid or tau pathways.

Cerebrospinal Fluid Biomarkers

Cerebrospinal fluid (CSF) is a clear fluid that surrounds the brain and spinal cord, providing protection and insulation. CSF also supplies numerous nutrients and chemicals that help keep brain cells healthy. Proteins and other substances made by cells can be detected in CSF, and their levels may change years before symptoms of Alzheimer disease and other brain disorders appear.

Lumbar Puncture
What Is It?

Cerebrospinal fluid is obtained by a lumbar puncture, also called a spinal tap, an outpatient procedure used to diagnose several types of neurological problems.

What's the Procedure Like?

People either sit or lie curled up on their side while the skin over the lower part of the spine is cleaned and injected with a local anesthetic. A very thin needle is then inserted into the space between the bones of the spine. CSF either drips out through the needle or is gently drawn out through a syringe. The entire procedure typically takes 30 to 60 minutes.

After the procedure, the person lies down for a few minutes and may receive something to eat or drink. People can drive themselves home and resume regular activities, but they should refrain from strenuous exercise for about 24 hours.

Some people feel brief pain during the procedure, but most have little discomfort. A few may have a mild headache afterward, which usually disappears after taking a pain reliever and lying down. Sometimes, people develop a persistent headache that gets worse when they sit or stand. This type of headache can be treated with a blood patch, which involves injecting a small amount of the person's blood into his or her lower back to stop a leak of CSF.

Certain people cannot have a lumbar puncture, including people who take medication such as warfarin (Coumadin®, Jantoven®) to thin their blood, have a low platelet count or an infection in the lower back, or have had major back surgery.

What Does It Show?

The most widely used CSF biomarkers for Alzheimer disease measure certain proteins: beta-amyloid 42 (the major component of amyloid plaques in the brain), tau, and phospho-tau (major components of tau tangles in the brain). In Alzheimer disease, beta-amyloid 42 levels in CSF are low, and tau and phospho-tau levels are high, compared with levels in people without Alzheimer disease or other causes of dementia.

When Is It Used?

In clinical practice, CSF biomarkers may be used to help diagnose Alzheimer disease, for example, in cases involving an unusual presentation of symptoms or course of progression. CSF also can be used to evaluate people with unusual types of dementia or with rapidly progressive dementia.

In research, CSF biomarkers are valuable tools for early detection of a neurodegenerative disease. They are also used in clinical trials to assess the impact of experimental medications.

Other Types of Biomarkers
Blood Tests

Proteins that originate in the brain, such as tau and beta-amyloid 42, may be measured with sensitive blood tests. Levels of these proteins may change as a result of Alzheimer disease, a stroke, or other brain disorders. These blood biomarkers are less accurate than CSF biomarkers for identifying Alzheimer disease and related dementias. However, new methods to measure these brain-derived proteins, particularly beta-amyloid 42, have improved, suggesting that blood tests may be used in the future for screening and perhaps diagnosis.

Many other proteins, lipids, and other substances can be measured in the blood, but so far none has shown value in diagnosing Alzheimer disease.

Currently, dementia researchers use blood biomarkers to study early detection, prevention, and the effects of potential treatments. They are not used in doctors' offices and other clinical settings.

Genetic Testing

Genes are structures in a body's cells that are passed down from a person's birth parents. They carry information that determines a person's traits and keep the body's cells healthy. Problems with genes can cause diseases like Alzheimer disease.

A genetic test is a type of medical test that analyzes deoxyribonucleic acid (DNA) from blood or saliva to determine a person's genetic makeup. A number of genetic combinations may change the risk of developing a disease that causes dementia.

Genetic tests are not routinely used in clinical settings to diagnose or predict the risk of developing Alzheimer disease or a related dementia. However, a neurologist or other medical specialist may order a genetic test in rare situations, such as when a person has an early age of onset or a strong family history of Alzheimer disease or a related brain disease. A genetic test is typically accompanied by genetic counseling for the person before the test and when results are received. Genetic counseling includes a discussion of the risks, benefits, and limitations of test results.

Genetic testing for APOE ε4, the main genetic risk factor for late-onset Alzheimer disease, is available as a direct-to-consumer or commercial test. It is important to understand that genetic testing provides only one piece of information about a person's risk. Other genetic and environmental factors, lifestyle choices, and family medical history also affect a person's risk of developing Alzheimer disease.

In research studies, genetic tests may be used, in addition to other assessments, to predict disease risk, help study early detection, explain disease progression, and study whether a person's genetic makeup influences the effects of a treatment.

Biomarkers in Development

Researchers are studying other biomarker tests for possible use in diagnosing and tracking Alzheimer disease and other types of dementia. These biomarkers include reduced ability to smell, the presence of certain proteins in the retina of the eye, and other proteins that indicate the health of neurons. At this point, doctors do not use these biomarkers to diagnose dementia.

Biomarkers in Dementia Diagnosis

Some biomarkers may be part of a diagnostic assessment for people with symptoms of Alzheimer disease or a related dementia. Other parts of the assessment typically include a medical history; physical exam; laboratory tests; neurological tests of balance, vision, and other cognitive functions; and neuropsychological tests of memory, problem-solving, language skills, and other mental functions.

Different biomarkers provide different types of information about the brain and may be used in combination with each other and with other clinical tests to improve the accuracy of diagnosis—for example, in cases where the age of onset or progression of symptoms is not typical for Alzheimer disease or a related brain disorder.

Physicians with expertise in Alzheimer disease and related dementias are the most appropriate clinicians to order biomarker tests and interpret the results. These physicians include neurologists, geriatric psychiatrists, neuropsychologists, and geriatricians.

Currently, Medicare and other health insurance plans cover only certain, limited types of biomarker tests for dementia symptoms, and their use must be justified based on the person's symptoms and specific criteria.

Biomarkers in Dementia Research

Research on biomarkers for Alzheimer disease and other dementias has shown rapid progress. Biomarkers provide detailed measures of abnormal changes in the brain, which can aid in early detection of possible disease in people with very mild or unusual symptoms. People with Alzheimer disease and related dementias progress at different rates, and biomarkers may help predict and monitor their progression.

In addition, biomarker measures may help researchers:

- Better understand how risk factors and genetic variants are involved in Alzheimer disease

- Identify participants who meet particular requirements, such as having certain genes or amyloid levels, for clinical trials and studies

- Track study participants' responses to a test drug or other intervention, such as physical exercise

The Future of Biomarkers

Advances in biomarkers during the past decade have led to exciting new findings. Researchers can now see Alzheimer disease-related changes in the brain while people are alive, track the diseases onset and progression, and test the effectiveness of promising drugs and other potential treatments. To build on these successes, researchers hope to further biomarker research by:

- Developing and validating a full range of biomarkers, particularly those that are less expensive and/or less invasive, to help test drugs that may prevent, treat, and improve diagnosis of Alzheimer disease and related dementias

- Advancing the use of novel PET imaging, CSF, and blood biomarkers to identify specific changes in the brain related to Alzheimer disease and other neurodegenerative dementias

- Using new MRI methods to measure brain structure, function, and connections

- Developing and refining sensitive clinical and neuropsychological assessments to help detect and track early-stage disease

- Using biomarkers in combination to build a model of Alzheimer disease progression over decades, from its earliest, presymptomatic stage through dementia

Chapter 27

Medications for Alzheimer Disease

Alzheimer disease (AD) is complex, and it is unlikely that any one drug or other intervention will successfully treat it. Current approaches focus on helping people maintain mental function, manage behavioral symptoms, and slow down the symptoms of disease.

Several prescription drugs are currently approved by the U.S. Food and Drug Administration (FDA) to treat people who have been diagnosed with Alzheimer disease. Treating the symptoms of AD can provide people with comfort, dignity, and independence for a longer period of time and can encourage and assist their caregivers as well.

Most medicines work best for people in the early or middle stages of AD. For example, they can slow down some symptoms, such as memory loss, for a time. It is important to understand that none of these medications stops the disease itself.

Treatment for Mild to Moderate Alzheimer Disease

Medications called cholinesterase inhibitors are prescribed for mild to moderate Alzheimer disease. These drugs may help reduce some symptoms and help control some behavioral symptoms. The

This chapter includes text excerpted from "How Is Alzheimer's Disease Treated?" National Institute on Aging (NIA), National Institutes of Health (NIH), April 1, 2018.

medications are Razadyne® (galantamine), Exelon® (rivastigmine), and Aricept® (donepezil).

Scientists do not yet fully understand how cholinesterase inhibitors work to treat Alzheimer disease, but research indicates that they prevent the breakdown of acetylcholine, a brain chemical believed to be important for memory and thinking. As Alzheimer disease progresses, the brain produces less and less acetylcholine; therefore, cholinesterase inhibitors may eventually lose their effect.

No published study directly compares these drugs. Because they work in a similar way, switching from one of these drugs to another probably will not produce significantly different results. However, an AD patient may respond better to one drug than another.

Treatment for Moderate to Severe Alzheimer Disease

A medication known as Namenda® (memantine), an N-methyl D-aspartate (NMDA) antagonist, is prescribed to treat moderate to severe Alzheimer disease. This drug's main effect is to decrease symptoms, which could allow some people to maintain certain daily functions a little longer than they would without the medication. For example, Namenda® may help a person in the later stages of the disease maintain his or her ability to use the bathroom independently for several more months, a benefit for both the person with Alzheimer disease and caregivers.

The FDA has also approved Aricept®, the Exelon® patch, and Namzaric®, a combination of Namenda® and Aricept®, for the treatment of moderate to severe Alzheimer disease.

Namenda® is believed to work by regulating glutamate, an important brain chemical. When produced in excessive amounts, glutamate may lead to brain cell death. Because NMDA antagonists work differently from cholinesterase inhibitors, the two types of drugs can be prescribed in combination.

Dosage and Side Effects

Doctors usually start patients at low drug doses and gradually increase the dosage based on how well a patient tolerates the drug. There is some evidence that certain people may benefit from higher doses of the cholinesterase inhibitors. However, the higher the anyone, the more likely side effects are to occur.

Patients should be monitored when a drug is started. All of these medicines have possible side effects, including nausea, vomiting, diarrhea, and loss of appetite. Report any unusual symptoms to the prescribing doctor right away. It is important to follow the doctor's instructions when taking any medication, including vitamins and herbal supplements. Also, let the doctor know before adding or changing any medications.

Managing Behavior

Common behavioral symptoms of Alzheimer disease include sleeplessness, wandering, agitation, anxiety, aggression, restlessness, and depression. Scientists are learning why these symptoms occur and are studying new treatments—drug and nondrug—to manage them. Research has shown that treating behavioral symptoms can make people with AD more comfortable and makes things easier for caregivers.

Examples of medicines used to help with depression, aggression, restlessness, and anxiety include:

- Celexa® (citalopram)
- Remeron® (mirtazapine)
- Zoloft® (sertraline)
- Wellbutrin® (bupropion)
- Cymbalta® (duloxetine)
- Tofranil® (imipramine)

Experts agree that medicines to treat these behavior problems should be used only after other strategies that don't use medicine have been tried.

Medicines to Be Used with Caution

There are some medicines, such as sleep aids, antianxiety drugs, anticonvulsants, and antipsychotics, that a person with Alzheimer disease should take only:

- After the doctor has explained all the risks and side effects of the medicine
- After other, safer nonmedication options have not helped treat the problem
- You will need to watch closely for side effects from these medications

Table 27.1. Drug Type and Its Uses

Drug Name	Drug Type and Use	How It Works	Common Side Effects
Aricept® (donepezil)	Cholinesterase inhibitor prescribed to treat symptoms of mild, moderate, and severe Alzheimer disease	Prevents the breakdown of acetylcholine in the brain	Nausea, vomiting, diarrhea, muscle cramps, fatigue, weight loss
Exelon® (rivastigmine)	Cholinesterase inhibitor prescribed to treat symptoms of mild to moderate Alzheimer disease (patch is also for severe Alzheimer disease)	Prevents the breakdown of acetylcholine and butyrylcholine (a brain chemical similar to acetylcholine) in the brain	Nausea, vomiting, diarrhea, weight loss, indigestion, muscle weakness
Namenda® (memantine)	N-methyl D-aspartate (NMDA) antagonist prescribed to treat symptoms of moderate to severe Alzheimer disease	Blocks the toxic effects associated with excess glutamate and regulates glutamate activation	Dizziness, headache, diarrhea, constipation, confusion
Namzaric® (memantine and donepezil)	NMDA antagonist and cholinesterase inhibitor prescribed to treat symptoms of moderate to severe Alzheimer disease	Blocks the toxic effects associated with excess glutamate and prevents the breakdown of acetylcholine in the brain	Headache, nausea, vomiting, diarrhea, dizziness, anorexia
Razadyne® (galantamine)	Cholinesterase inhibitor prescribed to treat symptoms of mild to moderate Alzheimer disease	Prevents the breakdown of acetylcholine and stimulates nicotinic receptors to release more acetylcholine in the brain	Nausea, vomiting, diarrhea, decreased appetite, dizziness, headache

Table 27.2. Drug and Recommended Dosage

Drug Name	Manufacturer's Recommended Dosage	For More Information
Aricept® (donepezil)	**Tablet***: Initial dose of 5 mg once a day; may increase dose to 10 mg/day after 4 to 6 weeks if well tolerated, then to 23 mg/day after at least 3 months Orally disintegrating tablet*: Same dosage as above (not available in 23 mg)	For more information about this drug's safety and use, visit www.aricept.com.
Exelon® (rivastigmine)	**Capsule***: Initial dose of 3 mg/day (1.5 mg twice a day); may increase dose to 6 mg/day (3 mg twice a day), 9 mg/day (4.5 mg twice a day), and 12 mg/day (6 mg twice a day) at minimum 2-week intervals if well-tolerated Patch*: Initial dose of 4.6 mg once a day; may increase dose to 9.5 mg once a day and 13.3 mg once a day at minimum 4-week intervals if well tolerated	For more information about this drug's safety and use, visit the www.fda.gov/Drugs. Click on "Search Drugs@FDA," search for Exelon, and click on drug-name links to see label information.
Namenda® (memantine)	**Tablet***: Initial dose of 5 mg once a day; may increase dose to 10 mg/day (5 mg twice a day), 15 mg/day (5 mg and 10 mg as separate doses), and 20 mg/day (10 mg twice a day) at minimum 1-week intervals if well tolerated Oral solution*: Same dosage as above Extended-release capsule*: Initial dose of 7 mg once a day; may increase dose to 14 mg/day, 21 mg/day, and 28 mg/day at minimum 1-week intervals if well tolerated	For more information about this drug's safety and use, visit www.namenda.com and www.namendaxr.com. Click on "Full Prescribing Information" to see the drug label.
Razadyne® (galantamine)	**Tablet***: Initial dose of 8 mg/day (4 mg twice a day); may increase dose to 16 mg/day (8 mg twice a day) and 24 mg/day (12 mg twice a day) at minimum 4-week intervals if well tolerated Extended-release capsule*: Same dosage as above but taken once a day	For more information about this drug's safety and use, visit www.janssenmd.com/razadyne. Click on "Full Prescribing Information" to see the drug label.

**Available as a generic drug.*

Sleep aids are used to help people get to sleep and stay asleep. People with Alzheimer disease should NOT use these drugs regularly because they make the person more confused and more likely to fall. Examples of these medicines include:

- Ambien® (zolpidem)

- Lunesta® (eszopiclone)

- Sonata® (zaleplon)

Antianxiety drugs are used to treat agitation. These drugs can cause sleepiness, dizziness, falls, and confusion any one, doctors recommend using them only for short periods of time. Examples of these medicines include:

- Ativan® (lorazepam)

- Klonopin® (clonazepam)

Anticonvulsants are drugs sometimes used to treat severe aggression. Side effects may cause sleepiness, dizziness, mood swings, and confusion. Examples of these medicines include:

- Depakote® (sodium valproate)

- Tegretol® (carbamazepine)

- Trileptal® (oxcarbazepine)

Antipsychotics are drugs used to treat paranoia, hallucinations, agitation, and aggression. Side effects of using these drugs can be serious, including increased risk of death in some older people with dementia. They should only be given to people with Alzheimer disease when the doctor agrees that the symptoms are severe. Examples of these medicines include:

- Risperdal® (risperidone)

- Seroquel® (quetiapine)

- Zyprexa® (olanzapine)

Looking for New Treatments

Alzheimer disease research has developed to a point where scientists can look beyond treating symptoms to think about addressing underlying disease processes. In ongoing clinical trials, scientists are developing and testing several possible interventions, including immunization therapy, drug therapies, cognitive training, physical activity, and treatments for cardiovascular disease (CVD) and diabetes.

Chapter 28

Participating in Alzheimer Disease Clinical Trials and Studies

Clinical research is medical research involving people. There are two types, clinical studies and clinical trials.

Clinical studies (sometimes called observational studies) observe people in normal settings. Researchers gather information, group volunteers according to broad characteristics, and compare changes over time. For example, researchers may collect data through medical exams, tests, or questionnaires about a group of older adults over time to learn more about the effects of different lifestyles on cognitive health. Clinical studies may help identify new possibilities for clinical trials.

Clinical trials are research studies performed in people that are aimed at evaluating a medical, surgical, or behavioral intervention.

This chapter contains text excerpted from the following sources: Text in this chapter begins with excerpts from "What Are Clinical Trials and Studies?" National Institute on Aging (NIA), National Institutes of Health (NIH), May 17, 2017; Text under the heading "Participating in Alzheimer Disease Research" is excerpted from "Participating in Alzheimer's Disease Research," National Institute on Aging (NIA), National Institutes of Health (NIH), May 23, 2017; Text beginning with the heading "How Can I Find out about Alzheimer Disease Trials and Studies?" is excerpted from "Common Questions about Participating in Alzheimer's and Related Dementias Research," National Institute on Aging (NIA), National Institutes of Health (NIH), November 15, 2018.

They are the primary way that researchers find out if a new treatment, like a new drug or diet or medical device (for example, a pacemaker) is safe and effective in people. Often a clinical trial is used to learn if a new treatment is more effective and/or has less harmful side effects than the standard treatment.

Other clinical trials test ways to find a disease early, sometimes before there are symptoms. Still, others test ways to prevent a health problem. A clinical trial may also look at how to make life better for people living with a life-threatening disease or a chronic health problem. Clinical trials sometimes study the role of caregivers or support groups.

Before the U.S. Food and Drug Administration (FDA) approves a clinical trial to begin, scientists perform laboratory tests and studies in animals to test a potential therapy's safety and efficacy. If these studies show favorable results, the FDA gives approval for the intervention to be tested in humans.

Phases of Clinical Trials

Clinical trials advance through four phases to test a treatment, find the appropriate dosage, and look for side effects. If, after the first three phases, researchers find a drug or other intervention to be safe and effective, the FDA approves it for clinical use and continues to monitor its effects.

Clinical trials of drugs are usually described based on their phase. The FDA typically requires Phase I, II, and III trials to be conducted to determine if the drug can be approved for use.

- A Phase I trial tests an experimental treatment on a small group of often healthy people (20 to 80) to judge its safety and side effects and to find the correct drug dosage.

- A Phase II trial uses more people (100 to 300). While the emphasis in Phase I is on safety, the emphasis in Phase II is on effectiveness. This phase aims to obtain preliminary data on whether the drug works in people who have a certain disease or condition. These trials also continue to study safety, including short-term side effects. This phase can last several years.

- A Phase III trial gathers more information about safety and effectiveness, studying different populations and different dosages, using the drug in combination with other drugs. The number of subjects usually ranges from several hundred to about 3,000 people. If the FDA agrees that the trial results are positive, it will approve the experimental drug or device.

- A Phase IV trial for drugs or devices takes place after the FDA approves their use. A device or drug's effectiveness and safety are monitored in large, diverse populations. Sometimes, the side effects of a drug may not become clear until more people have taken it over a longer period of time.

Participating in Alzheimer Disease Research

This is an exciting time for Alzheimer disease (AD) and related dementias clinical research. Thanks to advances in our understanding of this brain disorder and powerful new tools for "seeing" and diagnosing it in people, scientists are making great strides in identifying potential new ways to help diagnose, treat, and even prevent Alzheimer disease. These advances are possible because thousands of people have participated in Alzheimer disease clinical trials and other studies to learn more about the disease and test treatments. We know what we know because of them.

When you choose to participate in research, you become a partner in scientific discovery. Your contribution can help future generations lead healthier lives. Major medical breakthroughs could not happen without the generosity of clinical trial participants—young and old. You can make a difference by participating in research.

How Can I Find about Alzheimer Disease Trials and Studies?

Check the resources below:

- Ask your doctor, who may know about local research studies that may be right for you

- Sign up for a registry or a matching service to be invited to participate in studies or trials when they are available in your area

- Contact Alzheimer disease research centers or memory or neurology clinics in your community. They may be conducting trials.

- Visit the Alzheimer and related Dementias Education and Referral (ADEAR) Center clinical trials finder (www.nia.nih.gov/alzheimers/clinical-trials)

- Look for announcements in newspapers and other media
- Search www.clinicaltrials.gov

Why Would I Participate in a Clinical Trial?

There are many reasons why you might choose to join an Alzheimer disease or dementia clinical trial. You may want to:

- Help others, including future family members, who may be at risk for Alzheimer disease or a related dementia
- Receive regular monitoring by medical professionals
- Learn about Alzheimer disease and your health
- Test new treatments that might work better than those currently available
- Get information about support groups and resources

What Else Should I Consider?

Consider both benefits and risks when deciding whether to volunteer for a clinical trial. While there are benefits to participating in a clinical trial or study, there are some risks and other issues to consider as well.

Risk

Researchers make every effort to ensure participants' safety. But, all clinical trials have some risk. Before joining a clinical trial, the research team will explain what you can expect, including possible side effects or other risks. That way, you can make an informed decision about joining the trial.

Expectations and Motivations

Single clinical trials and studies generally do not have miraculous results, and participants may not benefit directly. With a complex disease like Alzheimer disease, it is unlikely that one drug will cure or prevent the disease.

Uncertainty

Some people are concerned that they are not permitted to know whether they are getting the experimental treatment or a placebo (inactive treatment), or may not know the results right away. Open communication with study staff can help you understand why the study is set up this way and what you can expect.

Time Commitment and Location

Clinical trials and studies last days to years. They usually require multiple visits to study sites, such as private research facilities, teaching hospitals, AD research centers, or doctors' offices. Some studies pay participants a fee and/or reimburse travel expenses.

Study Partner Requirement

Many Alzheimer disease trials require a caregiver or family member who has regular contact with the person to accompany the participant to study appointments. This study partner can give insight into changes in the person over time.

What Happens When a Person Joins a Clinical Trial or Study?

Once you identify a trial or study you are interested in, contact the study site or coordinator. You can usually find this contact information in the description of the study, or you can contact the Alzheimer Disease Education and Referral (ADEAR) Center. Study staff will ask a few questions on the phone to determine if you meet basic qualifications for the study. If so, they will invite you to come to the study site. If you do not meet the criteria for the study, don't give up! You may qualify for a future study.

What Is Informed Consent?

It is important to learn as much as possible about a study or trial to help you decide if you would like to participate. Staff members at the research center can explain the study in detail, describe possible risks and benefits, and clarify your rights as a participant. You and your family should ask questions and gather information until you understand it fully.

After the research is explained and you decide to participate, you will be asked to sign an informed consent form, which states that you understand and agree to participate. You are free to withdraw from the study at any time if you change your mind or your health status changes.

Researchers must consider whether the person with Alzheimer disease or another dementia is able to understand and consent to participate in research. If the person cannot provide informed consent because of problems with memory and thinking, an authorized legal representative, or proxy (usually a family member), may give permission for the person to participate, particularly if the person's durable power of attorney gives the proxy that authority. If possible, the person with Alzheimer disease should also agree to participate.

How Do Researchers Decide Who Will Participate?

Researchers carefully screen all volunteers to make sure they meet a study's criteria.

After you consent, you will be screened by clinical staff to see if you meet the criteria to participate in the trial or if anything would exclude you. The screening may involve cognitive and physical tests.

Inclusion criteria for a trial might include age, stage of dementia, gender, genetic profile, family history, and whether or not you have a study partner who can accompany you to future visits. Exclusion criteria might include factors such as specific health conditions or medications that could interfere with the treatment being tested.

Many volunteers must be screened to find enough people for a study. Generally, you can participate in only one trial or study at a time. Different trials have different criteria, so being excluded from one trial does not necessarily mean exclusion from another.

Chapter 29

Can Alzheimer Disease Be Prevented?

Will doing crossword puzzles prevent memory loss as we age? Does exercise delay or prevent Alzheimer disease (AD)? Will adding fish oil to a diet help keep our brains healthy as we age? National Institutes of Health (NIH) convened a conference to answer these and other questions. The conclusion? Research so far has offered good leads about preventing Alzheimer disease and age-related cognitive decline. Still, more research is needed before we can be sure what's effective.

"Scientists are actively investigating a wide range of strategies," says Dr. Richard J. Hodes, director of NIH's National Institute on Aging (NIA). "Before we can tell the public that something will prevent Alzheimer disease or cognitive decline, we want to make sure that the intervention is tested as rigorously as possible."

Alzheimer disease usually affects people 60 and older, but people with a rare form of the illness can develop the disease in their thirties or forties.

"The biggest risk factor for Alzheimer disease is age, and the number of Americans over the age of 65 is expected to double to 70 million by 2050," Hodes says. "We must find ways to prevent or delay this terrible disease."

This chapter includes text excerpted from "Can We Prevent Alzheimer's Disease?" *NIH News in Health*, National Institutes of Health (NIH), July 2010. Reviewed December 2018.

While aging brains may not store memories or recall information as easily as they once did, many older people function well despite these changes. In fact, experience can help some older people perform certain tasks as well or better than younger ones. Alzheimer disease and other dementias are definitely not, as people once thought, a normal part of aging.

The science of Alzheimer disease has come a long way since 1906, when a German neurologist and psychiatrist named Dr. Alois Alzheimer first described the key features of the disease now named after him. He noticed abnormal deposits in the brain of a 51-year old woman who had dementia. Researchers now know that Alzheimer disease is characterized by brain abnormalities called plaques and tangles. Plaques are clumps of protein in the spaces between the brain's nerve cells. Tangles are masses of twisted protein threads found inside nerve cells. Scientists know what these plaques and tangles are made of. But they still don't know what causes them to form, or how to stop the process.

During the three-day meeting—called the State-of-the-Science Conference on Preventing Alzheimer Disease and Cognitive Decline—an independent panel of 15 medical, science, and healthcare experts heard talks from leading scientists and reviewed the available evidence.

The panel noted the challenges in diagnosing and treating these complex disorders. It's hard to measure them in their earliest stages. There are no agreed-upon tests that doctors can use in their offices. Scientists are continuing to investigate methods for early detection.

A handful of approved medications are available to help treat the symptoms of Alzheimer disease. One, donepezil (Aricept), was found to delay the development of Alzheimer disease for about a year in people with mild impairment. None of the approved medications, however, appears to affect the underlying causes of the disease.

The panel reviewed a range of observational studies and a few short-term clinical trials looking at different prevention strategies. For example, these studies have suggested that physical activity, social engagement, and intellectual activity all may help prevent Alzheimer disease and cognitive decline. Controlling high blood pressure and diabetes may help. So may omega 3 fatty acids, which are found in salmon and other fish. Many of these strategies have already been shown to promote healthy aging and reduce the risk for other diseases.

However, none of the studies to date has given conclusive answers when it comes to preventing AD or cognitive decline. These strategies and many others are under further study. In addition, many drugs are now being tested in clinical trials.

"We wish we could tell people that taking a pill or doing a puzzle every day would prevent this terrible disease, but current evidence doesn't support this," says Dr. Martha L. Daviglus, panel chair and professor of preventive medicine at Northwestern University in Chicago.

Still, many of the healthy habits under study, like exercise, usually do no harm and likely benefit overall health. Smoking has been linked to a greater risk for dementia and cognitive decline, so if you smoke, try to quit. Chronic diseases, such as diabetes and depression, may also raise your risk, so be sure to address any long-term health problems.

Despite all the challenges, Hodes says, there are reasons to be optimistic. "Technology is advancing our ability to identify the gene mutations that may place some people at greater risk for developing Alzheimer disease. Scientists are developing new imaging tools to allow us to map the changes taking place in living brains. And we are moving closer to identifying the markers in blood that may signal disease onset, track its progress and test whether or not a medicine is working."

Whether you have memory problems or not, you can take an important step: You can volunteer to participate in research. NIA is now funding six clinical trials to examine the effects of exercise or other lifestyle changes on people with mild to severe Alzheimer disease. Another 14 clinical trials are testing ways to prevent cognitive decline in healthy older adults.

Chapter 30

Recent Alzheimer Disease Research

Chapter Contents

Section 30.1

Researchers Map How Alzheimer Disease Pathology Spreads across Brain Networks

This section includes text excerpted from "Researchers Map How Alzheimer's Pathology Spreads across Brain Networks," National Institute on Aging (NIA), National Institutes of Health (NIH), November 2, 2018.

Capitalizing on recent advances in neuroimaging and genetic biomarker research, scientists have been able to identify specific pathways by which tau and beta-amyloid (Aβ), two proteins that are hallmarks of Alzheimer disease (AD), accumulate in the brain over time. The National Institute on Aging (NIA)-supported researchers also found that the patterns of tau and beta-amyloid accumulation were related to specific genetic profiles, providing better understanding of AD risk and possible new avenues for diagnosis and monitoring of the disease.

Improved technology makes possible for intensive, side-by-side comparisons of how tau and beta-amyloid spread in the brain in distinctive patterns. Using this technology, researchers were able to reveal nuances into how, even in disease, the brain follows a dynamic and complex network of circuits and connections.

The study was led by Dr. Jorge Sepulcre and Dr. Keith Johnson of The Gordon Center for Medical Imaging at Massachusetts General Hospital (MGH) and Harvard Medical School (HMS), and Dr. Reisa Sperling, director of the Center for Alzheimer Research and Treatment at the Brigham (CART) and Women's Hospital and professor of Neurology at Harvard Medical School (HMS). The team used data from the Harvard Aging Brain Study (HABS) and the Allen Human Brain Atlas.

In a brain with Alzheimer disease, abnormal deposits of tau and beta-amyloid do not randomly appear, but instead show unique spatial patterns that follow the brain's existing connected neural networks. To better understand how tau and beta-amyloid interact with and influence each other, the researchers looked closely at 3-D brain network and gene maps and found that both tau and beta-amyloid were associated with genes devoted to lipid metabolism, and that the *APOE* E4 gene—a risk factor for Alzheimer disease—played a central role in the relationships of these genetic networks.

The scientists found common genetic background for the malfunction of both proteins. The findings showed that in addition to *APOE*, other variations in genetic pathways shared by tau and beta-amyloid could trigger their accumulation. The study also found that tau propagation was associated with an axon-related (parts of neurons that pass messages away from the cell body) genetic profile, while beta-amyloid's spread was connected with a dendrite-related (parts of neurons that receive messages from other cells) genetic profile.

The researchers hope this new understanding of tau and beta-amyloid's propagation patterns can be combined with a person's genetic profile to help develop precision medicine approaches for improved diagnosis, monitoring, and therapies for Alzheimer disease in the brain.

Section 30.2

NIH-Funded Study Finds New Evidence That Viruses May Play a Role in Alzheimer Disease

This section includes text excerpted from "NIH-Funded Study Finds New Evidence That Viruses May Play a Role in Alzheimer's Disease," National Institutes of Health (NIH), June 21, 2018.

Analysis of large data sets from postmortem brain samples of people with and without Alzheimer disease (AD) has revealed new evidence that viral species, particularly herpes viruses, may have a role in Alzheimer disease biology. Researchers funded by the National Institute on Aging (NIA), part of the National Institutes of Health (NIH), made the discovery by harnessing data from brain banks and cohort studies participating in the Accelerating Medicines Partnership—Alzheimer Disease (AMP-AD) consortium. Reporting in the June 21 issue of the journal *Neuron*, the authors emphasize that their findings do not prove that the viruses cause the onset or progression of AD. Rather, the findings show viral deoxyribonucleic acid (DNA) sequences and activation of biological networks—the interrelated systems of DNA, ribonucleic acid (RNA), proteins, and metabolites—may interact with molecular, genetic, and clinical aspects of Alzheimer disease.

"The hypothesis that viruses play a part in brain disease is not new, but this is the first study to provide strong evidence based on unbiased approaches and large data sets that lends support to this line of inquiry," said NIA Director Richard J. Hodes, M.D. "This research reinforces the complexity of Alzheimer disease, creates opportunities to explore Alzheimer disease more thoroughly, and highlights the importance of sharing data freely and widely with the research community."

Alzheimer disease is an irreversible, progressive brain disorder that slowly destroys memory and thinking skills and, eventually, the ability to carry out simple tasks. More evidence is accumulating to indicate that this loss of cognitive functioning is a mix of many different disease processes in the brain, rather than just one, such as buildup of amyloid or tau proteins. Identifying links to viruses may help researchers learn more about the complicated biological interactions involved in Alzheimer disease, and potentially lead to new treatment strategies.

The research group, which included experts from Icahn School of Medicine at Mount Sinai (ISMMS), New York City, and Arizona State University (ASU), Phoenix, originally set out to find whether drugs used to treat other diseases can be repurposed for treating AD. They designed their study to map and compare biological networks underlying Alzheimer disease. What they found is that Alzheimer disease biology is likely impacted by a complex constellation of viral and host genetic factors, adding that they identified specific testable pathways and biological networks.

"The robust findings by the Mount Sinai team would not have been possible without the open science data resources created by the Accelerating Medicines Partnership—Alzheimer Disease (AMP-AD) program—particularly the availability of raw genomic data," said NIA Program Officer Suzana Petanceska, Ph.D., who leads the AMP-AD Target Discovery and Preclinical Validation Project. "This is a great example of the power of open science to accelerate discovery and replication research."

The researchers used multiple layers of genomic and proteomic data from several the National Institute on Aging (NIA)-supported brain banks and cohort studies. They began their direct investigation of viral sequences using data from the Mount Sinai Brain Bank and were able to verify their initial observations using datasets from the Religious Orders Study (link is external), the Memory and Aging Project and the Mayo Clinic Brain Bank. They were then able to incorporate additional data from the Emory Alzheimer Disease Research Center (ADRC) to understand viral impacts on protein abundance. Through the application of sophisticated computational modeling the researchers made several key findings, including:

- Human herpesvirus 6A and 7 were more abundant in Alzheimer disease samples than non-Alzheimer disease.

- There are multiple points of overlap between virus-host interactions and genes associated with Alzheimer disease risk.

- Multiple viruses impact the biology of Alzheimer disease across domains such as DNA, RNA, and proteins.

Important roles for microbes and viruses in Alzheimer disease have been suggested and studied for decades, the authors noted. Since the 1980s, hundreds of reports have associated AD with bacteria and viruses. These studies combined suggest a viral contribution but have not explained how the connection works.

While the current findings are more specific, they do not provide evidence to change how risk and susceptibility are assessed, nor the diagnosis and treatment of Alzheimer disease, the authors said. Rather, the research gives scientists reason to revisit the old pathogen hypothesis and will be the basis for further work that will test whether herpes virus activity is one of the causes of AD.

Section 30.3

Lack of Sleep May Be Linked to Risk Factor for Alzheimer Disease

This section includes text excerpted from "Lack of Sleep May Be Linked to Risk Factor for Alzheimer's Disease," National Institutes of Health (NIH), April 13, 2018.

Losing just one night of sleep led to an immediate increase in beta-amyloid (Aβ), a protein in the brain associated with Alzheimer disease (AD), according to a small, new study by researchers at the National Institutes of Health (NIH). In Alzheimer disease, beta-amyloid proteins clump together to form amyloid plaques, a hallmark of the disease.

While acute sleep deprivation is known to elevate brain beta-amyloid levels in mice, less is known about the impact of sleep deprivation on beta-amyloid accumulation in the human brain. The study is among the first to demonstrate that sleep may play an important role in human beta-amyloid clearance.

"This research provides new insight about the potentially harmful effects of a lack of sleep on the brain and has implications for better characterizing the pathology of Alzheimer disease," said George F. Koob, Ph.D., director of the National Institute on Alcohol Abuse and Alcoholism (NIAAA), part of the National Institutes of Health (NIH), which funded the study.

Beta-amyloid is a metabolic waste product present in the fluid between brain cells. In Alzheimer disease, beta-amyloid clumps together to form amyloid plaques, negatively impacting communication between neurons.

Led by Drs. Ehsan Shokri-Kojori and Nora D. Volkow of the National Institute on Alcohol Abuse and Alcoholism (NIAAA) Laboratory of Neuroimaging (LONI), the study is now online in the Proceedings of the National Academy of Sciences (NAS). Dr. Volkow is also the director of the National Institute on Drug Abuse (NIDA) at NIH.

To understand the possible link between beta-amyloid accumulation and sleep, the researchers used positron emission tomography (PET) to scan the brains of 20 healthy subjects, ranging in age from 22 to 72, after a night of rested sleep and after sleep deprivation (being awake for about 31 hours). They found beta-amyloid increases of about five percent after losing a night of sleep in brain regions including the thalamus and hippocampus, regions especially vulnerable to damage in the early stages of Alzheimer disease.

In Alzheimer disease, beta-amyloid is estimated to increase about 43 percent in affected individuals relative to healthy older adults. It is unknown whether the increase in beta-amyloid in the study participants would subside after a night of rest.

The researchers also found that study participants with larger increases in beta-amyloid reported worse mood after sleep deprivation.

"Even though our sample was small, this study demonstrated the negative effect of sleep deprivation on beta-amyloid burden in the human brain. Future studies are needed to assess the generalizability to a larger and more diverse population," said Dr. Shokri-Kojori.

It is also important to note that the link between sleep disorders and Alzheimer disease risk is considered by many scientists to be "bidirectional," since elevated beta-amyloid may also lead to sleep disturbances.

Section 30.4

Clearing Senescent Cells from the Brain in Mice Preserves Cognition

This section contains text excerpted from the following sources: Text under the heading "What Are Senescent Cells?" is excerpted from "Senescent Cells: A Novel Therapeutic Target for Aging and Age-Related Diseases," National Center for Biotechnology Information (NCBI), June 10, 2014. Reviewed December 2018; Text under the heading "A Study on Clearing Senescent Cells from the Brain" is excerpted from "Clearing Senescent Cells from the Brain in Mice Preserves Cognition," National Institute on Aging (NIA), National Institutes of Health (NIH), October 19, 2018.

What Are Senescent Cells?

Aging is the main risk factor for most chronic diseases, disabilities, and declining health. It has been proposed that senescent cells—damaged cells that have lost the ability to divide—drive the deterioration that underlies aging and age-related diseases. Removal of senescent immune cells in the elderly may significantly boost their immune systems, extend their health spans, improve their quality of life, and reduce healthcare costs.

A Study on Clearing Senescent Cells from the Brain

Out-of-commission cells that clutter the brain may accelerate dementia, according to researchers who found that getting rid of such cells preserved cognitive function in mice. The National Institute on Aging (NIA)-funded research suggests that senescent cells—cells that are alive but no longer divide or perform their designated functions—in the brain play a role in the neurodegeneration associated with Alzheimer disease (AD) and other types of dementia. Eliminating these cells before they cause damage to neurons appears to preserve cognition. These results were reported in a letter published in *Nature*.

The study, led by Dr. Darren Baker of the Mayo Clinic, Rochester, MN, was conducted in mice bred to have the protein tau accumulate in the brain. In Alzheimer disease, tau turns into abnormal tangles that form inside neurons, disrupting normal communication among brain cells and contributing to cell death.

Researchers described a looping process of brain damage in which tau-producing neurons push glial cells (another type of brain cell) into senescence. The senescent glial cells in turn damage healthy neurons around them, and the damaged neurons produce toxic tau tangles.

The researchers found two methods to interrupt this sequence of events so that mice retained better short-term memory. In one method, they used a genetic tool to trigger expression of an enzyme that causes the glial cells to die as soon as they became senescent. In the mice that received this intervention, tau tangles did not build up as rapidly as in mice that did not receive the intervention.

In the second method, the researchers treated the mice with an anticancer drug, navitoclax, that can induce cell death and eliminate senescent cells. This, too, had protective effects against the accumulation of tau and short-term memory loss.

Future research questions include whether these findings apply to other mouse models of Alzheimer disease or to humans, and whether treatments to destroy or inhibit senescent cells can reverse cognitive damage that has already occurred.

Section 30.5

Higher Brain Glucose Levels May Mean More Severe Alzheimer Disease

This section includes text excerpted from "Higher Brain Glucose Levels May Mean More Severe Alzheimer's," National Institute on Aging (NIA), National Institutes of Health (NIH), November 6, 2017.

For the first time, scientists have found a connection between abnormalities in how the brain breaks down glucose and the severity of the signature amyloid plaques and tangles in the brain, as well as the onset of eventual outward symptoms, of Alzheimer disease (AD). The study was supported by the National Institute on Aging (NIA), part of the National Institutes of Health, and appears in the November 6, 2017 issue of *Alzheimer's & Dementia: the Journal of the Alzheimer's Association.*

Led by Madhav Thambisetty, M.D., Ph.D., investigator and chief of the Unit of Clinical and Translational Neuroscience in the NIA's

Laboratory of Behavioral Neuroscience, researchers looked at brain tissue samples at autopsy from participants in the Baltimore Longitudinal Study of Aging (BLSA), one of the world's longest-running scientific studies of human aging. The BLSA tracks neurological, physical, and psychological data on participants over several decades.

Researchers measured glucose levels in different brain regions, some vulnerable to Alzheimer disease pathology, such as the frontal and temporal cortex, and some that are resistant, like the cerebellum. They analyzed three groups of BLSA participants: those with Alzheimer disease symptoms during life and with confirmed Alzheimer disease pathology (beta-amyloid protein plaques and neurofibrillary tangles) in the brain at death; healthy controls; and individuals without symptoms during life but with significant levels of Alzheimer disease pathology found in the brain postmortem.

They found distinct abnormalities in glycolysis, the main process by which the brain breaks down glucose, with evidence linking the severity of the abnormalities to the severity of Alzheimer disease pathology. Lower rates of glycolysis and higher brain glucose levels correlated to more severe plaques and tangles found in the brains of people with the disease. More severe reductions in brain glycolysis were also related to the expression of symptoms of Alzheimer disease during life, such as problems with memory.

"For some time, researchers have thought about the possible links between how the brain processes glucose and Alzheimer's," said NIA Director Richard J. Hodes, M.D. "Research such as this involves new thinking about how to investigate these connections in the intensifying search for better and more effective ways to treat or prevent Alzheimer's disease."

While similarities between diabetes and Alzheimer disease have long been suspected, they have been difficult to evaluate, since insulin is not needed for glucose to enter the brain or to get into neurons. The team tracked the brain's usage of glucose by measuring ratios of the amino acids serine, glycine and alanine to glucose, allowing them to assess rates of the key steps of glycolysis. They found that the activities of enzymes controlling these key glycolysis steps were lower in Alzheimer disease cases compared to normal brain tissue samples. Furthermore, lower enzyme activity was associated with more severe Alzheimer disease pathology in the brain and the development of symptoms.

Next, they used proteomics—the large-scale measurement of cellular proteins—to tally levels of GLUT3, a glucose transporter protein, in neurons. They found that GLUT3 levels were lower in brains with

Alzheimer disease pathology compared to normal brains, and that these levels were also connected to the severity of tangles and plaques. Finally, the team checked blood glucose levels in study participants years before they died, finding that greater increases in blood glucose levels correlated with greater brain glucose levels at death.

"These findings point to a novel mechanism that could be targeted in the development of new treatments to help the brain overcome glycolysis defects in Alzheimer's disease," said Thambisetty.

The researchers cautioned that it is not yet completely clear whether abnormalities in brain glucose metabolism are definitively linked to the severity of Alzheimer disease symptoms or the speed of disease progression. The next steps for Thambisetty and his team include studying abnormalities in other metabolic pathways linked to glycolysis to determine how they may relate to Alzheimer disease pathology in the brain.

Section 30.6

Blood, Brain Metabolites Could Be Earlier Biomarkers of Alzheimer Disease

This section includes text excerpted from "Blood, Brain Metabolites Could Be Earlier Biomarkers of Alzheimer's Disease," National Institute on Aging (NIA), National Institutes of Health (NIH), March 12, 2018.

A panel of 26 metabolites that appear in the blood and brains of people with Alzheimer disease (AD) point to a potential new biomarker path to be pursued as future therapeutic targets.

A team of researchers from the National Institute on Aging's (NIA) Intramural Research Program (IRP), led by Dr. Madhav Thambisetty, Chief of the Clinical and Translational Neuroscience Unit of the NIA IRP, sought to clarify, with the use of advanced machine learning techniques, if brain metabolites associated with Alzheimer disease pathology could also be detected in blood and were related to progression of the disease.

Their results were published in the January 25, 2018, issue of *PLOS Medicine*. Previous biomarker studies for Alzheimer disease had not connected markers in the blood to those in the brain, as scientists have been trying to learn more about the long timeline between the start of Alzheimer disease brain pathology and the development of outward symptoms.

To attack this problem, first author Dr. Vijay Varma and colleagues performed metabolic analyses of brain and blood tissue samples from autopsies of three groups of participants in the Baltimore Longitudinal Study of Aging (BLSA): people who had Alzheimer disease, a normal control group, and a smaller group who had asymptomatic Alzheimer disease, meaning they had significant disease pathology at autopsy but showed no signs of cognitive impairment during life.

The team employed a computer system with machine learning techniques, which allowed them to use algorithms to more rapidly analyze metabolites and narrow them down to the most likely targets. With this approach, they used data patterns to identify a panel of 26 metabolites out of 180 studied that could accurately differentiate Alzheimer disease from control brain samples.

They then measured the same 26 metabolites in about 700 blood samples from the Alzheimer's Disease Neuroimaging Initiative and the BLSA, testing for relationships with known signs of Alzheimer disease, such as brain shrinkage on MRI scans, cerebrospinal fluid measures of abnormal proteins linked to Alzheimer disease, and cognitive test results.

The researchers found that altered blood concentrations of some of the 26 metabolites were consistently associated with brain atrophy, cerebrospinal fluid measures of Alzheimer disease pathology, cognitive performance and risk of Alzheimer disease before established symptoms developed.

The analysis zeroed in specifically on sphingolipids—common parts of cell membranes known to play a part in a variety of human diseases. These were found to be connected to several known Alzheimer disease biological mechanisms, such as tau phosphorylation (the precursor of tau tangles in the brain), beta-amyloid metabolism, problems with calcium regulation in neurons, production of the neurotransmitter acetylcholine, and brain cell death. While sphingolipids emerged from this study as one of the major types of metabolites for further exploration, the researchers also want to do more in-depth analyses of other metabolite classes.

Part Five

Living with Alzheimer Disease and Dementias

Chapter 31

Talking about Your Diagnosis

Chapter Contents

Section 31.1

Telling Others about an Alzheimer Disease Diagnosis

This section includes text excerpted from "Helping Family and Friends Understand Alzheimer's Disease," National Institute on Aging (NIA), National Institutes of Health (NIH), May 17, 2017.

When you learn that someone has Alzheimer disease (AD), you may wonder when and how to tell your family and friends. You may be worried about how others will react to or treat the person. Realize that family and friends often sense that something is wrong before they are told. Alzheimer disease is hard to keep secret.

There's no single right way to tell others about Alzheimer disease. When the time seems right, be honest with family, friends, and others. Use this as a chance to educate them about Alzheimer disease. You can:

- Tell friends and family about Alzheimer disease and its effects

- Share articles, websites, and other information about the disease

- Tell them what they can do to help. Let them know you need breaks.

When a family member has Alzheimer disease, it affects everyone in the family, including children and grandchildren. It's important to talk to them about what is happening.

Tips for Communicating

You can help family and friends understand how to interact with the person with Alzheimer disease. Here are some tips:

- Help family and friends realize what the person can still do and how much she or he still can understand.

- Give visitors suggestions about how to start talking with the person. For example, make eye contact and say, "Hello George, I'm John. We used to work together."

- Help them avoid correcting the person with Alzheimer disease if she or he makes a mistake or forgets something. Instead, ask visitors to respond to the feelings expressed or talk about something different.

- Help family and friends plan fun activities with the person, such as going to family reunions or visiting old friends. A photo album or other activity can help if the person is bored or confused and needs to be distracted.

Remind visitors to:

- Visit at times of day when the person with Alzheimer disease is at her or his best.

- Be calm and quiet. Don't use a loud voice or talk to the person as if she or he were a child.

- Respect the person's personal space, and don't get too close.

- Not take it personally if the person does not recognize you, is unkind, or gets angry. She or he is acting out of confusion.

When You're out in Public

Some caregivers carry a card that explains why the person with Alzheimer disease might say or do odd things. For example, the card could read, "My family member has Alzheimer disease. She or he might say or do things that are unexpected. Thank you for your understanding."

The card allows you to let others know about the person's Alzheimer disease without the person hearing you. It also means you don't have to keep explaining things.

Section 31.2

Talking to Children about Alzheimer Disease

This section includes text excerpted from "Helping Kids Understand Alzheimer's Disease," National Institute on Aging (NIA), National Institutes of Health (NIH), May 17, 2017.

When a family member has Alzheimer disease (AD), it affects everyone in the family, including children and grandchildren. It's important to talk to them about what is happening. How much and what kind of information you share depends on the child's age and relationship to the person with Alzheimer disease.

Helping Kids Cope

Here are some tips to help kids understand what is happening:

- Answer their questions simply and honestly. For example, you might tell a young child, "Grandma has an illness that makes it hard for her to remember things."

- Help them know that their feelings of sadness and anger are normal.

- Comfort them. Tell them no one caused the disease. Young children may think they did something to hurt their grandparent.

Talk with kids about their concerns and feelings. Some may not talk about their negative feelings, but you may see changes in how they act. Problems at school, with friends, or at home can be a sign that they are upset. A school counselor or social worker can help your child understand what is happening and learn how to cope.

A teenager might find it hard to accept how the person with Alzheimer disease has changed. She or he may find the changes upsetting or embarrassing and not want to be around the person. Don't force them to spend time with the person who has Alzheimer disease. This could make things worse.

Spending Time Together and Alone

It's important to show kids that they can still talk with the person with Alzheimer disease and help her or him enjoy activities. Many younger children will look to you to see how to act.

Doing fun things together can help both the child and the person with Alzheimer disease. Here are some things they might do:

- Do simple arts and crafts

- Play music or sing

- Look through photo albums

- Read stories out loud

If kids live in the same house as someone with Alzheimer disease:

- Don't expect a young child to help take care of or "babysit" the person.

- Make sure they have time for their own interests and needs, such as playing with friends, going to school activities, or doing homework.

- Make sure you spend time with them, so they don't feel that all your attention is on the person with Alzheimer disease.

- Be honest about your feelings when you talk with kids, but don't overwhelm them.

If the stress of living with someone who has Alzheimer disease becomes too great, think about placing the person with Alzheimer disease into a respite care facility. Then, both you and your kids can get a much-needed break.

Chapter 32

Getting Support for Alzheimer Disease and Dementia

Sometimes you can no longer care for a person with Alzheimer disease (AD) at home. The person may need around-the-clock care. Or, she or he may be incontinent, aggressive, or wander a lot. You may not be able to meet all of his or her needs at home anymore. When that happens, you may want to look for a long-term care facility for the person. Older woman with Alzheimer disease in a care facility with a caregiver.

You may feel guilty or upset about this decision, but moving the person to a facility may be the best thing to do. It will give you greater peace of mind knowing that the person is safe and getting good care.

Choosing the right place is a big decision. It's hard to know where to start. The following overview of options, along with questions to ask and other resources, can help you get started.

Residential Care

Residential care options include:

- **Continuing care retirement communities (CCRCs)**—a home, apartment, or room in a retirement community where

This chapter includes text excerpted from "Finding Long-Term Care for a Person with Alzheimer's," National Institute on Aging (NIA), National Institutes of Health (NIH), May 18, 2017.

people with Alzheimer disease can live and get care. Some of these places are for people who can care for themselves, while others are for people who need care around-the-clock. An advantage is that residents may move from one level of care to another—for example, from more independent living to more supervised care.

- **Assisted living facilities**—a facility with rooms or apartments for people who may need some help with daily tasks. Some assisted living facilities have special Alzheimer units. These units have staff who check on and care for people with Alzheimer disease. You will need to pay for the cost of the room or apartment, and you may need to pay extra for any special care.

- **Group homes**—a home where several people who can't care for themselves and two or more staff members live. At least one caregiver is on site at all times. You will need to pay the costs of the person with Alzheimer disease living in this kind of home. Remember that these homes may not be inspected or regulated, but may still provide good care.

- **Nursing homes**—a place for people who can't care for themselves anymore. Some nursing homes have special Alzheimer disease care units. These units are often in separate sections of the building where staff members have special training to care for people with Alzheimer disease. In many cases, you will have to pay for nursing home care. Most nursing homes accept Medicaid as payment. Also, long-term care insurance may cover some of the nursing home costs.

Next Steps: Gathering Information

Choosing the right place is a big decision. It's hard to know where to start. List of steps you can take to find the right place are as follows:

1. Gather Information

- Talk with your support group members, social worker, doctor of the person with Alzheimer disease, family members, and friends about facilities in your area.

- Check resources, such as Medicare's Nursing Home Compare (www.medicare.gov/nursinghomecompare/search.html), and the Joint Commission's Quality Check (www.qualitycheck.org).

- Make a list of questions to ask about the facility.
- Call to set up a time to visit.

2. *Visit Assisted Living Facilities and Nursing Homes*

Make several visits at different times of the day and evening. Ask yourself:

- How does the staff care for the residents?
- Is the staff friendly?
- Does the place feel comfortable?
- How do the people who live there look?
- Do they look clean and well cared for?
- Are mealtimes comfortable?
- Is the facility clean and well-maintained?
- Does it smell bad?
- How do staff members speak to residents—with respect?

Ask the staff:

- What activities are planned for residents?
- How many staff members are at the facility? How many of them are trained to provide medical care if needed?
- How many people in the facility have Alzheimer disease?
- Does the facility have a special unit for people with Alzheimer disease? If so, what kinds of services does it provide?
- Is there a doctor who checks on residents on a regular basis? How often?

You also may want to ask staff:

- What is a typical day like for the person with Alzheimer disease?
- Is there a safe place for the person to go outside?
- What is included in the fee?
- How does my loved one get to medical appointments?

Talk with other caregivers who have a loved one at the facility. Find out what they think about the place.

Find out about total costs of care. Each facility is different. You want to find out if long-term care insurance, Medicaid, or Medicare will pay for any of the costs. Remember that Medicare only covers nursing home costs for a short time after the person with Alzheimer disease has been in the hospital for a certain amount of time.

If you're asked to sign a contract, make sure you understand what you are agreeing to.

How to Make Moving Day Easier

Moving is very stressful. Moving the person with Alzheimer disease to an assisted living facility, group home, or nursing home is a big change for both the person and the caregiver. You may feel many emotions, from a sense of loss to guilt and sadness. You also may feel relieved. It is okay to have all these feelings. A social worker may be able to help you plan for and adjust to moving day. It's important to have support during this difficult step.

Here are some things that may help:

- Know that the day can be very stressful.

- Talk to a social worker about your feelings about moving the person into a new place. Find out how to help the person with Alzheimer disease adjust.

- Get to know the staff before the person moves into a facility.

- Talk with the staff about ways to make the change to the assisted living facility or nursing home go better.

- Don't argue with the person with Alzheimer disease about why she or he needs to be there.

Be an Advocate

Once the person has moved to his or her new home, check and see how the person is doing. As the caregiver, you probably know the person best. Look for signs that the person may need more attention, is taking too much medication, or may not be getting the care they need. Build a relationship with staff so that you work together as partners.

Chapter 33

Preventing Cognitive Decline If You Have Alzheimer Disease or Dementia

Dementia is a loss of cognitive abilities in multiple domains that results in impairment in normal activities of daily living and loss of independence. Alzheimer disease (AD) is the most common cause of dementia, responsible for 60 to 80 percent of all dementia. AD causes severe suffering for patients, including progressive functional impairment, loss of independence, emotional distress, and behavioral symptoms. Families and caregivers often experience emotional and financial stress.

The major risk factor for Alzheimer disease is age, with the prevalence doubling every five years after the age of 65. Most estimates of the prevalence of Alzheimer disease in the United States are about 2.3 million for individuals over age 70, but some estimates are as high as 5.3 million individuals over the age of 65. The number of individuals with mild cognitive impairment (MCI) exceeds the number with Alzheimer disease. These individuals have mild impairment in cognition or daily functions that does not meet the threshold for a diagnosis of dementia, but they are at increased risk for development of Alzheimer disease, which makes them a prime target for intervention protocols.

This chapter includes text excerpted from "Preventing Alzheimer's Disease and Cognitive Decline," Agency for Healthcare Research and Quality (AHRQ), U.S. Department of Health and Human Services (HHS), April 2010. Reviewed December 2018.

Studies of selected risk or protective factors for cognitive decline and Alzheimer disease have been published, but it is not clear whether the results of these previous studies are of sufficient strength to warrant specific recommendations for behavioral, lifestyle, or pharmaceutical interventions/modifications targeted to these endpoints.

As background for an upcoming State-of-the-Science Conference in April 2010, the National Institutes of Health (NIH) Office of Medical Applications of Research (OMAR) commissioned the evidence report on "Preventing Alzheimer disease and Cognitive Decline" through the Agency for Healthcare Research and Quality (AHRQ).

The existing literature on the following key questions were synthesized:

Key Question 1: What factors are associated with the reduction of risk of Alzheimer disease?

Key Question 2: What factors are associated with the reduction of risk of cognitive decline in older adults?

Key Question 3: What are the therapeutic and adverse effects of interventions to delay the onset of Alzheimer disease? Are there differences in outcomes among identifiable subgroups?

Key Question 4: What are the therapeutic and adverse effects of interventions to improve or maintain cognitive ability or function? Are there differences in outcomes among identifiable subgroups?

Key Question 5: What are the relationships between the factors that affect Alzheimer disease and the factors that affect cognitive decline?

Key Question 6: If recommendations for interventions cannot be made, what studies need to be done that could provide the quality and strength of evidence necessary to make such recommendations to individuals?

Methods

The researchers searched MEDLINE® using Medical Subject Heading (MeSH) search terms, supplemented by keyword searches. In addition to MEDLINE®, they manually searched reference lists and searched the Cochrane Database of Systematic Reviews (CDSR) to identify relevant systematic reviews. For topics with a good-quality systematic review, they updated the search by identifying relevant primary literature published from one year prior to the search date of the review through October 27, 2009. When they did not identify a relevant good-quality review, they searched the primary literature for studies from 1984 through October 27, 2009. Because of the large volume of literature and the availability of specialized registries for genetic studies, they developed a separate search strategy for this topic and limited our review to select genes of special interest.

They restricted our review to human studies conducted in economically developed countries and published in English. They considered studies with participants ≥ 50 years old, of both sexes, all racial and ethnic populations, and drawn from general populations. They limited the sample size to ≥ 50 for randomized controlled trials (RCTs) and ≥ 300 for observational studies. They required at least one year between exposure and outcomes assessment for studies of cognitive decline, and two years for studies of Alzheimer disease. For key questions 1 and 2, they evaluated studies using observational designs; for key questions 3 and 4, they evaluated RCTs. Two reviewers independently assessed study eligibility and study quality and abstracted data. For key questions 1 to 5, They considered factors identified by the Office of Medical Applications of Research (OMAR) planning committee in five major categories:

1. Nutritional factors

2. Medical factors (including medical conditions and prescription and nonprescription medications)

3. Social/economic/behavioral factors

4. Toxic and environmental factors

5. Genetics

Data were synthesized qualitatively and, when appropriate, using quantitative methods. They rated the overall level of evidence for each factor as high, moderate, or low using principles developed by the Grading of Recommendations Assessment, Development and Evaluation (GRADE) working group. The level of evidence is considered "high" when further research is very unlikely to change our confidence in the estimate of effect, and "low" when further research is very likely to have an important impact on our confidence in the estimate of effect and is likely to change the estimate.

Results

A total of 25 systematic reviews and 250 primary studies met our inclusion criteria. The number of included studies differed markedly across the factors considered. Results are summarized immediately below by key question. The summary focuses on the factors that showed an association with Alzheimer disease or cognitive decline.

Key Question 1—Factors Associated with Risk of Developing Alzheimer Disease

The results reported here are based on observational studies of Alzheimer disease (AD), but to fully understand the associations between factors and cognitive outcomes, it is important to consider the results from both observational studies and randomized controlled trials (RCTs) when the latter are available.

In the nutrition category, both higher levels of folic acid and higher adherence to a Mediterranean diet were associated with a small to moderate decrease in risk of Alzheimer disease. The level of evidence was low for both of these factors.

For medical conditions, diabetes, hyperlipidemia in mid-life, depression, and traumatic brain injury in males were all associated with increased risk of Alzheimer disease. The level of evidence was low for each of these factors. No other factors showed a consistent relation to AD.

In the medication category, use of statins showed an association with decreased risk of AD.

The observational studies for estrogen and antihypertensives showed a likely protective association with Alzheimer disease. The level of the evidence was low for these factors.

In the social, economic, and behavioral category, current smoking was associated with increased risk of AD. Moderate use of alcohol, more years of education, and higher levels of cognitive engagement showed an association with a moderately decreased risk of AD.

Participation in physical leisure activity was generally associated with decreased risk of AD. Limited data on marriage and social support suggest that never being married and having less social support are associated with a moderately increased risk of AD.

The level of evidence for all of these factors was low.

For the environmental exposure category, case-control studies were included for the subtopics reviewed (solvents, pesticides, lead, and aluminum) because there were few cohort studies that met inclusion criteria. Only pesticides showed a consistent and large association with higher risk of Alzheimer disease, but the level of the evidence was low.

For the review of genes, they identified 10 genes with the strongest and best quality evidence of an association with AD based on a systematic review and quality ratings conducted by *ALZ* Gene, an online database of genetic association studies performed on Alzheimer disease phenotypes. Based on the selection criteria, it is not surprising that all genes showed a significant association with AD. It is noteworthy that the epsilon 4 allele of the apolipoprotein E gene (*APOE* e4) allele showed the highest and most consistent risk for AD. The level of evidence was moderate for the *APOE* e4 allele.

Key Question 2—Factors Associated with Risk of Cognitive Decline

The results reported for this question are based on observational studies for cognitive decline.

Effect sizes in all cases were small to moderate. In the nutrition category, low plasma selenium showed an association with higher risk of cognitive decline. Higher amounts of vegetable intake, adherence to a Mediterranean diet, and higher levels of omega-3 fatty acids showed a likely association with decreased risk of cognitive decline, but evidence was limited for some of these factors. The level of evidence was low for all of these factors.

For the medical category, diabetes, metabolic syndrome, and depression showed fairly consistent associations with a small increased risk of cognitive decline. There were no studies that met inclusion criteria on cognitive decline and traumatic brain injury (TBI), sleep apnea, resiliency, or anxiety.

For the medication category, two types of medication nonsteroidal anti-inflammatory drugs (NSAIDs) and estrogen showed possibly decreased risk for cognitive decline in select subgroups, but the other medications evaluated (statins, antihypertensives, and cholinesterase inhibitors) showed no association or no consistent association with cognitive decline.

Among the social, economic, and behavioral factors, smoking showed an increased risk of cognitive decline. Participation in nonphysical/noncognitive leisure activities, cognitive engagement, and physical activity all showed a fairly consistent protective association against cognitive decline. For observational studies, the level of evidence was low for these factors.

There were no eligible studies identified for the environmental exposure category.

In the genetic category, only *APOE* has been assessed in relation to cognitive decline. The studies fairly consistently report that APOE e4 is associated with greater cognitive decline on selected cognitive measures that were not consistent across studies. The level of evidence was rated as low for this factor.

Key Question 3—Interventions to Delay the Onset of Alzheimer Disease

There were relatively few Randomized Controlled Trials (RCTs) assessing the association between the factors examined and AD. This is at least partially attributable to the fact that many of the factors are not amenable to testing in an RCT. There were also sparse, if any, data on differences in outcomes among subgroups because the few RCTs conducted have generally not been designed to assess such differences.

For the nutrition category, there was one RCT on vitamin E and one on gingko biloba that showed no association with Alzheimer disease. There were no other RCTs for nutritional factors, including folic acid and Mediterranean diet, factors suggested to decrease risk by observational studies.

The factors in the medical conditions category are not appropriate for randomization.

For the medications category, the three RCTs using antihypertensive medication showed no association with AD, but findings were limited by low power to detect a clinically important effect and assessment for all-cause dementia rather than Alzheimer disease. The eight RCTs using cholinesterase inhibitors showed no association with Alzheimer disease moderate level of evidence). The two RCTs assessing NSAIDs showed increased risk of Alzheimer disease with rofecoxib, a medication that was subsequently withdrawn from the market for safety reasons, and increased risk for nonspecific dementia with naproxen (HR 3.57; 95 percent CI 1.09 to 11.7) but the study was stopped early and findings were based on few cases. In intervention trials, estrogen alone showed no association, but estrogen combined with progesterone showed an increased risk of Alzheimer disease (HR 2.05; 5 95 percent CI 1.21 to 3.48). The level of evidence was rated as moderate for estrogen combined with progesterone and low for NSAIDs.

For the social, economic, and behavioral factors, there were no intervention trials for any factors, including physical activity and cognitive engagement, interventions suggested to be beneficial by observational studies.

Key Question 4—Interventions to Improve or Maintain Cognitive Ability or Function

There were few RCTs assessing the effect of the various factors on cognitive decline. Additionally, there was no information on differential outcomes by subgroups.

For the nutrition category, intervention trials of vitamin B_6 and B_{12}, vitamin E, and folic acid showed either no effect on cognitive decline or no consistent effect across trials. The level of evidence was judged to be high for vitamin E and moderate for the other supplements. They did not identify any trials that evaluated the Mediterranean diet or diets high in vegetables, practices that have been associated with lower risk of cognitive decline in observational studies.

The medical conditions were not appropriate for RCTs.

For the medication category, there was no effect of statins (level of evidence = high), antihypertensive medications (low), cholinesterase inhibitors (moderate), or estrogen (high). Some of the types of NSAIDs showed no effect, but one (naproxen) showed increased risk of cognitive decline. The level of evidence for NSAIDs was rated as low. Observational studies had suggested lower risk for both NSAIDs and estrogen.

For the social, economic, and behavioral categories, physical activity and cognitive training interventions showed a small protective association against cognitive decline. The level of the evidence for cognitive training was rated high, but that for physical activity was rated low.

Key Question 5—Relationships between Factors Affecting Alzheimer Disease and Cognitive Decline

To address this question, they used the results from key questions 1 to 4 to compare the evidence for the effects of each exposure on risk of AD and cognitive decline. For factors with both RCT and observational evidence, They first compared the consistency of findings across study designs for each outcome. RCTs were preferred when of high quality. When studies showed a consistent effect on risk that was in the same direction for both AD and cognitive decline, they judged the results concordant. For many factors, the available data are quite limited, and concordant evidence across outcomes should not necessarily be interpreted as a robust finding. For other factors, not only were data limited but there was also marked heterogeneity in exposure or outcome measures across studies, so it was not possible to draw a conclusion about concordance. It is important to note that risk modification was generally small to moderate when factors were associated with AD (i.e., odds ratios and relative risk ratios were often substantially < 2.0). For cognitive decline, it is more difficult to determine the threshold for a meaningful change due to the numerous cognitive measures used to assess cognitive decline. But generally the differences in annual rate of decline between the exposed and unexposed groups were quite small.

Chapter 34

Nutrition, Exercise, and Therapeutic Recommendations

Chapter Contents

Section 34.1

Questions and Answers about Alzheimer Disease Prevention

This section includes text excerpted from "Preventing Alzheimer's Disease: What Do We Know?" National Institute on Aging (NIA), National Institutes of Health (NIH), September 24, 2018.

Preventing Alzheimer Disease: What Do We Know?

As they get older, many people worry about developing Alzheimer disease (AD) or a related dementia. If they have a family member with Alzheimer disease, they may wonder about their family history and genetic risk. As many as 5.5 million Americans age 65 and older live with Alzheimer disease. Many more are expected to develop the disease as the population ages—unless ways to prevent or delay it are found.

Although scientists have conducted many studies, and more are ongoing, so far nothing has been proven to prevent or delay dementia caused by Alzheimer disease. But researchers have identified promising strategies and are learning more about what might—and might not—work.

We know that changes in the brain can occur many years before the first symptoms of Alzheimer disease appear. These early brain changes point to a possible window of opportunity to prevent or delay debilitating memory loss and other symptoms of dementia. While research may identify specific interventions that will prevent or delay the disease in some people, it's likely that many individuals may need a combination of treatments based on their own risk factors.

Researchers are studying many approaches to prevent or delay Alzheimer disease. Some focus on drugs, some on lifestyle or other changes. Let's look at the most promising interventions to date and what we know about them.

Evaluating the Latest Prevention Research

A review of research looked carefully at the evidence on ways to prevent or delay Alzheimer dementia or age-related cognitive decline. Led by a committee of experts from the National Academies of Sciences, Engineering, and Medicine (NASEM), the review found "encouraging but inconclusive" evidence for three types of interventions:

- Increased physical activity

- Blood pressure control for people with high blood pressure (also called hypertension)

- Cognitive training

The evidence for other interventions, such as medications and diet, was not as strong. However, scientists are continuing to explore these and other possible preventions.

Can Increasing Physical Activity Prevent Alzheimer Disease?

Physical activity has many health benefits, such as reducing falls, maintaining mobility and independence, and reducing the risk of chronic conditions like depression, diabetes, and older woman walking by lake with walking sticks high blood pressure. Based on research to date, there's not enough evidence to recommend exercise as a way to prevent Alzheimer dementia or mild cognitive impairment (MCI), a condition of mild memory problems that often leads to Alzheimer dementia.

Years of animal and human observational studies suggest the possible benefits of exercise for the brain. Some studies have shown that people who exercise have a lower risk of cognitive decline than those who don't. Exercise has also been associated with fewer Alzheimer plaques and tangles in the brain and better performance on certain cognitive tests.

While clinical trials suggest that exercise may help delay or slow age-related cognitive decline, there is not enough evidence to conclude that it can prevent or slow MCI or Alzheimer dementia. One study compared high-intensity aerobic exercises, such as walking or running on a treadmill, to low-intensity stretching and balance exercises in 65 volunteers with MCI and prediabetes. After six months, researchers found that the aerobic group had better executive function—the ability to plan and organize—than the stretching/balance group, but not better short-term memory.

Several other clinical trials are testing aerobic and nonaerobic exercise to see if they may help prevent or delay Alzheimer dementia. Many questions remain to be answered: Can exercise or physical activity prevent age-related cognitive decline, MCI, or Alzheimer dementia? If so, what types of physical activity are most beneficial? How much and how often should a person exercise? How does exercise affect the brains of people with no or mild symptoms?

Until scientists know more, experts encourage exercise for its many other benefits.

Can Controlling High Blood Pressure Prevent Alzheimer Disease?

Controlling high blood pressure is known to reduce a person's risk for heart disease and stroke. The NASEM committee of experts concluded that managing blood pressure when it's high, particularly for middle-aged adults, also might help prevent or delay Alzheimer dementia.

Many types of studies show a connection between high blood pressure, cerebrovascular disease (a disease of the blood vessels supplying the brain), and dementia. For example, it's older man getting blood pressure checked by doctor common for people with AD-related changes in the brain to also have signs of vascular damage in the brain, autopsy studies show. In addition, observational studies have found that high blood pressure in middle age, along with other cerebrovascular risk factors such as diabetes and smoking, increase the risk of developing dementia.

Clinical trials—the gold standard of medical proof—are underway to determine whether managing high blood pressure in individuals with hypertension can prevent Alzheimer dementia or cognitive decline. Further studies are needed to determine which people, at what age, might benefit most from particular blood pressure management approaches.

Researchers are comparing the effectiveness of different hypertension treatments, as well as the effect of different blood pressure levels on cognitive function. For example, a study called Memory and Cognition in Decreased Hypertension (MIND; an add-on to the Systolic Blood Pressure Intervention Trial, or SPRINT), is looking at any effects that lowering blood pressure below targets may have on cognitive function and dementia in middle-aged and older people. High blood pressure is now generally defined as 130 or higher for the first number, or 80 or higher for the second number.

While research continues, experts recommend that people control high blood pressure to lower their risk of serious health problems, including heart disease and stroke.

Can Cognitive Training Prevent Alzheimer Disease?

Cognitive training involves structured activities designed to enhance memory, reasoning, and speed of processing. There is encouraging but inconclusive evidence that a specific, computer-based cognitive training may help delay or slow age-related cognitive decline. However, there is no evidence that it can prevent or delay AD-related cognitive impairment.

Studies show that cognitive training can improve the type of cognition a person is trained in. For example, older adults who received ten hours of practice designed to enhance their Speedman in cap using computer with a group of people and accuracy in responding to pictures presented briefly on a computer screen ("speed of processing" training) got faster and better at this specific task and other tasks in which enhanced speed of processing is important. Similarly, older adults who received several hours of instruction on effective memory strategies showed improved memory when using those strategies. The important question is whether such training has long-term benefits or translates into improved performance on daily activities like driving and remembering to take medicine.

Some of the strongest evidence that this might be the case comes from the National Institute on Aging (NIA)-sponsored Advanced Cognitive Training for Independent and Vital Elderly (ACTIVE) trial. In this trial, healthy adults age 65 and older participated in ten sessions of memory, reasoning, or speed-of-processing training with certified trainers during five to six weeks, with "booster sessions" made available to some participants 11 months and 3 years after initial training. The sessions improved participants' mental skills in the area in which they were trained (but not in other areas), and improvements persisted years after the training was completed. In addition, participants in all three groups reported that they could perform daily activities with greater independence as many as ten years later, although there was no objective data to support this.

Findings from long-term observational studies—in which researchers observed behavior but did not influence or change it—also suggest that informal cognitively stimulating activities, such as reading or playing games, may lower risk of AD-related cognitive impairment and dementia. For example, a study of nearly 2,000 cognitively normal adults 70 and older found that participating in games, crafts, computer use, and social activities for about four years was associated with a lower risk of MCI.

Scientists think that some of these activities may protect the brain by establishing "reserve," the brain's ability to operate effectively even when it is damaged or some brain function is disrupted. Another theory is that such activities may help the brain become more adaptable in some mental functions so it can compensate for declines in others.

Scientists do not know if particular types of cognitive training—or elements of the training such as instruction or social interaction—work better than others, but many studies are ongoing.

Can Eating Certain Foods Prevent Alzheimer Disease?

People often wonder if a certain diet or specific foods can help prevent Alzheimer disease. The NASEM review of research did not find enough evidence to recommend a certain diet to prevent cognitive decline or Alzheimer disease. Despite observational studies that link Mediterranean-style diets to brain health, clinical trials have not shown strong evidence. Many trials have focused on individual foods rather than comprehensive diets. Newer studies of diets, such as the MIND diet—a combination of the Mediterranean and Dietary Approaches to Stop Hypertension (DASH) diets—are underway. In general, a healthy diet is an important part of healthy aging.

What Else Might Prevent Alzheimer Disease?

Researchers are exploring these and other interventions that may help prevent, delay, or slow Alzheimer dementia or age-related cognitive decline. Other research targets include:

- New drugs to delay onset or slow disease progression

- Diabetes treatment

- Depression treatment

- Blood pressure- and lipid-lowering treatments

- Sleep interventions

- Social engagement

- Vitamins such as B_{12} plus folic acid supplements and D

- Combined physical and mental exercises

A Word of Caution

Because Alzheimer disease is so devastating, some people are tempted by untried or unproven "cures." Check with your doctor before trying pills or any other treatment or supplement that promises to prevent Alzheimer disease. These "treatments" might be unsafe, a waste of money, or both. They might even interfere with other medical treatments that have been prescribed.

What's the Bottom Line on Alzheimer Disease Prevention?

Alzheimer disease is complex, and the best strategy to prevent or delay it may turn out to be a combination of measures. In the meantime, you can do many things that may keep your brain healthy and your body fit.

You also can help scientists by volunteering to participate in research. Clinical trials and studies are looking for all kinds of people—healthy volunteers, cognitively normal participants with a family history of Alzheimer disease, people with MCI, and people diagnosed with Alzheimer disease or a related dementia.

Section 34.2

Healthy Eating and Alzheimer Disease

This section includes text excerpted from "Healthy Eating and Alzheimer's Disease," National Institute on Aging (NIA), National Institutes of Health (NIH), May 18, 2017.

Eating healthy foods helps everyone stay well. It's even more important for people with Alzheimer disease (AD). Here are some tips for healthy eating.

Buying and Preparing Food

When the person with AD lives with you:

- Buy healthy foods such as vegetables, fruits, and whole-grain products. Be sure to buy foods that the person likes and can eat.

- Give the person choices about what to eat—for example, "Would you like green beans or salad?"

- Buy food that is easy to prepare, such as premade salads and single food portions.

It may be helpful to have someone else make meals or use a service such as Meals on Wheels, which brings meals right to your home.

When a person with early-stage Alzheimer disease lives alone, you can buy foods that the person doesn't need to cook. Call to remind him or her to eat.

Maintain Familiar Routines

Change can be difficult for a person with Alzheimer disease. Maintaining familiar routines and serving favorite foods can make mealtimes easier. They can help the person know what to expect and feel more relaxed. If a home health aide or other professional provides care, family members should tell this caregiver about the person's preferences.

Try these tips:

- View mealtimes as opportunities for social interaction. A warm and happy tone of voice can set the mood.

- Be patient and give the person enough time to finish the meal.

- Respect personal, cultural, and religious food preferences, such as eating tortillas instead of bread or avoiding pork.

- If the person has always eaten meals at specific times, continue to serve meals at those times.

- Serve meals in a consistent, familiar place and way whenever possible.

- Avoid new routines, such as serving breakfast to a person who has never routinely eaten breakfast.

As Alzheimer disease progresses, familiar routines and food choices may need to be adapted to meet the person's changing needs. For example, a family custom of serving appetizers before dinner can be preserved, but higher-calorie items might be offered to help maintain the person's weight.

Stay Safe

In the early stage of Alzheimer disease, people's eating habits usually do not change. When changes do occur, living alone may not be safe anymore. Look for these signs to see if living alone is no longer safe for the person with Alzheimer disease:

- The person forgets to eat.

- Food has burned because it was left on the stove.

- The oven isn't turned off.

Other difficulties, such as not sitting down long enough for meals and refusing to eat, can arise in the middle and late stages of the disease. These changes can lead to poor nourishment, dehydration, abnormally low blood pressure, and other problems.

Caregivers should monitor the person's weight and eating habits to make sure she or he is not eating too little or too much. Other things to look for include appetite changes, the person's level of physical activity, and problems with chewing or swallowing. Talk with the person's doctor about changes in eating habits.

Section 34.3

Physical Activity Benefits Nursing-Home Residents with Alzheimer Disease

This section contains text excerpted from the following sources: Text in this section begins with excerpts from "Staying Physically Active with Alzheimer's," National Institute on Aging (NIA), National Institutes of Health (NIH), May 18, 2017; Text under the heading "Physical Activity and Alzheimer's Hippocampal Atrophy" is excerpted from "Physical Activity and Alzheimer-Related Hippocampal Atrophy," National Institute on Aging (NIA), National Institutes of Health (NIH), August 4, 2014. Reviewed December 2018; Text under the heading "Moderate Physical Activity Linked to Increases in Metabolism across Brain Regions" is excerpted from "Moderate Physical Activity Linked to Increases in Metabolism across Brain Regions," National Institute on Aging (NIA), National Institutes of Health (NIH), September 7, 2017.

Being active and getting exercise helps people with Alzheimer disease (AD) feel better. Exercise helps keep their muscles, joints, and heart in good shape. It also helps people stay at a healthy weight and have regular toilet and sleep habits. You can exercise together to make it more fun.

You want someone with Alzheimer disease to do as much as possible for herself or himself. At the same time, you need to make sure that the person is safe when active. Group of older adults playing seated volleyball with a beach ball.

Getting Started

Here are some tips for helping the person with Alzheimer disease stay active:

- Help get the activity started or join in to make the activity more fun.

- Be realistic about how much activity can be done at one time. Several 10-minute "mini-workouts" may be best.

- Take a walk together each day. Exercise is good for caregivers, too!

- Make sure the person with Alzheimer disease has an ID bracelet with your phone number if she or he walks alone.

- Check your local TV guide to see if there is a program to help older adults exercise, or watch exercise videos made for older people.

- Add music to the exercises if it helps the person with Alzheimer disease. Dance to the music if possible.

- Break exercises into simple, easy-to-follow steps.

- Make sure the person wears comfortable clothes and shoes that fit well and are made for exercise.

- Make sure she or he drinks water or juice after exercise.

Gentle Exercise

Some people with Alzheimer disease may not be able to get around well. This is another problem that becomes more challenging to deal with as the disease gets worse. Some possible reasons for this include:

- Trouble with endurance

- Poor coordination

- Sore feet or muscles

- Illness

- Depression or general lack of interest

Even if people have trouble walking, they may be able to:

- Do simple tasks around the home, such as sweeping and dusting

- Use a stationary bike

- Use soft rubber exercise balls or balloons for stretching or throwing back and forth

- Use stretching bands, which you can buy in sporting goods stores. Be sure to follow the instructions.

- Lift weights or household items such as soup cans

Physical Activity and Alzheimer Disease-Related Hippocampal Atrophy

Physical activity may help prevent atrophy of the hippocampus, a brain region important for learning and memory that often shrinks in the brains of people with Alzheimer disease. A study that looked at the rate of atrophy over 18 months in cognitively normal older adults suggests that physical activity may help prevent or delay this AD-related change.

The National Institute of Aging (NIA)-funded study by researchers at the Cleveland Clinic's Schey Center for Cognitive Neuroimaging is the first to show the protective effects physical activity may have on the hippocampus in older adults at genetic risk for Alzheimer disease. It also adds to past findings that physical activity, from gardening to walking to structured exercise programs, may benefit cognitive function in older adults.

Researchers studied 97 cognitively normal adults, age 65 to 89, some of whom had a family history of dementia. They were divided into four groups based on their self-reported levels of physical activity (low or high) and the presence or absence of the apolipoprotein E (APOE) ε4 gene form, the strongest known genetic risk factor for Alzheimer disease. Individuals with low physical activity said they walked or did other low-intensity activities on two or fewer days per week; those with high activity said they engaged in moderate or vigorous activity, such as brisk walking or swimming, on three or more days per week.

All participants underwent magnetic resonance imaging (MRI) of the brain to measure the size of the hippocampus—a part of the brain that shrinks as Alzheimer disease progresses—and other brain structures, as well as neurobehavioral testing to measure cognition and daily functioning. MRIs scans were done at the beginning of the study and after 18 months. At the study end, researchers found the size of the hippocampus decreased by three percent in the group with high genetic risk and low physical activity. Hippocampal size remained stable in the group with low genetic risk and in participants with high genetic risk/high physical activity. Physical activity did not appear to affect several other brain areas, including the amygdala, thalamus, and cortical white matter.

While promising, more research is needed to confirm these findings. Researchers want to learn how physical activity influences hippocampal atrophy in people at high genetic risk of Alzheimer disease. Animal studies suggest several possibilities, including the impact of physical activity on cholinergic function, brain inflammation, and cerebral blood flow.

Moderate Physical Activity Linked to Increases in Metabolism across Brain Regions

Can exercise change how your brain works? A study suggests that how, and how often, older adults exercise could impact breakdown of glucose in the brain. Decreases in brain metabolism (hypometabolism) have been shown to be a characteristic of Alzheimer disease and predictive of cognitive decline and the conversion to Alzheimer disease in older adults. Physical activity has been shown to modulate brain glucose metabolism, but it is unclear what level of intensity and duration may be beneficial.

An NIA-supported study from the University of Wisconsin led by Dr. Ozioma Okonkwo found that even moderate physical activity may increase metabolism in brain regions important for learning and memory. The study asked cognitively normal, late-middle-age (average age 64 years old) participants to wear an accelerometer for 7 consecutive days to measure daily physical activity. Scientists were then able to determine the amount of time each individual engaged in light (e.g., a slow walk), moderate (e.g., a fast walk), and vigorous activities (e.g., run). The physical activity data were analyzed to determine how they corresponded with glucose metabolism within brain areas that have been demonstrated to be impacted in people with Alzheimer disease.

Increasing levels of engagement in moderate physical activity were associated with increases in cerebral glucose metabolism across all brain regions examined. Vigorous activity showed an increase in metabolism only in the hippocampus (an area important for learning and memory). Light physical activity was not associated with changes in metabolism in any of the brain regions examined. Further, how long one engaged in moderate physical activity impacted the amount of brain glucose metabolism. The more time spent performing moderate level of physical activity (average 43.3 min/day to average 68.1 min/day), the greater the increase in brain glucose metabolism.

Overall, this study adds to encouraging evidence that physical activity may be beneficial for neurometabolic function. Specifically, it makes a critical contribution to the efforts to identify the intensity and duration of physical activity that confer the most advantage for combating AD-related changes in mid-life.

Section 34.4

Dance Your Way to Better Brain Health

This section includes text excerpted from "Dance Your Way
to Better Brain Health," Centers for Disease Control
and Prevention (CDC), June 4, 2018.

Join a dance class to exercise your brain and body.

Exercise is not only good for your body, it's good for your brain! Sticking to a regular workout plan can be tough, but including activity in your routine doesn't need to be boring. Scientists have found that the areas of the brain that control memory and skills such as planning and organizing improve with exercise. Dance has the added dimensions of rhythm, balance, music, and a social setting that enhances the benefits of simple movement—and can be fun!

The Science of Dance

At the University of Illinois at Chicago (UIC), through the Centers for Disease Control and Prevention (CDC)-funded Prevention

Research Centers' (PRCs) Healthy Brain Research Network (HBRN), researchers designed a Latin ballroom dance program for older sedentary adults. Participants in the program, BAILAMOS©, reported improvements in memory, attention, and focus. In a separate ballroom dance program, older people experiencing mild cognitive impairment improved their thinking and memory after a 10-month-long ballroom dancing class.

So, how can you get moving?

- Sign up for a dance class and invite your friends to join. Find classes at your local community college, Young Men's Christian Association (YMCA), dance studio, or community center.

- Try dancing at home by following along with a DVD or videos on YouTube. Easy-to-follow, free exercise videos are available at the National Institute on Aging's (NIA) *Go4Life* YouTube channel (www.youtube.com/playlist?list=PLmk21KJuZUM4HTrJ7hrJ8yxhToKkJT8a8).

- For an extra challenge, try using small weights to build strength. Keep a 2-pound or 5-pound weight in each hand while doing your dance routine.

Help for Caregivers of People with Alzheimer Disease

Are you a caregiver for someone with Alzheimer disease or a related dementia? You can help the person you care for get moving, too.

- Split dance moves and exercises into small, easy-to-follow steps. Use exercise videos and follow along with the person you're caring for.

- At first, try shorter 5- or 10-minute mini dancing sessions to slowly build endurance.

- Take breaks when needed and make sure you are both drinking plenty of water.

Section 34.5

Complementary Health Approaches for Alzheimer Disease and Dementia

This section contains text excerpted from the following sources:
Text in this section begins with excerpts from "Alzheimer's Disease at a Glance," National Center for Complementary and Integrative Health (NCCIH), September 24, 2017; Text under the heading "Five Things to Know about Complementary Health Practices for Cognitive Function, Dementia, and Alzheimer Disease" is excerpted from "5 Things to Know about Complementary Health Practices for Cognitive Function, Dementia, and Alzheimer's Disease," National Center for Complementary and Integrative Health (NCCIH), March 14, 2018.

Researchers have explored many complementary health approaches for preventing or slowing dementia, including Alzheimer disease (AD). Currently, there is no strong evidence that any complementary health approach or diet can prevent cognitive impairment.

What the Science Says

Following are some of the complementary health approaches that have been studied.

- **Fish oil/omega-3s**. Among the nutritional and dietary factors studied to prevent cognitive decline in older adults, the most consistent positive research findings are for omega-3 fatty acids, often measured as how much fish people ate. However, taking omega-3 supplements did not have any beneficial effects on the cognitive functioning of older people without dementia.

- **Ginkgo**. A National Center for Complementary and Integrative Health (NCCIH)-funded study of the well-characterized ginkgo supplement EGb-761 found that it didn't lower the incidence of dementia, including Alzheimer disease, in older adults. Further analysis of the same data showed that ginkgo did not slow cognitive decline, lower blood pressure, or reduce the incidence of hypertension. In this clinical trial, known as the Ginkgo Evaluation of Memory study, researchers recruited more than 3,000 volunteers age 75 and older who took 240 mg of ginkgo daily. Participants were followed for an average of approximately 6 years.

- **B-vitamins**. Results of short-term studies suggest that B-vitamin supplements do not help cognitive functioning in adults age 50 or older with or without dementia. The vitamins studied were B_{12}, B_6, and folic acid, taken alone or in combination.

- **Curcumin**, which comes from turmeric, has anti-inflammatory and antioxidant properties that might affect chemical processes in the brain associated with Alzheimer disease, laboratory studies have suggested. However, the few clinical trials (studies done in people) that have looked at the effects of curcumin on Alzheimer disease have not found a benefit.

- **Melatonin**. People with dementia can become agitated and have trouble sleeping. Supplements of melatonin, which is a naturally occurring hormone that helps regulate sleep, are being studied to see if they improve sleep in some people with dementia. However, in one study researchers noted that melatonin supplements may worsen mood in people with dementia.

- For caregivers, taking a mindfulness meditation class or a caregiver education class reduced stress more than just getting time off from providing care, a small, 2010 NCCIH-funded study showed.

Side Effects and Risks

- Don't use complementary approaches as a reason to postpone seeing a healthcare provider about memory loss. Treatable conditions, such as depression, bad reactions to medications, or thyroid, liver, or kidney problems, can cause memory impairment.

- Keep in mind that although many dietary supplements (and some prescription drugs) come from natural sources, "natural" does not always mean "safe."

- Some dietary supplements have been found to interact with medications, whether prescription or over-the-counter (OTC). For example, the herbal supplement. St. John's wort interacts with many medications, making them less effective. Your healthcare provider can advise you.

Five Things to Know about Complementary Health Practices for Cognitive Function, Dementia, and Alzheimer Disease

Many people, particularly older individuals, worry about forgetfulness and whether it is the first sign of dementia or Alzheimer disease. In fact, forgetfulness has many causes. It can also be a normal part of aging, or related to various treatable health issues or to emotional problems, such as stress, anxiety, or depression. The National Institute on Aging (NIA) has a lot of information on the aging brain as well as cognitive function, dementia, and Alzheimer disease. Although no treatment is proven to stop dementia or Alzheimer disease, some conventional drugs may limit worsening of symptoms for a period of time in the early stages of the disease.

Many dietary supplements are marketed with claims that they enhance memory or improve brain function and health. To date, research has yielded no convincing evidence that any dietary supplement can reverse or slow the progression of dementia or Alzheimer disease. Additional research on dietary supplements, as well as several mind and body practices such as music therapy and mental imagery, which have shown promise in basic research or preliminary clinical studies, is underway.

Here are five things to know about the research on complementary health approaches for cognitive function, dementia, and Alzheimer disease.

1. To date there is no convincing evidence from a large body of research that any dietary supplement can prevent worsening of cognitive impairment associated with dementia or Alzheimer disease. This includes studies of ginkgo, omega-3 fatty acids/fish oil, vitamins B and E, Asian ginseng, grape seed extract, and curcumin. Additional research on some of these supplements is underway.

2. Preliminary studies of some mind and body practices such as music therapy suggest they may be helpful for some of the symptoms related to dementia, such as agitation and depression. Several studies on music therapy in people with Alzheimer disease have shown improvement in agitation, depression, and quality of life (QOL).

3. Mindfulness-based stress reduction programs may be helpful in reducing stress among caregivers of patients with dementia.

To reduce caregiver stress, studies suggest that a mindfulness-based stress reduction program is more helpful for improving mental health than attending an education and support program or just taking time off from providing care.

4. Don't use complementary health approaches as a reason to postpone seeing a healthcare provider about memory loss. Treatable conditions, such as depression, bad reactions to medications, or thyroid, liver, or kidney problems, can impair memory.

5. Some complementary health approaches interact with medications and can have serious side effects. If you are considering replacing conventional medications with other approaches, talk to your healthcare provider.

Chapter 35

Medications' Effects on Older Adults' Brain Functions

Medications and combinations of medicines can have side effects. Side effects are the unplanned symptoms or feelings a person has when taking a drug. Many side effects are not serious and either go away on their own or can be easily managed. However, some side effects can cause serious health problems, including effects on an older adult's cognition. Cognition is a person's ability to think, understand, learn, plan, and remember. Cognitive side effects include problems concentrating or paying attention, confusion, memory loss, and hallucinations or delusions. Older adults, their families, and Aging Network* staff that serve them sometimes mistake these side effects for dementia, such as Alzheimer disease (AD).

The Older Americans Act (OAA) of 1965 established a national network of federal, state, and local agencies to plan and provide services that help older adults to live independently in their homes and communities. This interconnected structure of agencies is known as the Aging Network.

This chapter includes text excerpted from "Brain Health: Medications' Effects on Older Adults' Brain Function," National Institute on Aging (NIA), National Institutes of Health (NIH), February 27, 2016.

What Happens as People Age?

As people age, their bodies change in ways that can influence how medications affect them. For example, older adults' brains begin to change in structure and ability. In addition, changes in older adults' digestive and circulatory systems, kidneys, and livers affect how fast medications enter and leave their bodies. Weight changes may also affect how much medication older adults need, and how long drugs stay in their bodies. As a result of these normal changes, reactions to medications can change as well. Chronic health conditions can further complicate the effects of medications. Eighty percent of older adults have at least one chronic health condition, and half have at least two. These health conditions can require medications that may interact with one another in harmful ways. An interaction occurs when one medication affects how another works when a person takes the two drugs together. In addition, medications can cause problems by interacting with food, supplements, natural products, alcohol, or other health conditions. For example, when mixed with some drugs, alcohol can cause dizziness, drowsiness, or changes in heartbeat.

What Groups of Medications Might Cause Trouble with Cognition?

In 2015, the National Academy of Medicine (NAM) published a report on cognitive aging. The report describes some groups of medications that may affect older adults' cognition. These groups include certain antihistamines, antianxiety and antidepressant medications, sleep aids, antipsychotics, muscle relaxants, antimuscarinics for urinary incontinence, and antispasmodics for relief of cramps or spasms of the stomach, intestines, and bladder. Some of the drugs that can cause cognitive problems in older adults are sold over-the-counter (OTC).

What Do Doctors Have to Say about Older Adults' Cognition and Use of Medications?

In 2015, the American Geriatrics Society (AGS), whose members are doctors, nurses, pharmacists, social workers, and other healthcare professionals serving older adults, updated its list of medications that older adults should avoid, or use with caution. The Society's list includes medications that have "anticholinergic" effects. These drugs block one of the chemicals (acetylcholine) that brain cells use to communicate with each other. A drug's anticholinergic effects can cause older adults to experience confusion, memory loss, and worsening of other mental functions, among other things. Several research reviews show links between drugs with anticholinergic effects and cognitive problems in older adults, such as delirium, cognitive impairment, and dementia. Older adults should get advice from a healthcare professional about use of prescription and OTC medications, especially before making any changes. Healthcare professionals can also provide information about alternatives to medications that may harm brain function. Some drugs with anticholinergic effects may be needed to treat allergies, nausea, depression, muscle spasm, and other medical conditions. However, sometimes these medications are used for the wrong reasons, or as substitutes for other medications that are more effective or have fewer side effects.

Another group of drugs, benzodiazepines, which treat anxiety, sleeplessness, and agitation, may increase older adults' risk for memory loss, delirium, cognitive impairment, falls, fractures, and motor vehicle accidents. The AGS says that healthcare professionals need to carefully consider these side effects when treating older adults, and limit the use of benzodiazepines to treating conditions such as seizures or other neurological conditions, alcohol withdrawal, severe generalized anxiety disorder, and anesthesia, as well as end-of-life care.

What Should Aging Network Staff Do?

Aging Network staff can:

- Educate older adults, their families, and others about the cognitive effects of certain types of drugs.

- Connect people with evidence-based resources, and encourage them to discuss their medications and any side effects with their healthcare professionals. This is especially important during care transitions, such as after having surgery or leaving a hospital.

When older adults talk to their healthcare professionals, they or their families need to describe any cognitive symptoms they may have, and provide a list of their medications, including OTC drugs, vitamins, natural products and supplements. Talking with their healthcare professionals can help older adults get the best and safest treatments possible.

Chapter 36

Common Medical Problems in People with Alzheimer Disease

A person with Alzheimer disease (AD) may have other medical problems over time, as we all do. These problems can cause more confusion and behavior changes. The person may not be able to tell you what is wrong. You need to watch for signs of illness and tell the doctor about what you see.

The most common medical problems:

Constipation

People can have constipation—trouble having a bowel movement—when they:

- Change what they eat
- Take certain medicines, including Namenda®
- Get less exercise than usual
- Drink less fluid than usual

Try to get the person to drink at least six glasses of liquid a day.

This chapter includes text excerpted from "Alzheimer's Disease: Common Medical Problems," National Institute on Aging (NIA), National Institutes of Health (NIH), May 18, 2017.

Besides water, other good sources of liquid include:

- Juice, especially prune juice
- Gelatin, such as Jell-O®
- Soup
- Milk or melted ice cream
- Decaffeinated coffee and tea
- Liquid cereal, such as Cream of Wheat®

Have the person eat foods high in fiber. Foods like dried apricots, raisins, or prunes; some dry cereals; or soybeans might help ease constipation. If possible, make sure that the person gets some exercise each day, such as walking. Call the doctor if you notice a change in the person's bowel habits.

Dehydration

Our bodies must have a certain amount of water to work well. If a person is sick or doesn't drink enough fluid, she or he may become dehydrated.

Signs of dehydration to look for include:

- Dry mouth
- Dizziness
- Hallucinations (Don't forget that hallucinations may be caused by the AD itself.)
- Rapid heart rate

Be aware of how much fluid the person is drinking. This is even more important during hot weather or in homes without air conditioning. Also, look for signs of dehydration during the winter months when heat in your home can create a lot of dry air.

Dental Problems

As AD gets worse, people need help taking care of their teeth or dentures.

Check the person's mouth for any problems such as:

- Sores
- Decayed teeth

- Food "pocketed" in the cheek or on the roof of the mouth

- Lumps

Be sure to take the person for dental checkups. Some people need medicine to calm them before they can see the dentist.

Diarrhea

Some medicines, including Alzheimer disease medications, may cause diarrhea—loose bowel movements. Certain medical problems also may cause diarrhea. Make sure the person takes in lots of fluids when she or he has diarrhea. Also, be sure to let the doctor know about this problem.

Falls

As Alzheimer disease gets worse, the person may have trouble walking and keeping his or her balance. She or he also may have changes in depth perception, which is the ability to understand distances. For example, someone with AD may try to step down when walking from a carpeted to a tile floor. This puts him or her at risk for falls.

To reduce the chance of a fall:

- Clean up clutter

- Remove throw rugs

- Use chairs with arms

- Put grab bars in the bathroom

- Use good lighting

- Make sure the person wears sturdy shoes with good traction

Fever

Having a fever means that the person's temperature is two degrees above his or her normal temperature.

A fever may be a sign of:

- Infection, caused by germs

- Dehydration, caused by a lack of fluids

- Heat stroke

- Constipation

Don't use a glass thermometer because the person might bite down on the glass. Use a digital thermometer, which you can buy at a grocery store or drugstore.

Flu and Pneumonia

These diseases spread quickly from one person to another, and people with AD are more likely to get them. Make sure that the person gets a flu shot each year and a pneumonia shot once after age 65. Some older people need to get more than one pneumonia vaccine. The shots lower the chances that the person will get flu or pneumonia.

Flu and pneumonia may cause:

- Fever (Not everyone with pneumonia has a fever).

- Chills

- Aches and pains

- Vomiting

- Coughing

- Breathing trouble

Incontinence

Incontinence means a person can't control his or her bladder and/ or bowels. This may happen at any stage of AD, but it is more often a problem in the later stages. Signs of this problem are leaking urine, problems emptying the bladder, and soiled underwear and bed sheets. Be sure to let the doctor know if this happens. She or he may be able to treat the cause of the problem.

Here are some examples of things that can be treated:

- Urinary tract infection

- Enlarged prostate gland

- Too little fluid in the body (dehydration)

- Diabetes that isn't being treated

- Taking too many water pills

- Drinking too much caffeine

- Taking medicines that make it hard to hold urine

When you talk to the doctor, be ready to answer the following questions:

- What medicines is the person taking?

- Does the person leak urine when she or he laughs, coughs, or lifts something?

- Does the person urinate often?

- Can the person get to the bathroom in time?

- Is the person urinating in places other than the bathroom?

- Is the person soiling his or her clothes or bed sheets each night?

- Do these problems happen each day or once in a while?

Here are some ways you can deal with incontinence:

- Remind the person to go to the bathroom every two to three hours.

- Show him or her the way to the bathroom, or take him or her.

- Make sure that the person wears loose, comfortable clothing that is easy to remove.

- Limit fluids after 6 p.m., if problems happen at night.

- Do not give the person fluids with caffeine, such as coffee or tea.

- Give the person fresh fruit before bedtime instead of fluids if she or he is thirsty.

- Mark the bathroom door with a big sign that reads "Toilet" or "Bathroom."

- Use a stable toilet seat that is at a good height. Using a colorful toilet seat may help the person identify the toilet. You can buy raised toilet seats at medical supply stores.

- Help the person when she or he needs to use a public bathroom. This may mean going into the stall with the person or using a family or private bathroom.

Things you may want to buy:

- Use adult disposable briefs or underwear, bed protectors, and waterproof mattress covers. You can buy these items at drugstores and medical supply stores.

- Use a drainable pouch for the person who can't control his or her bowel movements. Talk to the nurse about how to use this product.

Some people find it helpful to keep a record of how much food and fluid the person takes in and how often she or he goes to the bathroom. You can use this information to make a schedule of when she or he needs to go to the bathroom.

Other Medical Problems

People with AD can have the same medical problems as many older adults. Research suggests that some of these medical problems may be related to AD.

For example, some heart and blood circulation problems, stroke, and diabetes are more common in people who have AD than in the general population. Diseases caused by infections also are common.

Chapter 37

Alzheimer Disease and Hallucinations, Delusions, and Paranoia

Due to complex changes occurring in the brain, people with Alzheimer disease (AD) may see or hear things that have no basis in reality.

- Hallucinations involve hearing, seeing, smelling, or feeling things that are not really there. For example, a person with AD may see children playing in the living room when no children exist.

- Delusions are false beliefs that the person thinks are real. For example, the person may think his or her spouse is in love with someone else.

- Paranoia is a type of delusion in which a person may believe— without a good reason—that others are mean, lying, unfair, or "out to get me." She or he may become suspicious, fearful, or jealous of people.

If a person with AD has ongoing disturbing hallucinations or delusions, seek medical help. An illness or medication may cause these behaviors. Medicines are available to treat these behaviors but must

This chapter includes text excerpted from "Alzheimer's and Hallucinations, Delusions, and Paranoia," National Institute on Aging (NIA), National Institutes of Health (NIH), May 17, 2017.

be used with caution. The following tips may also help you cope with these behaviors.

Hallucinations and Delusions

Here are some tips for coping with hallucinations and delusions:

- Discuss with the doctor any illnesses the person with AD has and medicines she or he is taking. Sometimes an illness or medicine may cause hallucinations or delusions.

- Try not to argue with the person about what she or he sees or hears. Comfort the person if she or he is afraid.

- Distract the person. Sometimes moving to another room or going outside for a walk helps.

- Turn off the TV when violent or upsetting programs are on. Someone with AD may think these events are happening in the room.

- Make sure the person is safe and can't reach anything that could be used to hurt anyone or himself or herself.

Paranoia

In a person with Alzheimer disease, paranoia often is linked to memory loss. It can become worse as memory loss gets worse. For example, the person may become paranoid if she or he forgets:

- Where she or he put something. The person may believe that someone is taking his or her things

- That you are the person's caregiver. Someone with AD might not trust you if she or he thinks you are a stranger

- People to whom the person has been introduced. She or he may believe that strangers will be harmful.

- Directions you just gave. The person may think you are trying to trick him or her.

Paranoia may be the person's way of expressing loss. The person may blame or accuse others because no other explanation seems to make sense.

Here are some tips for coping with paranoia:

- Try not to react if the person blames you for something

- Don't argue with the person

- Let the person know that she or he is safe

- Use gentle touching or hugging to show you care

- Explain to others that the person is acting this way because she or he has Alzheimer disease

- Search for things to distract the person, then talk about what you found. For example, talk about a photograph or keepsake.

Also, keep in mind that someone with Alzheimer disease may have a good reason for acting a certain way. She or he may not be paranoid. There are people who take advantage of weak and elderly people. Find out if someone is trying to abuse or steal from the person with Alzheimer disease.

Chapter 38

Pain and Dementia

You've probably been in pain at one time or another. Maybe you've had a headache or bruise—pain that doesn't last too long. But, many older people have ongoing pain from health problems like arthritis, diabetes, shingles, or cancer.

Pain can be your body's way of warning you that something is wrong. Always tell the doctor where you hurt and exactly how it feels.

Alzheimer Disease and Pain

People who have Alzheimer disease (AD) may not be able to tell you when they're in pain. When you're caring for someone with Alzheimer disease, watch for clues. A person's face may show signs of being in pain or feeling ill. You may see a person frequently changing position or having trouble sleeping. You may also notice sudden changes in behavior such as increased agitation, crying, or moaning. Refusing to eat may be a sign that the person has tooth pain or other oral health issues. It's important to find out if there is something wrong. If you're not sure what to do, call the doctor for help.

Acute Pain and Chronic Pain

There are two kinds of pain. Acute pain begins suddenly, lasts for a short time, and goes away as your body heals. You might feel acute

This chapter includes text excerpted from "Pain: You Can Get Help," National Institute on Aging (NIA), National Institutes of Health (NIH), February 28, 2018.

pain after surgery or if you have a broken bone, infected tooth, or kidney stone.

Pain that lasts for three months or longer is called chronic pain. This pain often affects older people. For some people, chronic pain is caused by a health condition such as arthritis. It may also follow acute pain from an injury, surgery, or other health issue that has been treated, like postherpetic neuralgia (PHN) after shingles.

Living with any type of pain can be hard. It can cause many other problems. For instance, pain can:

- Get in the way of your daily activities

- Disturb your sleep and eating habits

- Make it difficult to continue working

- Be related to depression or anxiety

- Keep you from spending time with friends and family

Describing Pain

Many people have a hard time describing pain. Think about these questions when you explain how the pain feels:

- Where does it hurt?

- When did the pain start? Does it come and go?

- What does it feel like? Is the pain sharp, dull, or burning? Would you use some other word to describe it?

- Do you have other symptoms?

- When do you feel the pain? In the morning? In the evening? After eating?

- Is there anything you do that makes the pain feel better or worse? For example, does using a heating pad or ice pack help? Does changing your position from lying down to sitting up make it better?

- What medicines, including over-the-counter (OTC) medications and nonmedicine therapies have you tried, and what was their effect?

Your doctor or nurse may ask you to rate your pain on a scale of 0 to 10, with 0 being no pain and 10 being the worst pain you can imagine. Or, your doctor may ask if the pain is mild, moderate, or severe. Some doctors or nurses have pictures of faces that show different expressions of pain and ask you to point to the face that shows how you feel. Your doctor may ask you to keep a diary of when and what kind of pain you feel every day.

Attitudes about Pain

Everyone reacts to pain differently. Some people feel they should be brave and not complain when they hurt. Other people are quick to report pain and ask for help.

Worrying about pain is common. This worry can make you afraid to stay active, and it can separate you from your friends and family. Working with your doctor, you can find ways to continue to take part in physical and social activities despite having pain.

Some people put off going to the doctor because they think pain is part of aging and nothing can help. This is not true!

It is important to see a doctor if you have a new pain. Finding a way to manage pain is often easier if it is addressed early.

Treating Pain

Treating, or managing, chronic pain is important. Some treatments involve medications, and some do not. Your treatment plan should be specific to your needs.

Most treatment plans focus on both reducing pain and increasing ways to support daily function while living with pain.

Talk with your doctor about how long it may take before you feel better. Often, you have to stick with a treatment plan before you get relief. It's important to stay on a schedule. Sometimes this is called "staying ahead" or "keeping on top" of your pain. Be sure to tell your doctor about any side effects. You might have to try different treatments until you find a plan that works for you. As your pain lessens, you can likely become more active and will see your mood lift and sleep improve.

Medicines to Treat Pain

Your doctor may prescribe one or more of the following pain medications. Talk with your doctor about their safety and the right dose to take.

- **Acetaminophen** may help all types of pain, especially mild to moderate pain. Acetaminophen is found in OTC and prescription medicines. People who have more than three drinks per day or who have liver disease should not take acetaminophen.

- **Nonsteroidal anti-inflammatory drugs (NSAIDs)** include aspirin, naproxen, and ibuprofen. Long-term use of some NSAIDs can cause side effects, like internal bleeding or kidney problems, which make them unsafe for many older adults. You may not be able to take ibuprofen if you have high blood pressure.

- **Narcotics** (also called opioids) are used for moderate to severe pain and require a doctor's prescription. They may be habit-forming. They can also be dangerous when taken with alcohol or certain other drugs. Examples of narcotics are codeine, morphine, and oxycodone.

- **Other medications** are sometimes used to treat pain. These include antidepressants, anticonvulsive medicines, local painkillers like nerve blocks or patches, and ointments and creams.

As people age, they are at risk for developing more side effects from medications. It's important to take exactly the amount of pain medicine your doctor prescribes. Don't chew or crush your pills if they are supposed to be swallowed whole. Talk with your doctor or pharmacist if you're having trouble swallowing your pills.

Mixing any pain medication with alcohol or other drugs can be dangerous. Make sure your doctor knows all the medicines you take, including OTC drugs and dietary supplements, as well as the amount of alcohol you drink.

What Other Treatments Help with Pain?

In addition to drugs, there are a variety of complementary and alternative approaches that may provide relief. Talk to your doctor about these treatments. It may take both medicine and other treatments to feel better.

- **Acupuncture** uses hair-thin needles to stimulate specific points on the body to relieve pain.

- **Biofeedback** helps you learn to control your heart rate, blood pressure, muscle tension, and other body functions. This may help reduce your pain and stress level.

- **Cognitive behavioral therapy (CBT)** is a form of short-term counseling that may help reduce your reaction to pain.

- **Distraction** can help you cope with acute pain, taking your mind off your discomfort.

- **Electrical nerve stimulation** uses electrical impulses to relieve pain.

- **Guided imagery** uses directed thoughts to create mental pictures that may help you relax, manage anxiety, sleep better, and have less pain.

- **Hypnosis** uses focused attention to help manage pain.

- **Massage therapy** can release tension in tight muscles.

- **Mind-body stress reduction** combines mindfulness meditation, body awareness, and yoga* to increase relaxation and reduce pain.

- **Physical therapy** uses a variety of techniques to help manage everyday activities with less pain and teaches you ways to improve flexibility and strength.

A mind and body practice with origins in ancient Indian philosophy. The various styles of yoga typically combine physical postures, breathing techniques, and meditation or relaxation.

Helping Yourself

There are things you can do yourself that might help you feel better. Try to:

- **Keep a healthy weight.** Putting on extra pounds can slow healing and make some pain worse. A healthy weight might help with pain in the knees, back, hips, or feet.

- **Be physically active.** Pain might make you inactive, which can lead to more pain and loss of function. Activity can help.

- **Get enough sleep.** It can reduce pain sensitivity, help healing, and improve your mood.

- **Avoid tobacco, caffeine, and alcohol.** They can get in the way of treatment and increase pain.

- **Join a pain support group.** Sometimes, it can help to talk to other people about how they deal with pain. You can share your thoughts while learning from others.

Pain at the End of Life

Not everyone who is dying is in pain. But, if a person has pain at the end of life, there are ways to help. Experts believe it's best to focus on making the person comfortable, without worrying about possible addiction or drug dependence.

Some Facts about Pain

- **Most people don't have to live with pain.** There are pain treatments. While not all pain can be cured, most pain can be managed. If your doctor has not been able to help you, ask to see a pain specialist.

- **The side effects from pain medicine are often manageable.** Side effects from pain medicine like constipation, dry mouth, and drowsiness may be a problem when you first begin taking the medicine. These problems can often be treated and may go away as your body gets used to the medicine.

- **Your doctor will not think you're a sissy if you talk about your pain.** If you're in pain, tell your doctor so you can get help.

- **If you use pain medicine now, it will still work when you need it later.** Using medicine at the first sign of pain may help control your pain later.

- **Pain is not "all in your head."** No one but you know how your pain feels. If you're in pain, talk with your doctor.

Chapter 39

Sexuality and Alzheimer Disease

Alzheimer disease (AD) can cause changes in intimacy and sexuality in both a person with the disease and the caregiver. The person with AD may be stressed by the changes in his or her memory and behaviors. Fear, worry, depression, anger, and low self-esteem (how much the person likes herself or himself) are common. The person may become dependent and cling to you. She or he may not remember your life together and feelings toward one another. The person may even fall in love with someone else.

You, the caregiver, may pull away from the person in both an emotional and physical sense. You may be upset by the demands of caregiving. You also may feel frustrated by the person's constant forgetfulness, repeated questions, and other bothersome behaviors.

Most caregivers learn how to cope with these challenges, but it takes time. Some learn to live with the illness and find new meaning in their relationships with people who have AD.

How to Cope with Changes in Intimacy

Most people with Alzheimer disease need to feel that someone loves and cares about them. They also need to spend time with other people

This chapter includes text excerpted from "Changes in Intimacy and Sexuality in Alzheimer's Disease," National Institute on Aging (NIA), National Institutes of Health (NIH), May 17, 2017.

as well as you. Your efforts to take care of these needs can help the person with AD to feel happy and safe. It's important to reassure the person that:

- You love her or him
- You will keep her or him safe
- Others also care about her or him

The following tips may help you cope with your own needs:

- Talk with a doctor, social worker, or clergy member about these changes. It may feel awkward to talk about such personal issues, but it can help.
- Talk about your concerns in a support group
- Think more about the positive parts of the relationship

How to Cope with Changes in Sexuality

The well spouse/partner or the person with Alzheimer disease may lose interest in having sex. This change can make you feel lonely or frustrated. You may feel that:

- It's not okay to have sex with someone who has AD
- The person with AD seems like a stranger
- The person with AD seems to forget that the spouse/partner is there or how to make love

A person with Alzheimer disease may have side effects from medications that affect his or her sexual interest. She or he may also have memory loss, changes in the brain, or depression that affect her or his interest in sex.

Here are some tips for coping with changes in sexuality:

- Explore new ways of spending time together
- Focus on other ways to show affection, such as snuggling or holding hands
- Try other nonsexual forms of touching, such as massage, hugging, and dancing
- Consider other ways to meet your sexual needs. Some caregivers report that they masturbate.

Hypersexuality

Sometimes, people with Alzheimer disease are overly interested in sex. This is called hypersexuality. The person may masturbate a lot and try to seduce others. These behaviors are symptoms of the disease and don't always mean that the person wants to have sex.

To cope with hypersexuality, try giving the person more attention and reassurance. You might gently touch, hug, or use other kinds of affection to meet his or her emotional needs. Some people with this problem need medicine to control their behaviors. Talk to the doctor about what steps to take.

Chapter 40

Managing Sleep Problems in Alzheimer Disease

Alzheimer disease (AD) often changes a person's sleeping habits. Some people with AD sleep too much; others don't sleep enough. Some people wake up many times during the night; others wander or yell at night.

The person with AD isn't the only one who loses sleep. Caregivers may have sleepless nights, leaving them tired for the challenges they face.

If you're caring for someone with AD, take these steps to make him or her safer and help you sleep better at night:

- Make sure the floor is clear of objects

- Lock up any medicines

- Attach grab bars in the bathroom

- Place a gate across the stairs

This chapter contains text excerpted from the following sources: Text in this chapter begins with excerpts from "A Good Night's Sleep," National Institute on Aging (NIA), National Institutes of Health (NIH), May 1, 2016; Text under the heading "Six Tips for Managing Sleep Problems in Alzheimer Disease" is excerpted from "6 Tips for Managing Sleep Problems in Alzheimer's," National Institute on Aging (NIA), National Institutes of Health (NIH), May 17, 2017.

Six Tips for Managing Sleep Problems in Alzheimer Disease

Alzheimer disease often affects a person's sleeping habits. It may be hard to get the person to go to bed and stay there. Someone with Alzheimer may sleep a lot or not enough, and may wake up many times during the night.

Here are some tips that may help caregivers manage sleep problems in people with Alzheimer disease:

1. Help the person get exercise each day, limit naps, and make sure the person gets enough rest at night. Being overly tired can increase late-afternoon and nighttime restlessness.

2. Plan activities that use more energy early in the day. For example, try bathing in the morning or having the largest family meal in the middle of the day.

3. Set a quiet, peaceful mood in the evening to help the person relax. Keep the lights low, try to reduce the noise levels, and play soothing music if she or he enjoys it.

4. Try to have the person go to bed at the same time each night. A bedtime routine, such as reading out loud, also may help.

5. Limit caffeine.

6. Use nightlights in the bedroom, hall, and bathroom.

Chapter 41

Driving Safety and Alzheimer Disease

Good drivers are alert, think clearly, and make good decisions. When a person with Alzheimer disease (AD) is not able to do these things, she or he should stop driving. But, she or he may not want to stop driving or even think there is a problem.

As the caregiver, you will need to talk with the person about the need to stop driving. Do this in a caring way. Understand how unhappy the person may be to admit that she or he has reached this new stage.

Safety First

A person with some memory loss may be able to drive safely sometimes. But, she or he may not be able to react quickly when faced with a surprise on the road. Someone could get hurt or killed. If the person's reaction time slows, you need to stop the person from driving.

Here are some other things to know about driving and memory loss:

- The person may be able to drive short distances on local streets during the day but may not be able to drive safely at night or on a freeway. If this is the case, then limit the times and places the person can drive.

This chapter includes text excerpted from "Driving Safety and Alzheimer's Disease," National Institute on Aging (NIA), National Institutes of Health (NIH), May 18, 2017.

- Some people with memory problems decide on their own not to drive, while others may deny they have a problem.

Signs that the person should stop driving include new dents and scratches on the car. You may also notice that the person takes a long time to do a simple errand and cannot explain why, which may indicate that she or he got lost.

To find out if a person with Alzheimer disease (AD) is still competent to drive, watch him or her drive at different times of the day, in different types of traffic, and in different road conditions and weather. If riding with the driver is not possible, follow the driver in another vehicle. Over time, a picture will emerge of things the driver can and cannot do well.

When Driving Becomes Unsafe

Here are some ways to stop people with Alzheimer disease from driving:

- Try talking about your concerns with the person.

- Take him or her to get a driving test.

- Ask the doctor to tell him or her to stop driving. The doctor can write, "Do not drive" on a prescription pad, and you can show this to the person.

- Hide the car keys, move the car, take out the distributor cap, or disconnect the battery.

Finding Other Transportation Options

If a person with AD can no longer drive, find other ways that the person can travel on her or his own. Contact your local Area Agency on Aging (AAA) or Eldercare Locator for information about transportation services in your area. These services may include free or low-cost buses, taxi service, or carpools for older people. Some churches and community groups have volunteers who take seniors wherever they want to go. Family and friends are another great resource.

If the person with Alzheimer disease won't stop driving, ask your State Department of Motor Vehicles (DMV) about a medical review. The person may be asked to retake a driving test. In some cases, the person's license could be taken away.

Chapter 42

Living Alone with Alzheimer Disease or Dementia

People with Alzheimer disease (AD) and other dementias who live alone have care needs that differ and that are dependent on factors including the extent of their cognitive and functional abilities, availability of a caregiver, access to adequate care and services, and coordination of care. People with dementia generally report fewer unmet care needs than their caregivers. The number of reported unmet care needs is related to the severity of their dementia and their living situation. Some reasons for unmet needs in community-dwelling people with dementia, including those living alone, are lack of knowledge of existing services and that some of the services are insufficient and not customized to the person's needs or preferences.

Many people with dementia who live alone are at risk for self-neglect. Self-neglect is when a vulnerable adult is unable to practice basic self-care, including but not limited to provision of food, clothing, or shelter, and management of healthcare needs; physical and mental health maintenance, emotional well-being, and general safety; or manage financial affairs. Signs of self-neglect include dehydration, malnutrition, untreated medical conditions, poor personal hygiene, unsafe or unsanitary living conditions, inappropriate or inadequate

This chapter includes text excerpted from "Identifying and Meeting the Needs of Individuals with Dementia Who Live Alone," Administration for Community Living (ACL), September 2015. Reviewed December 2018.

clothing, and inadequate housing or homelessness. In a survey conducted by the National Association of Professional Geriatric Care Managers (NAPGCM), 92 percent of care managers said that elder self-neglect was a significant problem in their community and 94 percent of care managers indicated that elder self-neglect is a largely hidden problem with cases frequently going unreported. According to a national survey on vulnerable adult abuse conducted by the National Center on Elder Abuse (NCEA), self-neglect is the highest category of abuse investigated and substantiated by Adult Protective Services (APS).

Self-neglect in older adults includes both medical and social care needs and has implications for public health. Cases of self-neglect can be among the most difficult to address and manage. At times, a person will resist interventions, deny or underestimate the severity and importance of his or her cognitive deficits, and have little or no awareness regarding his or her circumstances thus placing them at greater risk for adverse outcomes. Service providers working with these individuals are presented with the ethical dilemma of balancing efforts to support individual autonomy with efforts to ensure safety, with the understanding that there is "no perfect environment" for someone with dementia living alone and that "a certain amount of risk is inevitable."

People with dementia who live alone may underuse needed long-term services and supports. In a study of African American older adults with dementia living in the community, social workers rated 61 percent of the persons with dementia living alone as receiving inadequate support and supervision, compared with 25 percent of persons with dementia living with others. A study from Sweden indicated that a large number of people with Alzheimer disease (AD) or other dementia living alone had severe cognitive and functional impairment, but use of home help services did not match the severity of cognitive impairment.

Ability to Manage Personal Care Needs and Daily Activities

Among individuals with dementia, the ability to live alone is dependent on their physical ability and cognitive capacity to perform daily activities independently. Miranda-Castillo reported that individuals with dementia who lived alone had significantly more unmet needs than those living with others, particularly in the areas of looking after the home, food, self-care, and accidental self-harm. One study indicated that activity of daily living impairment was more common among subjects who lived with others but nearly half of the individuals with dementia living alone were found to have two or more impairments in instrumental activities of daily living.

People living alone with dementia are also at greater risk for malnutrition than those living with others. A study of individuals with dementia and their caregivers (about half of whom lived separately from each other) showed that the nutritional status of older people with dementia is strongly and positively associated with the nutritional status of caregivers. Accordingly, it is recommended that nutritional interventions in the context of dementia should address the caregiving dyad and not strictly the person with dementia.

Medication nonadherence is a complex problem with various risk factors, particularly in older adults living alone. Accidental injuries from errors in medication self-administration are more likely for people with dementia than injury from fires/burns and wandering. According to one study, the majority of self-medication errors occurred in administering the medication, modifying the medication regimen, or not following clinical advice about medication use. These errors were attributed to cognitive deficits, sensory or physical problems with dispensers, or the complexity of the regimen.

In a study of 339 elderly participants with cognitive impairment who lived alone and took at least one medication, 17.4 percent had at least one report of medication nonadherence. The most frequently occurring medical consequences were essential hypertension (13.0%), exacerbation of diabetes mellitus (13.0%), complications of heart disease (8.7%), constipation (8.7%), and edema (8.7%). Eleven (47.8%) of the 23 who had a medical consequence also required an emergency medical service.

Indications that a person with dementia living alone is not able to adequately manage his or her personal care needs and daily activities include frequent emergency medical visits, little or no food in the home, unkempt appearance, dirty clothes, and inappropriate clothing for the weather. Intervention strategies include referral for pharmacist or nurse medication reconciliation, home-delivered meals, arranging for home care services, and notifying the police and fire departments of the person's condition and providing contact information.

Home Safety Issues

Alzheimer and other dementias result in deficiencies that can reduce an individual's ability to remain safe at home, such as impairments in balance and mobility, judgment, sense of time and place, orientation and recognition of environmental cues, and changes in vision or hearing. As a result of an impaired judgment, visual and spatial perception deficits, and disorientation, cognitive impairment increases the risk of falls by almost two-fold. Falls are the most common source of in-home accidents leading to morbidity and mortality. Falls are also the leading source of in-home injury in dementia. Signs that a person is at risk for falling include confusion, poor balance and unsteady gait, and four or more prescription medications.

Compulsive hoarding or extreme clutter and debris in the home can contribute to an individual's inability to manage his or her own daily activities and self-care. Food preparation becomes difficult if the person cannot access cooking appliances or even cupboards where food is stored. A significantly cluttered environment can lead to unsanitary living conditions and poses safety risks such as fire or falls/trips hazards. The living conditions affect not only the individual and family members but also neighbors and can become a public health concern.

Safety considerations and adaptations to the home to reduce safety risks include removal of throw rugs that may be a trip hazard, placement of latches on kitchen cabinets and drawers to keep knives and cleaning products out of reach, monitoring the environment for rearranging or removing furniture, removal of clutter and organization of areas of the home, installation of a ramp and grab bars in the bathroom, and widening doorways. Various types of assistive technology can also be used to prevent injuries in the home such as gas detectors, room air temperature monitors, and devices that monitor water levels to prevent accidents and damage from flooding. Technology is available to alert a caregiver or emergency response system when the person with dementia has fallen. These systems may monitor for activity in the home or may detect falls through a floor impact sensor.

Wandering

Wandering is a serious safety risk for people with dementia living alone because the likelihood of a person returning home safely largely depends on others recognizing that the person is missing or that something is unusual and reporting it to the appropriate authorities. Rowe and Glover define "unattended wandering" as forays into the community without the supervision of a caregiver. The professionals interviewed indicated that those at greatest risk are individuals with dementia living alone or living with a caregiver who leaves them alone while attending to other family or job responsibilities.

The Alzheimer Association suggests that families make a plan if someone with dementia goes missing. Strategies include keeping a list of people to call on for help, a recent close-up photo, a list of places where the person may wander, and enrolling the person in an identification program. A missing person report should be filed immediately so that police can begin to search for the individual.

Global positioning systems (GPS) and other assistive technologies are being used to monitor and locate people with dementia at risk of wandering. A person can wear a location device as a watch or pendant, carry it like a mobile phone, or even mount it to the car. As technology advances, people with dementia are being engaged in the process of design with the hope of leading to devices that are more acceptable, user-friendly, and relevant to their needs. There are some limitations to using these devices. GPS and other assistive technologies are dependent on transmission and reception capability to be effective and buildings or other objects can impede signal transmission. In addition, a person with dementia may not like wearing or carrying a device and may remove it.

Although a location device may increase personal freedom and provide peace of mind to the person with dementia and those close to her or him, the decision to use one raises ethical issues regarding personal autonomy and privacy. Some have also suggested that having a location device may lead family members or friends to check in with the person less often. Experts have also suggested that the person with dementia is involved in decision-making and that this decision should be made in a formal structured meeting facilitated by a professional team.

Ability to Respond to Emergencies

The ability of persons with dementia to respond to crisis situations in the home is another important safety concern. One study found that older people who die as a result of a fire are more likely to be living alone than other older people. Another study of 38 people with dementia who are living at home demonstrated that those living alone were perceived to be more at risk than those living with someone, and the most commonly reported risks included fire, nutrition, and medication management. Dementia increases the risk of fire-related death. Alden found that the majority of persons with burn injuries among persons with dementia were unsupervised at the time of injury and were burned while performing routine activities of daily living, such as cooking or bathing. The causes of burn injuries were predominantly bathroom or kitchen scalding and flame burns, suggesting that routine cooking and bathroom activities are of concern when an individual with dementia is alone.

Living alone with dementia increases the risk of mortality associated with accidental injuries because of impaired insight and problem-solving ability, the absence of a caregiver and delayed medical help. Difficulties in using the telephone are common among individuals with dementia living alone, so when emergencies do arise calling for help may not be possible.

Home and community-based services providers need to understand how to respond in an emergency, to the unique needs of someone with dementia who lives alone. Emergency personnel at the time of the crisis situation should have access to concise, accurate information about the person's medical conditions, medications and dosage, and other important information.

Home and community-based services providers should be trained on working with first responders such as fire personnel or police to assist with finding individuals in emergency situations, effective communication strategies for people with dementia, and effective approaches when offers of assistance meet resistance.

Financial Exploitation

According to the National Elder Abuse Incidence Study, financial exploitation is one of the most commonly reported types of elder abuse in people with dementia living alone. The perpetrators are often friends or family members who have a relationship of trust with the victim. The National Association of Adult Protective Services Administrators (NAAPSA) recommends that all professional financial service providers receive special training on identifying and reporting financial exploitation.

Marson defines financial capacity as the ability to independently manage one's financial affairs in a manner consistent with one's personal interests and values. Further, he notes that financial capacity has both a performance aspect and a judgment aspect. The person must be able to perform a variety of tasks and skills to meet his or her financial needs such as recognizing money and its value when paying for things at the store or understanding basic financial terms and concepts such as a mortgage, will, or annuity. In addition, the individual must be able to use appropriate judgment and decision-making regarding household budget and financial investments.

Individuals with dementia are at risk for financial exploitation or money mismanagement when they are unable to get to the bank without assistance; have multiple care providers; repeatedly targeted by cold callers and scams; or leave money, bills, and other financial information around the house. An individual with dementia is also at risk if they are socially isolated and have a propensity to talk about their financial situation with strangers; or feel pressured by family or friends for money. Care providers and family members can reduce the risk of exploitation by removing the person's name from telemarketer lists, checking their credit report yearly, enrolling in automatic bill payment, and notifying shopkeepers, bank tellers, and others of the person's difficulty with financial transactions.

Social Isolation and Loneliness

Relationships with others and having the support of family and friends are important to sustain people with dementia who live alone. In a qualitative study of 15 people with dementia who live alone, the participants indicated that having a strong social support network was the most important factor in helping them cope with living alone. The study participants were concerned about maintaining their independence, continuing to drive, and being involved in decision making for as long as possible. Most were comfortable living alone but they did experience feelings of loneliness. The author suggests that services for people with dementia living alone need to be sensitive to the person's needs and wishes, and not just about responding to safety concerns.

A study found that people with dementia who live alone with an unmet care need did not manage everyday life when they felt lonely. Feelings of loneliness may negatively impact a person's ability to act and engage in everyday activities. The presence of a homecare worker, for the purpose of performing a task, did not relieve feelings of loneliness. One of the participants in the study described the home care worker as being rushed and expressed a wish for a longer visit to allow for companionship and conversation. The authors also found that without the presence of others, the person with dementia seemed to lack initiative and experienced difficulties in managing everyday life. The importance of the presence of caregivers for those who live alone with dementia that addresses needs for socialization and not solely focus on specific tasks or physical needs.

If there is no one in the home to observe changes in the person's cognitive and functional abilities, the progressive decline associated with Alzheimer or related dementia may go unnoticed until it is a problem. Changes in the ability to plan, organize, and follow through with daily activities and personal care needs are likely to lead to self-neglect because of the individual's lack of insight and poor judgment.

Chapter 43

Financial Concerns and Alzheimer Disease

People with Alzheimer disease (AD) often have problems managing their money. In fact, money problems may be one of the first noticeable signs of the disease.

Early on, a person with AD may be able to perform basic tasks, such as paying bills, but she or he is likely to have problems with more complicated tasks, such as balancing a checkbook. As the disease gets worse, the person may try to hide financial problems to protect his or her independence. Or, the person may not realize that she or he is losing the ability to handle money matters.

Signs of Money Problems

Look for signs of money problems such as trouble counting change, paying for a purchase, calculating a tip, balancing a checkbook, or understanding a bank statement. The person may be afraid or worried when she or he talks about money. You may also find:

- Unpaid and unopened bills

This chapter contains text excerpted from the following sources: Text in this chapter begins with excerpts from "Managing Money Problems in Alzheimer's Disease," National Institute on Aging (NIA), National Institutes of Health (NIH), May 18, 2017; Text under the heading "Saving Money on Medicines" is excerpted from "Saving Money on Medicines," National Institute on Aging (NIA), National Institutes of Health (NIH), May 23, 2017.

- Lots of new purchases on a credit card bill
- Strange new merchandise
- Money missing from the person's bank account

A family member or trustee (someone who holds title to property and/or funds for the person) should check bank statements and other financial records each month to see how the person with Alzheimer disease is doing and step in if there are serious concerns. This can protect the person from becoming a victim of financial abuse or fraud.

Take Steps Early

Many older adults will be suspicious of attempts to take over their financial affairs. You can help the person with AD feel independent by:

- Giving him or her small amounts of cash or voided checks to have on hand
- Minimizing the spending limit on credit cards or having the cards canceled
- Telling the person that it is important to learn about finances, with his or her help

To prevent serious problems, you may have to take charge of the person's financial affairs through legal arrangements. It's important to handle the transfer of financial authority with respect and understanding.

You can get consent to manage the person's finances via a durable power of attorney for finances, preferably while the person can still understand and approve the arrangement. You can also ensure that the person finalizes trusts and estate arrangements.

Guard against Financial Abuse and Fraud

People with AD may be victims of financial abuse or scams by dishonest people. Sometimes, the person behind the scam is a "friend" or family member. Telephone, e-mail, or in-person scams can take many forms, such as:

- Identity theft
- Get-rich-quick offers
- Phony offers of prizes or home or auto repairs

- Insurance scams

- Health scams such as ads for unproven memory aids

- Threats

Look for signs that the person with AD may be a victim of financial abuse or fraud:

- There are signatures on checks or other papers don't look like the person's signature

- The person's will has been changed without permission

- The person's home is sold, and she or he did not agree to sell it

- The person has signed legal papers (such as a will, power of attorney, or joint deed to a house) without knowing what the papers mean

- Things that belong to you or the person with AD, such as clothes or jewelry, are missing from the home

Saving Money on Medicines

Medicines can be costly. If they are too expensive for you, the doctor may be able to suggest less expensive alternatives. If the doctor does not know the cost, ask the pharmacist before filling the prescription. You can ask your doctor if there is a generic or other less expensive choice. Your doctor may also be able to refer you to a medical assistance program that can help with drug costs.

Ask your insurance company for a copy of your drug plan "formulary"—the list of all medicines covered by your insurance company—and bring it to your doctors' appointments. Together, you and your doctor can evaluate the choice of medicines that will be most cost effective.

You might be thinking about buying your medicines online to save some money. It's important to know which websites are safe and reliable. The U.S. Food and Drug Administration (FDA) has safety tips for buying medicines and medical products online.

Some insurance drug plans offer special prices on medicines if you order directly from them rather than filling prescriptions at a pharmacy. Contact the Centers for Medicare & Medicaid Services (CMS) to learn about Medicare prescription drug plans that may help save you money, or visit www.medicare.gov/part-d. You can also contact your State Health Insurance Assistance Program. If you are a veteran, the

U.S. Department of Veterans Affairs (VA) may also be able to help with your prescriptions.

Here are some websites that can provide additional assistance:

- Medicare Extra Help Program (www.ssa.gov/benefits/medicare/ prescriptionhelp) provides information about the Social Security assistance program and application process for the Medicare Part D subsidy.

- State Pharmaceutical Assistance Program (SPAP) (www. medicare.gov/pharmaceutical-assistance-program/state-programs.aspx) provides information about any available state-funded assistance programs for prescription drug costs.

- Partnership for Prescription Assistance (www.pparx.org) helps connect underinsured people with patient assistance programs for which they may be eligible.

Chapter 44

Medicare and Alzheimer Disease

What's Medicare?

Medicare is the federal health insurance program for:

- People who are 65 or older
- Certain younger people with disabilities
- People with end-stage renal disease (permanent kidney failure requiring dialysis or a transplant, sometimes called ESRD)

The different parts of Medicare help cover specific services:

Medicare Part A (Hospital Insurance)

Part A covers inpatient hospital stays, care in a skilled nursing facility, hospice care, and some home healthcare.

This chapter contains text excerpted from the following sources: Text under the heading "What's Medicare?" is excerpted from "What's Medicare?" Centers for Medicare & Medicaid Services (CMS), September 14, 2018; Text beginning with the heading "How to Get Medicare Coverage" is excerpted from "Things to Think about When You Compare Medicare Drug Coverage," Centers for Medicare & Medicaid Services (CMS), December 2017.

Medicare Part B (Medical Insurance)

Part B covers certain doctors' services, outpatient care, medical supplies, and preventive services.

Medicare Part D (Prescription Drug Coverage)

Part D adds prescription drug coverage to:

- Original Medicare
- Some Medicare Cost Plans
- Some Medicare Private-Fee-for-Service (PFFS) Plans
- Medicare Medical Savings Account (MSA) Plans

These plans are offered by insurance companies and other private companies approved by Medicare. Medicare Advantage Plans may also offer prescription drug coverage that follows the same rules as Medicare Prescription Drug Plans.

How to Get Medicare Coverage

There are two ways to get Medicare prescription drug coverage. You can join a Medicare Prescription Drug Plan and keep your health coverage under Original Medicare. Or, you could join a Medicare Advantage Plan (like an health maintenance organization (HMO) or preferred provider organization (PPO) that offers prescription drug coverage to get your Medicare benefits through a private insurance company. Whichever you choose, prescription drug coverage can vary by cost, coverage, convenience, and quality. Some of these things might be more important to you than others, depending on your situation and prescription drug needs.

No matter which type of Medicare drug plan you join, your plan will send you information about plan changes each fall. You should review your prescription drug needs and compare Medicare drug plans during Medicare Open Enrollment, which runs between October 15 to December 7.

Cost

When you get Medicare prescription drug coverage, you pay part of the costs, and Medicare pays part of the costs. Your costs will vary depending on which drug plan you choose and whether or not you get Extra Help. You should look at your current prescription drug costs to find a drug plan that works with your financial situation.

Monthly Premium

Most drug plans charge a monthly fee that varies by plan. You pay this fee in addition to the Medicare Part B (Medical Insurance) premium. If you have the type of Medicare Advantage Plan or Medicare Cost Plan that includes Medicare prescription drug coverage, the monthly premium you pay to your plan may include an amount for prescription drug coverage.

Consider Automatic Premium Deduction

When you join a Medicare drug plan, think about having your premiums automatically deducted from your Social Security payment. Automatic premium deduction has many benefits:

- It takes the worry out of remembering to pay your premiums

- Your premiums will get paid on time

- You'll be helping the environment by not getting a paper bill from your plan

Yearly Deductible

This is the amount you must pay before your drug plan begins to pay its share of your covered drugs. Some drug plans don't have a deductible.

Copayment / Coinsurance

This is the amount you pay for each of your prescriptions after you've paid the deductible (if the plan has one). Some drug plans have different levels or "tiers" of coinsurance or copayments, with different costs for different types of drugs. Coinsurance means you pay a percentage (25%, for example) of the cost of the drug. With a copayment, you pay a set amount ($10, for example) for all drugs on a tier. For example, you might have to pay a lower copayment for generic drugs than brand-name drugs, or lower coinsurance for some brand-name drugs than for others.

Coverage Gap

Most drug plans have a coverage gap (also called the "donut hole"). This means that there's a temporary limit on what the drug plan will cover for drugs. The coverage gap begins after you and your drug plan have spent a certain amount for covered drugs. In 2018, once you enter the coverage gap, you pay 35 percent of the plan's cost for covered brand-name drugs and 44 percent of the plan's cost for covered generic drugs until you reach the end of the coverage gap. Not everyone will enter the coverage gap.

These amounts all count toward you getting out of the coverage gap:

- Your yearly deductible, coinsurance, and copayments

- The discount you get on brand-name drugs in the coverage gap

- What you pay in the coverage gap

These amounts don't count toward you getting out of the coverage gap:

- Your Medicare drug plan premium

- What you pay for noncovered drugs

- What's paid by other insurance

Some plans offer additional coverage during the gap, like for generic drugs, but they may charge a higher monthly premium. Check with the plan first to see if your drugs would be covered during the gap.

In addition to the discount on covered brand-name prescription drugs, there will be increasing coverage for drugs in the coverage gap each year until the gap closes in 2020.

Catastrophic Coverage

Once you get out of the coverage gap, you automatically get "catastrophic coverage." Catastrophic coverage means that you only pay a small coinsurance amount or copayment for covered drugs for the rest of the year.

Late Enrollment Penalty

If you don't join a Medicare drug plan when you're first eligible, and you don't have other creditable prescription drug coverage or get Extra Help, you'll likely pay a Part D late enrollment penalty. Creditable prescription drug coverage is coverage (for example, from an employer or union) that's expected to pay, on average, at least as much as Medicare's standard prescription drug coverage. If you're subject to the penalty, you may have to pay it each month for as long as you have Medicare drug coverage.

Coverage

Review your prescription drug needs, and look for a plan that meets these needs. Medicare drug plans may vary in what drugs they cover, and some may have special rules that you must follow before a drug is covered.

Formulary

A formulary is a list of the drugs that a drug plan covers. It includes how much you pay for each drug. If the plan uses tiers, the formulary lists which drugs are in each tier. Formularies include both generic and brand-name drugs. In general, each drug plan's formulary must include most types of drugs that people with Medicare use. However, each drug plan has its own formulary, so you should check to make sure your drugs are covered.

Coverage Rules

Drug plans may require "prior authorization." This means that before the drug plan will cover certain prescriptions, you must show the plan you meet certain criteria for you to have that particular drug. Your doctor may need to provide additional information about why the drug is medically necessary for you before you can fill the prescription. Plans may also require "step therapy" on certain drugs. This means you must try one or more similar, lower cost drugs before the plan will cover the prescribed drug. Plans may also set "quantity limits"—limits on how much medication you can get.

Convenience

Check with each drug plan you're considering to make sure your current pharmacy is in the plan's network or there are pharmacies convenient to you. Some drug plans charge lower copayments or coinsurance amounts at some pharmacies in their network than at others. Also, some drug plans may offer a mail-order program that will allow you to have drugs sent directly to your home. You should consider the most cost effective and convenient way to have your prescriptions filled.

Quality

In addition to a plan's costs, coverage, and convenience, you should also review the quality ratings for plans before you decide which one best meets your needs. Medicare uses information from member satisfaction surveys, plans, and healthcare providers to give overall performance star ratings to plans. A plan can get a rating between one to five stars. A five-star rating is considered excellent. These ratings are listed on the Medicare Plan Finder at Medicare.gov/find-a-plan.

Five-Star Special Enrollment Period

You can switch to a Medicare Advantage Plan or a Medicare Prescription Drug Plan that has Five stars for its overall plan rating once from December 8, 2017 to November 30, 2018. The overall plan ratings are available at Medicare.gov/find-a-plan. Medicare updates these ratings each fall for the following year. These ratings can change each year.

You can only switch to a Five-star Medicare drug plan if one is available in your area.

You can only use this Special Enrollment Period once during the above timeframe.

What Should I Do before Making a Decision?

Each year, you have the opportunity to join or switch Medicare drug plans during Medicare Open Enrollment, which runs from October 15 to December 7. If you switch plans during this time, your coverage with the new plan will start on January 1. As you make a decision about your health and prescription drug coverage, remember to review your current health and prescription drug plans. Health and drug plan benefits and costs can change each year. Look at other plans in your area to see if one may better meet your needs. If you want to keep your current plan, and it's still being offered next year, you don't need to do anything for your enrollment to continue.

Where Can I Get Help?

To help you compare drug plans, think about what you need in terms of cost, coverage, convenience, and quality. Then, visit Medicare. gov/find-a-plan to see which plans are available in your area. To get personalized information, you need:

Table 44.1. Some Common Situations to Consider

If You...	You Might Want to...
...currently take specific prescription drugs.	...look at drug plans that have included your drugs on their formularies. Then, compare costs
...want extra protection from high prescription drug costs.	...look for plans that offer coverage in the coverage gap, and then check with those plans to be sure your drugs would be covered during the gap. (The plans may charge a higher monthly premium.)
...want your drug expenses to be balanced throughout the year	...want your drug expenses to be balanced throughout the year
...take a lot of generic prescriptions.	...look at plans with tiers that charge you nothing or low copayments for generic prescriptions.
...don't have many drug costs now, but want coverage for peace of mind and to avoid future penalties.	...look for plans with low monthly premiums for drug coverage. If you need prescriptions in the future, all plans still must cover most drugs used by people with Medicare.
...like the extra benefits and lower costs that are available by getting your healthcare and prescription drug coverage from one plan and are willing to accept the plan's restrictions on what doctors, hospitals, and other healthcare providers you can use.	...look for Medicare Advantage Plans with prescription drug coverage.

- Your Medicare card that has your Medicare number and Medicare effective date (Medicare Part A [Hospital Insurance] or Medicare Part B [Medical Insurance])
- Date of birth (DOB)
- Last name
- ZIP (zone improvement plan) code

To get general drug plan information or to find out what plans are available in your area, just answer a few simple questions. You can also enter your current prescription drug information to get more detailed cost information.

Chapter 45

Getting Your Affairs in Order

Chapter Contents

Section 45.1

Planning for the Future

This section includes text excerpted from "Getting Your Affairs in Order," National Institute on Aging (NIA), National Institutes of Health (NIH), June 1, 2018.

No one ever plans to be sick or disabled. Yet, it's this kind of planning that can make all the difference in an emergency.

What Exactly Is an "Important Paper"?

The answer to this question may be different for every family. Remember, this is a starting place. You may have other information to add. For example, if you have a pet, you will want to include the name and address of your veterinarian. Include complete information about:

Personal Records

- Full legal name

- Social Security number (SSN)

- Legal residence

- Date and place of birth

- Names and addresses of spouse and children

- Location of birth and death certificates and certificates of marriage, divorce, citizenship, and adoption

- Employers and dates of employment

- Education and military records

- Names and phone numbers of religious contacts

- Memberships in groups and awards received

- Names and phone numbers of close friends, relatives, doctors, lawyers, and financial advisors

- Medications taken regularly (be sure to update this regularly)

- Location of living will and other legal documents

Financial Records

- Sources of income and assets (pension from your employer, IRAs, 401(k)s, interest, etc.)

- Social Security and Medicare/Medicaid information

- Insurance information (life, health, long-term care, home, car) with policy numbers and agents' names and phone numbers

- Names of your banks and account numbers (checking, savings, credit union)

- Investment income (stocks, bonds, and property) and stockbrokers' names and phone numbers

- Copy of most recent income tax return

- Location of most up-to-date will with an original signature

- Liabilities, including property tax—what is owed, to whom, and when payments are due

- Mortgages and debts—how and when they are paid

- Location of original deed of trust for home

- Car title and registration

- Credit and debit card names and numbers

- Location of safe deposit box and key

Steps for Getting Your Affairs in Order

- Put your important papers and copies of legal documents in one place. You can set up a file, put everything in a desk or dresser drawer, or list the information and location of papers in a notebook. If your papers are in a bank safe deposit box, keep copies in a file at home. Check each year to see if there's anything new to add.

- Tell a trusted family member or friend where you put all your important papers. You don't need to tell this friend or family member about your personal affairs, but someone should know where you keep your papers in case of an emergency. If you don't have a relative or friend you trust, ask a lawyer to help.

- Discuss your end-of-life preferences with your doctor. She or he can explain what health decisions you may have to make in the future and what treatment options are available. Talking with your doctor can help ensure your wishes are honored, and the visit may be covered by insurance.

- Give permission in advance for your doctor or lawyer to talk with your caregiver as needed. There may be questions about your care, a bill, or a health insurance claim. Without your consent, your caregiver may not be able to get needed information. You can give your okay in advance to Medicare, a credit card company, your bank, or your doctor. You may need to sign and return a form.

Legal Documents

There are many different types of legal documents that can help you plan how your affairs will be handled in the future. Many of these documents have names that sound alike, so make sure you are getting the documents you want. Also, state laws vary, so find out about the rules, requirements, and forms used in your state.

Wills and trusts let you name the person you want your money and property to go to after you die.

Advance directives let you make arrangements for your care if you become sick. Two common types of advance directives are:

- A living will gives you a say in your healthcare if you become too sick to make your wishes known. In a living will, you can state what kind of care you do or don't want. This can make it easier for family members to make tough healthcare decisions for you.

- A durable power of attorney for healthcare lets you name the person you want to make medical decisions for you if you can't make them yourself. Make sure the person you name is willing to make those decisions for you.

For legal matters, there are ways to give someone you trust the power to act in your place.

- A general power of attorney lets you give someone else the authority to act on your behalf, but this power will end if you are unable to make your own decisions.

- A durable power of attorney allows you to name someone to act on your behalf for any legal task, but it stays in place if you become unable to make your own decisions.

Help for Getting Your Papers in Order

You may want to talk with a lawyer about setting up a general power of attorney, durable power of attorney, joint account, trust, or advance directive. Be sure to ask about the lawyer's fees before you make an appointment.

You should be able to find a directory of local lawyers on the Internet or at your local library, or you can contact your local bar association for lawyers in your area. Your local bar association can also help you find what free legal aid options your state has to offer. An informed family member may be able to help you manage some of these issues.

Section 45.2

Legal and Healthcare Planning Document

This section includes text excerpted from "Legal and Financial Planning for People with Alzheimer's," National Institute on Aging (NIA), National Institutes of Health (NIH), November 15, 2017.

Many people are unprepared to deal with the legal and financial consequences of a serious illness such as Alzheimer disease (AD). Legal and medical experts encourage people recently diagnosed with a serious illness—particularly one that is expected to cause declining mental and physical health—to examine and update their financial and healthcare arrangements as soon as possible. Basic legal and financial documents, such as a will, a living trust, and advance directives, are available to ensure that the person's late-stage or end-of-life healthcare and financial decisions are carried out.

A complication of diseases such as AD is that the person may lack or gradually lose the ability to think clearly. This change affects his or her ability to make decisions and participate in legal and financial planning.

People with early-stage Alzheimer disease (EOAD) can often understand many aspects and consequences of legal decision making. However, legal and medical experts say that many forms of planning can

345

help the person and his or her family even if the person is diagnosed with later-stage Alzheimer disease.

There are good reasons to retain a lawyer when preparing advance planning documents. For example, a lawyer can help interpret different state laws and suggest ways to ensure that the person's and family's wishes are carried out. It's important to understand that laws vary by state, and changes in a person's situation—for instance, a divorce, relocation, or death in the family—can influence how documents are prepared and maintained.

Legal, Financial, and Healthcare Planning Documents

Families beginning the legal planning process should discuss a number of strategies and legal documents. Depending on the family situation and the applicable state laws, a lawyer may introduce some or all of the following terms and documents to assist in this process:

- Documents that communicate the healthcare wishes of someone who can no longer make healthcare decisions

- Documents that communicate the financial management and estate plan wishes of someone who can no longer make financial decisions

Advance Directives for Healthcare

Advance directives for healthcare are documents that communicate the healthcare wishes of a person with Alzheimer disease. These decisions are then carried out after the person no longer can make decisions. In most cases, these documents must be prepared while the person is legally able to execute them.

A living will records a person's wishes for medical treatment near the end-of-life or if the person is permanently unconscious and cannot make decisions about emergency treatment.

A durable power of attorney for healthcare designates a person, sometimes called an agent or proxy, to make healthcare decisions when the person with Alzheimer disease no longer can do so.

A do not resuscitate (DNR) order instructs healthcare professionals not to perform cardiopulmonary resuscitation (CPR) if a person's heart stops or if she or he stops breathing. A DNR order is signed by a doctor and put in a person's medical chart.

In addition to these, there may be other documents discussing organ and tissue donation, dialysis, and blood transfusions.

Advance Directives for Financial and Estate Management

Advance directives for financial and estate management must be created while the person with Alzheimer disease still can make these decisions (sometimes referred to as "having legal capacity" to make decisions). These directives may include the following:

A will indicates how a person's assets and estate will be distributed upon death. It also can specify:

- Arrangements for care of minors

- Gifts

- Trusts to manage the estate

- Funeral and/or burial arrangements

- Medical and legal experts say that the newly diagnosed person with Alzheimer disease and his or her family should move quickly to make or update a will and secure the estate

A durable power of attorney for finances names someone to make financial decisions when the person with Alzheimer disease no longer can. It can help people with the disease and their families avoid court actions that may take away control of financial affairs.

A living trust provides instructions about the person's estate and appoints someone, called the trustee, to hold title to property and funds for the beneficiaries. The trustee follows these instructions after the person with Alzheimer disease no longer can manage his or her affairs.

The person with Alzheimer disease also can name the trustee as the healthcare proxy through the durable power of attorney for healthcare.

A living trust can:

- Include a wide range of property

- Provide a detailed plan for property disposition

- Avoid the expense and delay of probate (in which the courts establish the validity of a will)

- State how property should be distributed when the last beneficiary dies and whether the trust should continue to benefit others

Who Can Help?

Healthcare providers cannot act as legal or financial advisers, but they can encourage planning discussions between patients and their families. Qualified clinicians can also guide patients, families, the care team, attorneys, and judges regarding the patient's ability to make decisions. Medicare covers advance care planning discussions between doctors and their patients.

An elder law attorney helps older people and families interpret state laws, plan how their wishes will be carried out, understand their financial options, and learn how to preserve financial assets while caring for a loved one.

The National Academy of Elder Law Attorneys (NAELA) and the American Bar Association (ABA) can help families find qualified attorneys.

Geriatric care managers are trained social workers or nurses who can help people with Alzheimer disease and their families.

Table 45.1. Overview of Medical Documents

Medical Document	How It Is Used
Living Will	Describes and instructs how the person wants end-of-life healthcare managed
Durable Power of Attorney for Healthcare	Gives a designated person the authority to make healthcare decisions on behalf of the person with AD
Do Not Resuscitate (DNR) Order	Instructs healthcare professionals not to perform CPR in case of stopped heart or stopped breathing

Table 45.2. Overview of Legal and Financial Documents

Legal/Financial Document	How It Is Used
Will	Indicates how a person's assets and estate will be distributed among beneficiaries after his/her death
Durable Power of Attorney for Finances	Gives a designated person the authority to make legal/financial decisions on behalf of the person with AD
Living Trust	Gives a designated person (trustee) the authority to hold and distribute property and funds for the person with AD

Other Planning Advice

Start discussions early. The rate of decline differs for each person with Alzheimer disease, and his or her ability to be involved in planning will decline over time. People in the early stages of the disease may be able to understand the issues, but they may also be defensive or emotionally unable to deal with difficult questions. Remember that not all people are diagnosed at an early stage. Decision making already may be difficult when AD is diagnosed.

Review plans over time. Changes in personal situations—such as a divorce, relocation, or death in the family—and in state laws can affect how legal documents are prepared and maintained. Review plans regularly, and update documents as needed.

Reduce anxiety about funeral and burial arrangements. Advance planning for the funeral and burial can provide a sense of peace and reduce anxiety for both the person with AD and the family.

Resources for Low-Income Families

Families who cannot afford a lawyer still can do advance planning. Samples of basic health planning documents are available online. Area Agency on Aging (AAA) officials may provide legal advice or help. Other possible sources of legal assistance and referral include state legal aid offices, state bar associations, local nonprofit agencies, foundations, and social service agencies.

Section 45.3

Healthcare Decisions at the End of Life

This section includes text excerpted from "Understanding Healthcare Decisions at the End of Life," National Institute on Aging (NIA), National Institutes of Health (NIH), May 17, 2017.

It can be overwhelming to be asked to make healthcare decisions for someone who is dying and is no longer able to make his or her own decisions. It is even more difficult if you do not have written or verbal guidance. How do you decide what type of care is right for someone? Even when you have written documents, some decisions still might not be clear since the documents may not address every situation you could face.

Two approaches might be useful. One is to put yourself in the place of the person who is dying and try to choose as she or he would. This is called substituted judgment. Some experts believe that decisions should be based on substituted judgment whenever possible.

Another approach, known as best interests, is to decide what would be best for the dying person. This is sometimes combined with substituted judgment.

If you are making decisions for someone at the end-of-life and are trying to use one of these approaches, it may be helpful to think about the following questions:

- Has the dying person ever talked about what she or he would want at the end-of-life?

- Has she or he expressed an opinion about how someone else was being treated?

- What were his or her values in life? What gave meaning to life? Maybe it was being close to family—watching them grow and making memories together. Perhaps just being alive was the most important thing.

As a decision-maker without specific guidance from the dying person, you need as much information as possible on which to base your actions. You might ask the doctor:

- What might we expect to happen in the next few hours, days, or weeks if we continue our current course of treatment?

- Why is this new test being suggested?

- Will it change the current treatment plan?

- Will a new treatment help my relative get better?

- How would the new treatment change his or her quality of life (QOL)?

- Will it give more quality time with family and friends?

- How long will this treatment take to make a difference?

- If we choose to try this treatment, can we stop it at any time? For any reason?

- What are the side effects of the approach you are suggesting?

- If we try this new treatment and it doesn't work, what then?

- If we don't try this treatment, what will happen?

- Is the improvement we saw today an overall positive sign or just something temporary?

It is a good idea to have someone with you when discussing these issues with medical staff. Having someone take notes or remember details can be very helpful. If you are unclear about something you are told, don't be afraid to ask the doctor or nurse to repeat it or to say it another way that does make sense to you. Keep asking questions until you have all the information you need to make decisions. Make sure you know how to contact a member of the medical team if you have a question or if the dying person needs something.

Sometimes, the whole family wants to be involved in every decision. Maybe that is the family's cultural tradition. Or, maybe the person dying did not pick one person to make healthcare choices before becoming unable to do so. That is not unusual, but it makes sense to choose one person to be the contact when dealing with medical staff. The doctors and nurses will appreciate having to phone only one person.

Even if one family member is named as the decision-maker, it is a good idea, as much as possible, to have family agreement about the care plan. If you can't agree on a care plan, a decision-maker, or even a spokesperson, the family might consider a mediator, someone trained to bring people with different opinions to a common decision.

In any case, as soon as it is clear that the patient is nearing the end of life, the family should try to discuss with the medical team which end-of-life care approach they want for their family member. That way, decision making for crucial situations can be planned and may feel less rushed.

Issues You May Face

Maybe you are now faced with making end-of-life choices for someone close to you. You've thought about that person's values and opinions, and you've asked the healthcare team to explain the treatment plan and what you can expect to happen.

But, there are other issues that are important to understand in case they arise. What if the dying person starts to have trouble breathing and a doctor says a ventilator might be needed? Maybe one family member wants the healthcare team to do everything possible to keep this relative alive. What does that involve? Or, what if family members can't agree on end-of-life care or they disagree with the doctor? What happens then?

Here are some other common end-of-life issues. They will give you a general understanding and may help your conversations with the doctors.

If We Say Do Everything Possible, What Does That Mean?

This means that if someone is dying, all measures that might keep vital organs working will be tried—for example, using a ventilator to support breathing or starting dialysis for failing kidneys. Such life support can sometimes be a temporary measure that allows the body to heal itself and begin to work normally again. It is not intended to be used indefinitely in someone who is dying.

What Can Be Done If Someone's Heart Stops Beating (Cardiac Arrest)?

Cardiopulmonary resuscitation (CPR) can sometimes restart a stopped heart. It is most effective in people who were generally healthy before their heart stopped. During CPR, the doctor repeatedly pushes on the chest with great force and periodically puts air into the lungs. Electric shocks (called defibrillation) may also be used to correct an abnormal heart rhythm, and some medicines might also be given. Although not usually shown on television, the force required for CPR can cause broken ribs or a collapsed lung. Often, CPR does not succeed in older adults who have multiple chronic illnesses or who are already frail.

What If Someone Needs Help Breathing or Completely Stops Breathing (Respiratory Arrest)?

If a patient has very severe breathing problems or has stopped breathing, a ventilator may be needed. A ventilator forces the lungs to work. Initially, this involves intubation, putting a tube attached to a ventilator down the throat into the trachea or windpipe. Because this tube can be quite uncomfortable, people are often sedated with very strong intravenous medicines. Restraints may be used to prevent them from pulling out the tube. If the person needs ventilator support for more than a few days, the doctor might suggest a tracheotomy, sometimes called a "trach" (rhymes with "make"). This tube is then attached to the ventilator. This is more comfortable than a tube down the throat and may not require sedation. Inserting the tube into the trachea is a bedside surgery. A tracheotomy can carry risks, including a collapsed lung, a plugged tracheotomy tube, or bleeding.

How Can I Be Sure the Medical Staff Knows That We Don't Want Efforts to Restore a Heartbeat or Breathing?

Tell the doctor in charge as soon as the patient or person making healthcare decisions decides that CPR or other life-support procedures should not be performed. The doctor will then write this on the patient's chart using terms such as do not resuscitate (DNR), do not attempt to resuscitate (DNAR), allow natural death (AND), or do not intubate (DNI). DNR forms vary by state and are usually available online.

If end-of-life care is given at home, a special nonhospital DNR, signed by a doctor, is needed. This ensures that if emergency medical technicians (EMTs) are called to the house, they will respect your wishes. Make sure it is kept in a prominent place so EMTs can see it. Without a nonhospital DNR, in many states EMTs are required to perform CPR and similar techniques. Hospice staff can help determine whether a medical condition is part of the normal dying process or something that needs the attention of EMTs.

DNR orders do not stop all treatment. They only mean that CPR and a ventilator will not be used. These orders are not permanent—they can be changed if the situation changes.

What about Pacemakers (Or Similar Devices)—Should They Be Turned Off?

A pacemaker is a device implanted under the skin on the chest that keeps a heartbeat regular. It will not keep a dying person alive. Some people have an implantable cardioverter defibrillator (ICD) under the skin. An ICD shocks the heart back into regular rhythm when needed. The ICD should be turned off at the point when life support is no longer wanted. This can be done at the bedside without surgery.

What If the Doctor Suggests a Feeding Tube?

If a patient can't or won't eat or drink, the doctor might suggest a feeding tube. While a patient recovers from an illness, getting nutrition temporarily through a feeding tube can be helpful. But, at the end-of-life, a feeding tube might cause more discomfort than not eating. For people with dementia, tube feeding does not prolong life or prevent aspiration.

As death approaches, loss of appetite is common. Body systems start shutting down, and fluids and food are not needed as before. Some experts believe that at this point few nutrients are absorbed from any type of nutrition, including those received through a feeding tube. Further, after a feeding tube is inserted, the family might need to make a difficult decision about when, or if, to remove it.

If tube feeding will be tried, there are two methods that could be used. In the first, a feeding tube, known as a nasogastric or NG tube, is threaded through the nose down to the stomach to give nutrition for a short time. Sometimes, the tube is uncomfortable. Someone with an NG tube might try to remove it. This usually means the person has to be restrained, which could mean binding his or her hands to the bed.

If tube feeding is required for an extended time, then a gastric or G tube is put directly into the stomach through an opening made in the side or abdomen. This second method is sometimes called a percutaneous endoscopic gastrostomy (PEG) tube. It carries risks of infection, pneumonia, and nausea.

Hand feeding (sometimes called assisted oral feeding) is an alternative to tube feeding. This approach may have fewer risks, especially for people with dementia.

Should Someone Who Is Dying Be Sedated?

Sometimes, for patients very near the end-of-life, the doctor might suggest sedation to manage symptoms that are not responding to other treatments and are still making the patient uncomfortable. This means using medicines to put the patient in a sleep-like state. Many doctors suggest continuing to use comfort care measures like pain medicine even if the dying person is sedated. Sedatives can be stopped at any time. A person who is sedated may still be able to hear what you are saying—so try to keep speaking directly to, not about, him or her. Do not say things you would not want the patient to hear.

What about Antibiotics?

Antibiotics are medicines that fight infections caused by bacteria. Lower respiratory infections (such as pneumonia) and urinary tract infections (UTIs) are often caused by bacteria and are common in older people who are dying. Many antibiotics have side effects, so the value of trying to treat an infection in a dying person should be weighed against any unpleasant side effects. If someone is already dying when the infection began, giving antibiotics is probably not going to prevent death but might make the person feel more comfortable.

Is Refusing Treatment Legal?

Choosing to stop treatment that is not curing or controlling an illness, or deciding not to start a new treatment, is completely legal— whether the choice is made by the person who is dying or by the person making healthcare decisions. Some people think this is like allowing death to happen. The law does not consider refusing such treatment to be either suicide or euthanasia, sometimes called mercy killing.

What Happens If the Doctor and I Have Different Opinions about Care for Someone Who Is Dying?

Sometimes medical staff, the patient, and family members disagree about a medical care decision. This can be especially problematic when the dying person can't tell the doctors what kind of end-of-life care she or he wants. For example, the family might want more active treatment, like chemotherapy, than the doctors think will be helpful. If there is an advance directive explaining the patient's preferences, those guidelines should determine care.

Without the guidance of an advance directive, if there is a disagreement about medical care, it may be necessary to get a second opinion from a different doctor or to consult the ethics committee or patient representative, also known as an ombudsman, of the hospital or facility. Palliative care consultation may also be helpful. An arbitrator (mediator) can sometimes assist people with different views to agree on a plan.

The Doctor Does Not Seem Familiar with Our Family's Views about Dying. What Should We Do?

America is a rich melting pot of religions, races, and cultures. Ingrained in each tradition are expectations about what should happen as a life nears its end. It is important for everyone involved in a patient's care to understand how each family background may influence expectations, needs, and choices.

Your background may be different from that of the doctor with whom you are working. Or, you might be used to a different approach to making healthcare decisions at the end of life than your medical team. For example, many healthcare providers look to a single person—the dying person or his or her chosen representative—for important healthcare decisions at the end of life. But, in some cultures, the entire immediate family takes on that role.

It is helpful to discuss your personal and family traditions with your doctors and nurses. If there are religious or cultural customs surrounding death that are important to you, make sure to tell your healthcare providers.

Knowing that these practices will be honored could comfort the dying person. Telling the medical staff ahead of time may also help avoid confusion and misunderstanding when death occurs. Make sure you understand how the available medical options presented by the healthcare team fit into your family's desires for end-of-life care.

Questions to Ask about Healthcare Decisions

Here are some questions you might want to ask the medical staff:

- What is the care plan? What are the benefits and risks?

- How often should we reassess the care plan?

- If we try using the ventilator to help with breathing and decide to stop, how will that be done?

- If my family member is dying, why does she or he have to be connected to all those tubes and machines? Why do we need more tests?

- What is the best way for our family to work with the care staff?

- How can I make sure I get a daily update on my family member's condition?

- Will you call me if there is a change in his or her condition?

Thoughts to Share

Make sure the healthcare team knows what is important to your family surrounding the end-of-life. You might say:

- In my religion, we . . . (then describe your religious traditions regarding death)

- Where we come from . . . (tell what customs are important to you at the time of death)

- In our family when someone is dying, we prefer . . . (describe what you hope to have happen)

Part Six

Caregiver Concerns

Chapter 46

Caring for a Person with Alzheimer Disease or Dementia

Understanding How Alzheimer Disease Changes People—Challenges and Coping Strategies

Alzheimer disease (AD) is an illness of the brain. It causes large numbers of nerve cells in the brain to die. This affects a person's ability to remember things and think clearly. People with AD become forgetful and easily confused. They may have a hard time concentrating and behave in odd ways. These problems get worse as the illness gets worse, making your job as caregiver harder.

It's important to remember that the disease, not the person with AD, causes these changes. Also, each person with AD may not have all the problems we talk about in this chapter.

This chapter contains text excerpted from the following sources: Text beginning with the heading "Understanding How Alzheimer Disease Changes People— Challenges and Coping Strategies" is excerpted from "Caring for a Person with Alzheimer's Disease," National Institute on Aging (NIA), National Institutes of Health (NIH), January 2017; Text under the heading "Getting Help with Alzheimer Disease Caregiving" is excerpted from "Getting Help with Alzheimer's Disease Caregiving," National Institute on Aging (NIA), National Institutes of Health (NIH), May 18, 2017.

The following sections describe the three main challenges that you may face as you care for someone with AD:

1. Challenge: Changes in Communication Skills

Communication is hard for people with AD because they have trouble remembering things. They may struggle to find words or forget what they want to say. You may feel impatient and wish they could just say what they want, but they can't.

It may help you to know more about common communication problems caused by AD. Once you know more, you'll have a better sense of how to cope.

Here are some communication problems caused by AD:

- Trouble finding the right word when speaking

- Problems understanding what words mean

- Problems paying attention during long conversations

- Loss of train-of-thought when talking

- Trouble remembering the steps in common activities, such as cooking a meal, paying bills, getting dressed, or doing laundry

- Problems blocking out background noises from the radio, TV, telephone calls, or conversations in the room

- Frustration if communication isn't working

- Being very sensitive to touch and to the tone and loudness of voices

Also, AD causes some people to get confused about language. For example, the person might forget or no longer understand English if it was learned as a second language. Instead, she or he might understand and use only the first language learned, such as Spanish.

How to Cope with Changes in Communication Skills

The first step is to understand that the disease causes changes in these skills. The second step is to try some tips that may make communication easier. For example, keep the following suggestions in mind as you go about day-to-day care.

To connect with a person who has AD:

- Make eye contact to get his or her attention, and call the person by name.

- Be aware of your tone and how loud your voice is, how you look at the person, and your "body language." Body language is the message you send just by the way you hold your body. For example, if you stand with your arms folded very tightly, you may send a message that you are tense or angry.

- Encourage a two-way conversation for as long as possible. This helps the person with AD feel better about himself or herself.

- Use other methods besides speaking to help the person, such as gentle touching to guide her or him.

- Try distracting someone with AD if communication creates problems. For example, offer a fun activity such as a snack or a walk around the neighborhood.

To encourage the person with AD to communicate with you:

- Show a warm, loving, matter-of-fact manner

- Hold the person's hand while you talk

- Be open to the person's concerns, even if she or he is hard to understand

- Let her or him make some decisions and stay involved

- Be patient with angry outbursts. Remember, it's the illness "talking"

- If you become frustrated, take a "timeout" for yourself

To speak effectively with a person who has AD:

- Offer simple, step-by-step instructions

- Repeat instructions and allow more time for a response. Try not to interrupt.

- Don't talk about the person as if she or he isn't there

- Don't talk to the person using "baby talk" or a "baby voice"

Here are some examples of what you can say:

- "Let's try this way," instead of pointing out mistakes

- "Please do this," instead of "Don't do this"

- "Thanks for helping," even if the results aren't perfect

You also can:

- Ask questions that require a yes or no answer. For example, you could say, "Are you tired?" instead of "How do you feel?"

- Limit the number of choices. For example, you could say, "Would you like a hamburger or chicken for dinner?" instead of "What would you like for dinner?"

- Use different words if she or he doesn't understand what you say the first time. For example, if you ask the person whether she or he is hungry and you don't get a response, you could say, "Dinner is ready now. Let's eat."

- Try not to say, "Don't you remember?" or "I told you."

2. Challenge: Changes in Personality and Behavior

Because AD causes brain cells to die, the brain works less well over time. This changes how a person acts. You will notice that she or he will have good days and bad days.

Here are some common personality changes you may see:

- Getting upset, worried, and angry more easily
- Acting depressed or not interested in things
- Hiding things or believing other people are hiding things
- Imagining things that aren't there
- Wandering away from home
- Pacing a lot of the time
- Showing unusual sexual behavior
- Hitting you or other people
- Misunderstanding what she or he sees or hears

Also, you may notice that the person stops caring about how she or he looks, stops bathing, and wants to wear the same clothes every day.

Other Factors That May Affect How People with AD Behave

In addition to changes in the brain, the following things may affect how people with AD behave.
How they feel:

- Sadness, fear, or a feeling of being overwhelmed

- Stress caused by something or someone
- Confusion after a change in routine, including travel
- Anxiety about going to a certain place

Health-related problems:

- Illness or pain
- New medications
- Lack of sleep
- Infections, constipation, hunger, or thirst
- Poor eyesight or hearing
- Alcohol abuse
- Too much caffeine

Problems in their surroundings:

- Being in a place she or he doesn't know well
- Too much noise, such as TV, radio, or many people talking at once. Noise can cause confusion or frustration.
- Stepping from one type of flooring to another. The change in texture or the way the floor looks may make the person think she or he needs to take a step down.
- Misunderstanding signs. Some signs may cause confusion. For example, one person with AD thought a sign reading "Wet Floor" meant he should urinate on the floor.
- Mirrors. Someone with AD may think that a mirror image is another person in the room.

How to Cope with Personality and Behavior Changes

Here are some ways to cope with changes in personality and behavior:

- Keep things simple. Ask or say one thing at a time.
- Have a daily routine, so the person knows when certain things will happen.
- Reassure the person that she or he is safe and you are there to help.

- Focus on his or her feelings rather than words. For example, say, "You seem worried."

- Don't argue or try to reason with the person.

- Try not to show your anger or frustration. Step back. Take deep breaths, and count to 10. If safe, leave the room for a few minutes.

- Use humor when you can.

- Give people who pace a lot a safe place to walk. Provide comfortable, sturdy shoes. Give them light snacks to eat as they walk, so they don't lose too much weight, and make sure they have enough to drink.

Use distractions:

- Try using music, singing, or dancing to distract the person. One caregiver found that giving her husband chewing gum stopped his cursing.

- Ask for help. For instance, say, "Let's set the table" or "I really need help folding the clothes."

Other ideas:

Enroll the person in the MedicAlert®+Alzheimer's Association Safe Return® Program. If people with AD wander away from home, this program can help get them home safely (www.alz.org or 888-572-8566).

Talk to the doctor about any serious behavior or emotional problems, such as hitting, biting, depression, or hallucinations.

How to Cope with Sleep Problems

Evenings are hard for many people with AD. Some may become restless or irritable around dinnertime. This restlessness is called "sundowning." It may even be hard to get the person to go to bed and stay there.

Here are some tips that may help:

- Help the person get exercise each day, limit naps, and make sure the person gets enough rest at night. Being overly tired can increase late-afternoon and nighttime restlessness.

- Plan activities that use more energy early in the day. For example, try bathing in the morning or having the largest family meal in the middle of the day.

- Set a quiet, peaceful mood in the evening to help the person relax. Keep the lights low, try to reduce the noise levels, and play soothing music if she or he enjoys it.

- Try to have the person go to bed at the same time each night. A bedtime routine, such as reading out loud, also may help.

- Limit caffeine.

- Use nightlights in the bedroom, hall, and bathroom.

How to Cope with Hallucinations and Delusions

As the disease progresses, the person with AD may have hallucinations. During a hallucination, a person sees, hears, smells, tastes, or feels something that isn't there. For example, the person may see his or her dead mother in the room. She or he also may have delusions. Delusions are false beliefs that the person thinks are real. For example, the person may think his or her spouse is in love with someone else.

Here are some things you can do:

- Tell the doctor or AD specialist about the delusions or hallucinations.

- Discuss with the doctor any illnesses the person has and medicines she or he is taking. Sometimes an illness or medicine may cause hallucinations or delusions.

- Try not to argue about what the person with AD sees or hears. Comfort the person if she or he is afraid.

- Distract the person. Sometimes moving to another room or going outside for a walk helps.

- Turn off the TV when violent or upsetting programs are on. Someone with AD may think these events are really going on in the room.

- Make sure the person is safe and can't reach anything that could be used to hurt anyone or himself or herself.

How to Cope with Paranoia

Paranoia is a type of delusion in which a person may believe—without a good reason—that others are mean, lying, unfair, or "out to get him or her." She or he may become suspicious, fearful, or jealous of people.

In a person with AD, paranoia often is linked to memory loss. It can become worse as memory loss gets worse. For example, the person may become paranoid if she or he forgets:

- Where she or he put something. The person may believe that someone is taking his or her things.

- That you are the person's caregiver. Someone with AD might not trust you if she or he thinks you are a stranger.

- People to whom she or he has been introduced. The person may believe that strangers will be harmful.

- Directions you just gave. The person may think you are trying to trick her or him.

Paranoia may be the person's way of expressing loss. The person may blame or accuse others because no other explanation seems to make sense.

Here are some tips for dealing with paranoia:

- Try not to react if the person blames you for something

- Don't argue with her or him

- Let the person know that she or he is safe

- Use gentle touching or hugging to show the person you care

- Explain to others that the person is acting this way because she or he has AD

- Search for missing things to distract the person; then talk about what you found. For example, talk about a photograph or keepsake.

- Have extra sets of keys or eyeglasses in case they are lost

How to Cope with Agitation and Aggression

Agitation means that a person is restless and worried. She or he doesn't seem to be able to settle down. Agitated people may pace a lot, not be able to sleep, or act aggressively toward others. They may verbally lash out or try to hit or hurt someone. When this happens, try to find the cause. There is usually a reason.

For example, the person may have:

- Pain, depression, or stress

- Too little rest or sleep

- Constipation

- Soiled underwear or diaper

Here are some other causes of agitation and aggression:

- Sudden change in a well-known place, routine, or person

- A feeling of loss—for example, the person with AD may miss driving or caring for children

- Too much noise or confusion or too many people around

- Being pushed by others to do something—for example, to bathe or remember events or people—when AD has made the activity very hard or impossible

- Feeling lonely and not having enough contact with other people

- Interaction of medicines

Here are suggestions to help you cope with agitation and aggression:

- Look for the early signs of agitation or aggression. Then you can deal with the cause before the problem behaviors start.

- Doing nothing can make things worse. Try to find the causes of the behavior. If you deal with the causes, the behavior may stop.

- Slow down and try to relax if you think your own worries may be affecting the person with AD. Try to find a way to take a break from caregiving.

- Allow the person to keep as much control in his or her life as possible.

- Try to distract the person with a favorite snack, object, or activity.

You also can:

- Reassure her or him. Speak calmly. Listen to the person's concerns and frustrations. Try to show that you understand if the person is angry or fearful.

- Keep well-loved objects and photographs around the house. This can make the person feel more secure.

- Reduce noise, clutter, or the number of people in the room.

- Try gentle touching, soothing music, reading, or walks.

- Build quiet times into the day, along with activities.

- Limit the amount of caffeine, sugar, and "junk food" the person drinks and eats.

Here are things the doctor can do:

- Give the person a medical exam to find any problems that may cause the behavior. These problems might include pain, depression, or the effects of certain medicines.

- Check the person's vision and hearing each year.

Here are some important things to do when the person is aggressive:

- Protect yourself and your family members from aggressive behavior. If you have to, stay at a safe distance from the person until the behavior stops.

- As much as possible, protect the person from hurting himself or herself.

- Ask the doctor or AD specialist if medicine may be needed to prevent or reduce agitation or aggression.

How to Cope with Wandering

Many people with AD wander away from their home or caregiver. As the caregiver, you need to know how to limit wandering and prevent the person from becoming lost. This will help keep the person safe and give you greater peace of mind.

Try to follow these tips before the person with AD wanders:

- Make sure the person carries some kind of ID or wears a medical bracelet. If the person gets lost, an ID will let others know about his or her illness. It also shows where the person lives.

- Consider enrolling the person in the MedicAlert®+ Alzheimer Association Safe Return® Program (www.alz.org or call 888-572-8566 to find the program in your area). This service is not affiliated with the National Institute on Aging (NIA). There may be a charge for this service.

- Let neighbors and the local police know that the person with AD tends to wander.

- Keep a recent photograph or video recording of the person to help police if the person becomes lost.

- Keep the doors locked. Consider a keyed deadbolt, or add another lock placed up high or down low on the door. If the person can open a lock, you may need to get a new latch or lock.

- Install an "announcing system" that chimes when a door is opened.

How to Cope with Rummaging and Hiding Things

Someone with AD may start rummaging or searching through cabinets, drawers, closets, the refrigerator, and other places where things are stored. She or he also may hide items around the house. This behavior can be annoying or even dangerous for the caregiver or family members. If you get angry, try to remember that this behavior is part of the disease.

In some cases, there might be a logical reason for this behavior. For instance, the person may be looking for something specific, although she or he may not be able to tell you what it is. She or he may be hungry or bored. Try to understand what is causing the behavior so you can fit your response to the cause.

Here are some other steps to take:

- Lock up dangerous or toxic products, or place them out of the person's sight and reach.

- Remove spoiled food from the refrigerator and cabinets. Someone with AD may look for snacks, but lack the judgment or sense of taste to stay away from spoiled foods.

- Remove valuable items that could be misplaced or hidden by the person, like important papers, checkbooks, charge cards, jewelry, and keys.

- People with AD often hide, lose, or throw away mail. If this is a serious problem, consider getting a post office box. If you have a yard with a fence and a locked gate, place your mailbox outside the gate.

- Keep the person with AD from going into unused rooms. This limits his or her rummaging through and hiding things.

- Search the house to learn where the person often hides things. Once you find these places, check them often, out of sight of the person.

- Keep all trash cans covered or out of sight. People with AD may not remember the purpose of the container or may rummage through it.

- Check trash containers before you empty them, in case something has been hidden there or thrown away by accident.

You also can create a special place where the person with AD can rummage freely or sort things. This could be a chest of drawers, a bag of objects, or a basket of clothing to fold or unfold. Give her or him a personal box, chest, or cupboard to store special objects. You may have to remind the person where to find his or her personal storage place.

3. Challenge: Changes in Intimacy and Sexuality

Intimacy is the special bond we share with a person we love and respect. It includes the way we talk and act toward one another. This bond can exist between spouses or partners, family members, and friends. AD often changes the intimacy between people.

Sexuality is one type of intimacy. It is an important way that spouses or partners express their feelings physically for one another.

AD can cause changes in intimacy and sexuality in both the person with AD and the caregiver. The person with AD may be stressed by the changes in his or her memory and behaviors. Fear, worry, depression, anger, and low self-esteem (how much the person likes himself or herself) are common. The person may become dependent and cling to you. She or he may not remember your life together and feelings toward one another. Sometimes the person may even fall in love with someone else.

You, the caregiver, may pull away from the person in both an emotional and physical sense. You may be upset by the demands of caregiving. You also may feel frustrated by the person's constant forgetfulness, repeated questions, and other bothersome behaviors.

Most caregivers learn how to cope with these challenges, but it takes time. Some learn to live with the illness and find new meaning in their relationships with people who have AD.

How to Cope with Changes in Intimacy

Remember that most people with AD need to feel that someone loves and cares about them. They also need to spend time with other people as well as you. Your efforts to take care of these needs can help the person with AD to feel happy and safe.

It's important to reassure the person that:

- You love her or him

- You will keep her or him safe

- Others also care about her or him

When intimacy changes, the following tips may help you cope with your own needs:

- Talk with a doctor, social worker, or clergy member about these changes. It may feel awkward to talk about such personal issues, but it can help.

- Talk about your concerns in a support group.

- Think more about the positive parts of the relationship.

How to Cope with Changes in Sexuality

The well spouse/partner or the person with AD may lose interest in having sex. This change can make you feel lonely or frustrated. Here are some possible reasons for changes in sexual interest.

The well spouse/partner may feel that:

- It's not okay to have sex with someone who has AD.

- The person with AD seems like a stranger.

- The person with AD seems to forget that the spouse/partner is there or how to make love.

A person with AD may have:

- Side effects from medications that affect his or her sexual interest

- Memory loss, changes in the brain, or depression that affects his or her interest in sex

Here are some suggestions for coping with changes in sexuality:

- Explore new ways of spending time together.

- Focus on other ways to show affection. Some caregivers find that snuggling or holding hands reduces their need for a sexual relationship.

- Try other nonsexual forms of touching, such as giving a massage, hugging, and dancing.

- Consider other ways to meet your sexual needs. Some caregivers report that they masturbate to meet their needs.

Helping a Person Who Is Aware of Memory Loss

AD is being diagnosed at earlier stages. This means that many people are aware of how the disease is affecting their memory. Here are tips on how to help someone who knows that she or he has memory problems:

- Take time to listen. The person may want to talk about the changes she or he is noticing.

- Be as sensitive as you can. Don't just correct the person every time she or he forgets something or says something odd. Try to understand that it's a struggle for the person to communicate.

- Be patient when someone with AD has trouble finding the right words or putting feelings into words.

- Help the person find words to express thoughts and feelings.

- For example, Mrs. D cried after forgetting her garden club meeting. She finally said, "I wish they stopped." Her daughter said, "You wish your friends had stopped by for you." Mrs. D nodded and repeated some of the words. Then Mrs. D said, "I want to go." Her daughter said, "You want to go to the garden club meeting." Again, Mrs. D nodded and repeated the words.

- Be careful not to put words in the person's mouth or "fill in the blanks" too quickly.

- As people lose the ability to talk clearly, they may rely on other ways to communicate their thoughts and feelings.

- For example, their facial expressions may show sadness, anger, or frustration. Grasping at their undergarments may tell you they need to use the bathroom.

Getting Help with Alzheimer Disease Caregiving

Some caregivers need help when the person is in the early stages of Alzheimer disease. Other caregivers look for help when the person is in the later stages of AD. It's okay to seek help whenever you need it.

As the person moves through the stages of AD, she or he will need more care. One reason is that medicines used to treat Alzheimer disease can only control symptoms; they cannot cure the disease. Symptoms, such as memory loss and confusion, will get worse over time.

Because of this, you will need more help. You may feel that asking for help shows weakness or a lack of caring, but the opposite is true. Asking for help shows your strength. It means you know your limits and when to seek support.

Build a Support System

According to many caregivers, building a local support system is a key way to get help. Your support system might include a caregiver support group, the local chapter of the Alzheimer's Association, family, friends, and faith groups.

Direct Services: Groups That Help with Everyday Care in the Home

Here is a list of services that can help you care for the person with AD at home. Find out if these services are offered in your area. Also, contact Medicare to see if they cover the cost of any of these services. See below for Medicare contact information.

Home Healthcare Services

Home healthcare services send a home health aide to your home to help you care for a person with AD. These aides provide care and/or company for the person. They may come for a few hours or stay for 24 hours. Some home health aides are better trained and supervised than others.

What to know about costs:

- Home health services charge by the hour.

- Medicare covers some home health service costs.

- Most insurance plans do not cover these costs.

- You must pay all costs not covered by Medicare, Medicaid, or insurance.

How to find them:

- Ask your doctor or other healthcare professional about good home healthcare services in your area.

- Search the Internet for "home healthcare" in your area.

Here are some questions you might ask before signing a home healthcare agreement:

- Is your service licensed and accredited?

- What is the cost of your services?

- What is included and not included in your services?

- How many days a week and hours a day will an aide come to my home?

- Is there a minimum number of hours required?

- How do you check the background and experience of your home health aides?

- How do you train your home health aides?

- Can I get special help in an emergency?

- What types of emergency care can you provide?

- Whom do I contact if there is a problem?

Meal Services

Meal services bring hot meals to the person's home or your home. The delivery staff do not feed the person.

What to know about costs:

- The person with AD must qualify for the service based on local guidelines.

- Some groups do not charge for their services. Others may charge a small fee.

How to find them:

The Eldercare Locator can help at 800-677-1116 or www.eldercare. acl.gov. Or, contact the Meals on Wheels organization at 888-998-6325 or www.mealsonwheelsamerica.org

Adult Day Care Services

Adult day care services provide a safe environment, activities, and staff who pay attention to the needs of the person with AD in an adult day care facility. They also provide transportation. The facility may pick up the person with AD, take her or him to daycare, and then return the person home. Adult day care services provide a much-needed break for you.

What to know about costs:

- Adult day care services charge by the hour.

- Most insurance plans don't cover these costs. You must pay all costs not covered by insurance.

How to find them:

- Call the National Adult Day Services Association (NADSA) at 877-745-1440, or visit www.nadsa.org/consumers/choosing-a-center. You can contact the Eldercare Locator at 800-677-1116 or at www.eldercare.acl.gov.

Respite Services

Respite services provide short-term care for the person with AD at home, in a healthcare facility, or at an adult day center. The care may last for as short as a few hours or as long as several weeks. These services allow you to get a break to rest or go on a vacation.

What to know about costs:

- Respite services charge by the hour or by the number of days or weeks that services are provided.

- Most insurance plans do not cover these costs. You must pay all costs not covered by insurance or other funding sources.

- Medicare will cover most of the cost of up to five days in a row of respite care in a hospital or skilled nursing facility for a person receiving hospice care.

- Medicaid also may offer assistance.

- There may be other sources of funding in your state.

How to find them:

- Visit the ARCH National Respite Locator at archrespite.org/respitelocator.

Geriatric Care Managers

Geriatric care managers make a home visit and suggest needed services. They also can help you get needed services.

What to know about costs:

- Geriatric care managers charge by the hour.

- Most insurance plans don't cover these costs.

- Medicare does not pay for this service.

- You will probably have to pay for this service.

How to find them:

- Call the Aging Life Care Association at 520-881-8008, or visit www.aginglifecare.org.

Counseling from a Mental Health or Social Work Professional

Mental health or social work professionals help you understand your feelings, such as anger, sadness, or feeling out of control and overwhelmed, and help you deal with any stress you may be feeling. They also help develop plans for unexpected or sudden events.

What to know about costs:

- Professional mental health counselors charge by the hour. There may be big differences in the rates you would be charged from one counselor to another.

- Some insurance companies will cover some of these costs.

- Medicare or Medicaid may cover some of these costs.

- You must pay all costs not covered by Medicare, Medicaid, or insurance.

How to find them:

- It's a good idea to ask your health insurance staff which counselors and services, if any, your insurance plan covers. Then check with your doctor, local family service agencies, and community mental health agencies for referrals to counselors.

Hospice Services

Hospice services provide care for a person who is near the end of life. They keep the person who is dying as comfortable and pain-free as possible, and provide care in the home or in a hospice facility. They also support the family in providing in-home or end-of-life care.

What to know about costs:

- Hospice services charge by the number of days or weeks that services are provided.

- Medicare or Medicaid may cover hospice costs.

- Most insurance plans do not cover these costs.

- You must pay all costs not covered by Medicare, Medicaid, or insurance.

How to find them:

- National Association for Home Care & Hospice (NAHC) at 202-547-7424 or agencylocator.nahc.org

- Hospice Foundation of America (HFA) at 800-854-3402 or www.hospicefoundation.org

- National Hospice and Palliative Care Organization (NHPCO) at 800-658-8898 or www.nhpco.org/find-hospice

Chapter 47

Helping Family Members and Others Understand Alzheimer Disease

Deciding When and How to Tell Family Members and Friends

When you learn that someone you love has Alzheimer disease (AD), you may wonder when and how to tell your family and friends. You may be worried about how others will react to or treat the person. While there is no single right way to tell others, we've listed some things to think about.

Think about the following questions:

- Are others already wondering what is going on?

- Do you want to keep this information to yourself?

- Are you embarrassed?

- Do you want to tell others so that you can get support from family members and friends?

- Are you afraid that you will burden others?

This chapter includes text excerpted from "Caring for Persons with Alzheimer's Disease," National Institute on Aging (NIA), National Institutes of Health (NIH), January 2017.

- Does keeping this information secret take too much of your energy?

- Are you afraid others won't understand?

Realize that family and friends often sense that something is wrong before they are told. AD is hard to keep secret. When the time seems right, it is best for you to be honest with family, friends, and others. Use this as a chance to educate them about AD.

For example, you can:

- Tell them about the disease and its effects

- Share books and information to help them understand what you and the person with AD are going through

- Tell them how they can learn more

- Tell them what they can do to help. Let them know you need breaks.

Help family and friends understand how to interact with the person who has AD. You can:

- Help them realize what the person still can do and how much she or he still can understand

- Give them suggestions about how to start talking with the person. For example, "Hello George, I'm John. We used to work together."

- Help them avoid correcting the person with AD if she or he makes a mistake or forgets something

- Help them plan fun activities with the person, such as going to family reunions; church, temple, or mosque gatherings; other community activities; or visiting old friends

Communicate with others when you're out in public. Some caregivers carry a card that explains why the person with AD might say or do odd things. For example, the card could read, "My family member has Alzheimer disease. She or he might say or do things that are unexpected. Thank you for your understanding."

The card allows you to let others know about the person's AD without the person hearing you. It also means that you don't have to keep explaining things.

Helping Children Understand Alzheimer Disease

When a family member has AD, it affects everyone in the family, including children and grandchildren. It's important to talk to them about what is happening. How much and what kind of information you share depends on the child's age. It also depends on her or his relationship to the person with AD.

Give children information about AD that they can understand. There are good books about AD for children of all ages. Some are listed on the Alzheimer and related Dementias Education and Referral (ADEAR) Center website (www.nia.nih.gov/health/alzheimers/caregiving).

Here are some other suggestions to help children understand what is happening:

- Answer their questions simply and honestly. For example, you might tell a young child, "Grandma has an illness that makes it hard for her to remember things."

- Help them know that their feelings of sadness and anger are normal.

- Comfort them. Tell them no one caused the disease. Young children may think they did something to hurt their grandparent.

If the child lives in the same house as someone with AD:

- Don't expect a young child to help take care of or "babysit" the person with AD.

- Make sure the child has time for his or her own interests and needs, such as playing with friends, going to school activities, or doing homework.

- Make sure you spend time with your child, so she or he doesn't feel that all your attention is on the person with AD.

- Help the child understand your feelings. Be honest about your feelings when you talk with a child, but don't overwhelm him or her.

Many younger children will look to you to see how to act around the person with AD. Show children they can still talk with the person, and help them enjoy things each day. Doing fun things together can help both the child and the person with AD.

Here are some things they might do:

- Do simple arts and crafts
- Play music
- Sing
- Look through photo albums
- Read stories out loud

Some children may not talk about their negative feelings, but you may see changes in how they act. Problems at school, with friends, or at home can be a sign that they are upset. You may want to ask a school counselor or a social worker to help your child understand what is happening and learn how to cope. Be sure to check with your child often to see how she or he is feeling.

A teenager might find it very hard to accept how the person with AD has changed. She or he may find the changes upsetting or embarrassing and not want to be around the person. It's a good idea to talk with teenagers about their concerns and feelings. Don't force them to spend time with the person who has AD. This could make things worse.

If the stress of living with someone who has AD becomes too great for a child, think about placing the person with AD into a respite care facility. Then, both you and your child can get a much-needed break.

Chapter 48

Long-Distance Caregiving

Who Is a Long-Distance Caregiver?

Anyone, anywhere, can be a long-distance caregiver, no matter your gender, income, age, social status, or employment. If you are living an hour or more away from a person who needs your help, you're probably a long-distance caregiver.

What Can I Really Do from Far Away?

Long-distance caregivers take on different roles. You may:

- Help with finances, money management, or bill paying.

- Arrange for in-home care—hire professional caregivers or home health or nursing aides and help get needed durable medical equipment.

- Locate care in an assisted living facility or nursing home. (also known as a skilled nursing facility)

- Provide emotional support and occasional respite care for a primary caregiver, the person who takes on most of the everyday caregiving responsibilities.

This chapter includes text excerpted from "Getting Started with Long-Distance Caregiving," National Institute on Aging (NIA), National Institutes of Health (NIH), May 2, 2017.

- Serve as an information coordinator—research health problems or medicines, help navigate through a maze of new needs, and clarify insurance benefits and claims.

- Keep family and friends updated and informed.

- Create a plan and get paperwork in order in case of an emergency.

- Evaluate the house and make sure it's safe for the older person's needs.

Over time, as your family members need change, so will your role as a long-distance caregiver.

I'm New to Long-Distance Caregiving—What Should I Do First?

To get started:

- Ask the primary caregiver, if there is one, and the care recipient how you can be most helpful.

- Talk to friends who are caregivers to see if they have suggestions about ways to help.

- Find out more about local resources that might be useful.

- Develop a good understanding of the person's health issues and other needs.

- Visit as often as you can; not only might you notice something that needs to be done and can be taken care of from a distance, but you can also relieve a primary caregiver for a short time.

Many of us don't automatically have a lot of caregiver skills. Information about training opportunities is available. Some local chapters of the American Red Cross (ARC) (www.redcross.org/take-a-class) might offer courses, as do some nonprofit organizations focused on caregiving. Medicare and Medicaid will sometimes pay for this training.

As a Caregiver, What Do I Need to Know about My Family Members Health?

Learn as much as you can about your family members condition and any treatment. This can help you understand what is going on, anticipate the course of an illness, prevent crises, and assist in health-care management. It can also make talking with the doctor easier.

Get written permission, as needed under the Health Insurance Portability and Accountability Act (HIPAA) Privacy Rule, to receive medical and financial information. To the extent possible, the family member with permission should be the one to talk with all healthcare providers. Try putting together a notebook, on paper or online, that includes all the vital information about medical care, social services, contact numbers, financial issues, and so on. Make copies for other caregivers, and keep it up-to-date.

How Can I Be Most Helpful during My Visit?

Talk to the care recipient ahead of time and find out what she or he would like to do during your visit. Also check with the primary caregiver, if appropriate, to learn what she or he needs, such as handling some caregiving responsibilities while you are in town. This may help you set clear-cut and realistic goals for the visit. Decide on the priorities and leave other tasks to another visit.

Remember to actually spend time visiting with your family member. Try to make time to do things unrelated to being a caregiver, like watching a movie, playing a game, or taking a drive. Finding time to do something simple and relaxing can help everyone—it can be fun and build family memories. And, try to let outside distractions wait until you are home again.

How Can I Stay Connected from Far Away?

Try to find people who live near your loved one and can provide a realistic view of what is going on. This may be your other parent. A social worker may be able to provide updates and help with making decisions. Many families schedule conference calls with doctors, the assisted living facility team, or nursing home staff so that several relatives can be in one conversation and get the same up-to-date information about health and progress.

Don't underestimate the value of a phone and e-mail contact list. It is a simple way to keep everyone updated on your parents' needs.

You may also want to give the person you care for a cell phone (and make sure she or he knows how to use it). Or, if your family member lives in a nursing home, consider having a private phone line installed in his or her room. Program telephone numbers of doctors, friends, family members, and yourself into the phone, and perhaps provide a list of the speed-dial numbers to keep with the phone. Such simple strategies can be a lifeline. But try to be prepared should you find yourself inundated with calls from your parent.

Where Can I Find Local Resources for My Family Member?

Searching online is a good way to start collecting resources. Here are a few potentially helpful places to look:

- Eldercare Locator (eldercare.acl.gov/Public/Index.aspx), 800-677-1116 (toll-free)
- National Institute on Aging (NIA) website (www.nia.nih.gov/health/caregiving)
- Family Care Navigator (www.caregiver.org/family-care-navigator)
- Your state government's website

You might also check with local senior centers.

Chapter 49

Coping with Challenging Behaviors

Chapter Contents

Section 49.1

Personality and Behavior Changes in Alzheimer Disease

This section includes text excerpted from "Managing Personality and Behavior Changes in Alzheimer's," National Institute on Aging (NIA), National Institutes of Health (NIH), May 17, 2017.

Alzheimer disease (AD) causes brain cells to die, so the brain works less well over time. This changes how a person acts. This section has suggestions that may help you understand and cope with changes in personality and behavior in a person with Alzheimer disease.

Common Changes in Personality and Behavior

Common personality and behavior changes you may see include:

- Getting upset, worried, and angry more easily
- Acting depressed or not interested in things
- Hiding things or believing other people are hiding things
- Imagining things that aren't there
- Wandering away from home
- Pacing a lot
- Showing unusual sexual behavior
- Hitting you or other people
- Misunderstanding what she or he sees or hears

You also may notice that the person stops caring about how she or he looks, stops bathing, and wants to wear the same clothes every day.

Other Factors That Can Affect Behavior

In addition to changes in the brain, other things may affect how people with Alzheimer behave:

- Feelings such as sadness, fear, stress, confusion, or anxiety
- Health-related problems, including illness, pain, new medications, or lack of sleep

• Other physical issues like infections, constipation, hunger or thirst, or problems seeing or hearing

Other problems in their surroundings may affect behavior for a person with Alzheimer disease. Too much noise, such as television (TV), radio, or many people talking at once can cause frustration and confusion. Stepping from one type of flooring to another or the way the floor looks may make the person think she or he needs to take a step down. Mirrors may make them think that a mirror image is another person in the room.

If you don't know what is causing the problem, call the doctor. It could be caused by a physical or medical issue.

Keep Things Simple. . . and Other Tips

Caregivers cannot stop Alzheimer-related changes in personality and behavior, but they can learn to cope with them. Here are some tips:

• Keep things simple. Ask or say one thing at a time.

• Have a daily routine, so the person knows when certain things will happen.

• Reassure the person that she or he is safe and you are there to help.

• Focus on his or her feelings rather than words. For example, say, "You seem worried."

• Don't argue or try to reason with the person.

• Try not to show your frustration or anger. If you get upset, take deep breaths and count to 10. If it's safe, leave the room for a few minutes.

• Use humor when you can.

• Give people who pace a lot a safe place to walk. Provide comfortable, sturdy shoes. Give them light snacks to eat as they walk, so they don't lose too much weight, and make sure they have enough to drink.

• Try using music, singing, or dancing to distract the person.

• Ask for help. For instance, say, "Let's set the table" or "I need help folding the clothes."

Talk with the person's doctor about problems like hitting, biting, depression, or hallucinations. Medications are available to treat some behavioral symptoms.

Section 49.2

Agitation and Aggression in Alzheimer Disease

This section includes text excerpted from "Coping with Agitation
and Aggression in Alzheimer's Disease," National Institute on Aging
(NIA), National Institutes of Health (NIH), May 17, 2017.

People with Alzheimer disease (AD) may become agitated or aggressive as the disease gets worse. Agitation means that a person is restless or worried. She or he doesn't seem to be able to settle down. Agitation may cause pacing, sleeplessness, or aggression, which is when a person lashes out verbally or tries to hit or hurt someone.

Causes of Agitation and Aggression

Most of the time, agitation and aggression happen for a reason. When they happen, try to find the cause. If you deal with the causes, the behavior may stop. For example, the person may have:

- Pain, depression, or stress

- Too little rest or sleep

- Constipation

- Soiled underwear or diaper

- Sudden change in a well-known place, routine, or person

- A feeling of loss—for example, the person may miss the freedom to drive

- Too much noise or confusion or too many people in the room

- Being pushed by others to do something—for example, to bathe or to remember events or people—when Alzheimer has made the activity very hard or impossible

- Feeling lonely and not having enough contact with other people

- Interaction of medicines

Look for early signs of agitation or aggression. If you see the signs, you can deal with the cause before problem behaviors start. Try not to ignore the problem. Doing nothing can make things worse.

A doctor may be able to help. She or he can give the person a medical exam to find any problems that may cause agitation and aggression. Also, ask the doctor if a medicine is needed to prevent or reduce agitation or aggression.

Tips for Coping with Agitation or Aggression

Here are some ways you can cope with agitation or aggression:

- Reassure the person. Speak calmly. Listen to his or her concerns and frustrations. Try to show that you understand if the person is angry or fearful.

- Allow the person to keep as much control in his or her life as possible.

- Try to keep a routine, such as bathing, dressing, and eating at the same time each day.

- Build quiet times into the day, along with activities.

- Keep well-loved objects and photographs around the house to help the person feel more secure.

- Try gentle touching, soothing music, reading, or walks.

- Reduce noise, clutter, or the number of people in the room.

- Try to distract the person with a favorite snack, object, or activity.

- Limit the amount of caffeine, sugar, and "junk food" the person drinks and eats.

Here are some things you can do:

- Slow down and try to relax if you think your own worries may be affecting the person with Alzheimer.

- Try to find a way to take a break from caregiving.

Safety Concerns

When the person is aggressive, protect yourself and others. If you have to, stay at a safe distance from the person until the behavior stops. Also, try to protect the person from hurting himself or herself.

Section 49.3

When a Person with Alzheimer Disease Rummages and Hides Things

This section includes text excerpted from "When a Person with Alzheimer's Rummages and Hides Things," National Institute on Aging (NIA), National Institutes of Health (NIH), May 17, 2017.

Someone with Alzheimer disease (AD) may start rummaging or searching through cabinets, drawers, closets, the refrigerator, and other places where things are stored. She or he also may hide items around the house. This behavior can be annoying or even dangerous for the caregiver or family members. If you get angry, try to remember that this behavior is part of the disease.

In some cases, there might be a logical reason for this behavior. For instance, the person may be looking for something specific, although she or he may not be able to tell you what it is. She or he may be hungry or bored. Try to understand what is causing the behavior so you can fit your response to the cause.

Rummaging—with Safety

You can take steps that allow the person with Alzheimer disease to rummage while protecting your belongings and keeping the person safe. Try these tips:

- Lock up dangerous or toxic products, or place them out of the person's sight and reach.

- Remove spoiled food from the refrigerator and cabinets. Someone with Alzheimer may look for snacks but lack the judgment or sense of taste to stay away from spoiled foods.

- Remove valuable items that could be misplaced or hidden by the person, like important papers, checkbooks, charge cards, jewelry, and keys.

- People with Alzheimer often hide, lose, or throw away mail. If this is a serious problem, consider getting a post office box. If you have a yard with a fence and a locked gate, place your mailbox outside the gate.

You also can create a special place where the person with Alzheimer can rummage freely or sort things. This could be a chest of drawers, a bag of objects, or a basket of clothing to fold or unfold. Give him or her a personal box, chest, or cupboard to store special objects. You may have to remind the person where to find his or her personal storage place.

More Tips for Rummaging and Hiding Behavior

Here are some more suggestions:

- Keep the person with Alzheimer from going into unused rooms. This limits his or her rummaging through and hiding things.

- Search the house to learn where the person often hides things. Once you find these places, check them often, out of sight of the person.

- Keep all trash cans covered or out of sight. People with Alzheimer may not remember the purpose of the container or may rummage through it.

- Check trash containers before you empty them, in case something has been hidden there or thrown away by accident.

Section 49.4

Coping with Sundowning

This section includes text excerpted from "Tips for Coping with Sundowning," National Institute on Aging (NIA), National Institutes of Health (NIH), May 17, 2017.

Late afternoon and early evening can be difficult for some people with Alzheimer disease (AD). They may experience sundowning—restlessness, agitation, irritability, or confusion that can begin or worsen as daylight begins to fade—often just when tired caregivers need a break. Sundowning can continue into the night, making it hard for people with AD to fall asleep and stay in bed. As a result, they and their caregivers may have trouble getting enough sleep and functioning well during the day.

Possible Causes

The causes of sundowning are not well understood. One possibility is that Alzheimer disease-related brain changes can affect a person's "biological clock," leading to confused sleep-wake cycles. This may result in agitation and other sundowning behaviors.

Other possible causes of sundowning include:

- Being overly tired
- Unmet needs such as hunger or thirst
- Depression
- Pain
- Boredom

Tips for Coping with Sundowning

Look for signs of sundowning in the late afternoon and early evening. These signs may include increased confusion or anxiety and behaviors such as pacing, wandering, or yelling. If you can, try to find the cause of the person's behavior.

If the person with Alzheimer disease becomes agitated, listen calmly to his or her concerns and frustrations. Try to reassure the person that everything is OK and distract him or her from stressful or upsetting events.

You can also try these tips:

- Reduce noise, clutter, or the number of people in the room.
- Try to distract the person with a favorite snack, object, or activity. For example, offer a drink, suggest a simple task like folding towels, or turn on a familiar TV show (but not the news or other shows that might be upsetting).
- Make early evening a quiet time of day. You might play soothing music, read, or go for a walk. You could also have a family member or friend call during this time.
- Close the curtains or blinds at dusk to minimize shadows and the confusion they may cause. Turn on lights to help minimize shadows.

Preventing Sundowning

Being too tired can increase late-afternoon and early-evening restlessness. Try to avoid this situation by helping the person:

- Go outside or at least sit by the window—exposure to bright light can help reset the person's body clock

- Get physical activity or exercise each day

- Get daytime rest if needed, but keep naps short and not too late in the day

- Get enough rest at night

Avoid things that seem to make sundowning worse:

- Do not serve coffee, cola, or other drinks with caffeine late in the day.

- Do not serve alcoholic drinks. They may add to confusion and anxiety.

- Do not plan too many activities during the day. A full schedule can be tiring.

If Problems Persist

If sundowning continues to be a problem, seek medical advice. A medical exam may identify the cause of sundowning, such as pain, a sleep disorder or other illness, or a medication side effect.

If medication is prescribed to help the person relax and sleep better at night, be sure to find out about possible side effects. Some medications can increase the chances of dizziness, falls, and confusion. Doctors recommend using them only for short periods of time.

Chapter 50

Coping with Late-Stage Alzheimer Disease

When a person moves to the later stages of Alzheimer disease, caregiving may become even harder. This article offers ways to cope with changes that take place during severe or late-stage Alzheimer disease.

When the Person with Alzheimer Disease Can't Move

If the person with AD can't move around on his or her own, contact a home health aide, physical therapist, or nurse. Ask the doctor for a referral to one of these health professionals. They can show you how to move the person safely, such as changing his or her position in bed or in a chair.

Also, a physical therapist can show you how to move the person's body joints using range-of-motion exercises. During these exercises, you hold the person's arms or legs, one at a time, and move and bend it several times a day. Movement prevents stiffness of the arms, hands, and legs. It also prevents pressure or bedsores.

This chapter includes text excerpted from "Coping with Late-Stage Alzheimer's Disease," National Institute on Aging (NIA), National Institutes of Health (NIH), May 18, 2017.

How to Make Someone with Alzheimer Disease More Comfortable

Here are some ways to make the person with Alzheimer disease more comfortable:

- Buy special mattresses and wedge-shaped seat cushions that reduce pressure sores. You can purchase these at a medical supply store or drugstore or online. Ask the home health aide, nurse, or physical therapist how to use the equipment.

- Move the person to a different position at least every two hours.

- Use a lap board to rest the person's arms and support the upper body when she or he is sitting up.

- Give the person something to hold, such as a washcloth, while being moved. The person will be less likely to grab onto you or the furniture. If she or he is weak on one side, stand on the weak side to support the stronger side and help the person change positions.

How to Keep from Hurting Yourself When Moving the Person

To keep from hurting yourself when moving someone with AD disease:

- Know your strength when lifting or moving the person; don't try to do too much. Also, be aware of how you position your body.

- Bend at the knees and then straighten up by using your thigh muscles, not your back.

- Keep your back straight, and don't bend at the waist.

- Hold the person as close as possible to avoid reaching away from your body.

- Place one foot in front of the other, or space your feet comfortably apart for a wide base of support.

- Use little steps to move the person from one seat to another. Don't twist your body.

- Use a transfer or "Posey" belt. You can buy this belt at a medical supply store or drugstore. To move the person, wrap the transfer belt around the person's waist and slide him or her to the edge of the chair or bed. Face the person and place your hands under the belt on either side of his or her waist. Then bend your knees, and pull up by using your thigh muscles to raise the person from a seated to a standing position.

How to Make Sure the Person Eats Well

Here are specific suggestions about foods to eat and liquids to drink:

- Give the person finger foods to eat such as cheese, small sandwiches, small pieces of chicken, fresh fruits, or vegetables. Sandwiches made with pita bread are easier to handle.

- Give him or her high-calorie, healthy foods to eat or drink, such as protein milkshakes. You can buy high-protein drinks and powders at grocery stores, drugstores, or discount stores. Also, you can mix healthy foods in a blender and let the person drink his or her meal. Use diet supplements if she or he is not getting enough calories. Talk with the doctor or nurse about what kinds of supplements are best.

- Try to use healthy fats in cooking, such as olive oil. Also, use extra cooking oil, butter, and mayonnaise to cook and prepare food if the person needs more calories. If the person has heart disease check with the doctor about how much and what kinds of fat to use.

- If the person has diabetes or high blood pressure, check with the doctor or a nutrition specialist about which foods to limit.

- Have the person take a multivitamin—a tablet, capsule, powder, liquid, or injection that adds vitamins, minerals, and other important things to a person's diet.

- Serve bigger portions at breakfast because it's the first meal of the day.

What to Do about Swallowing Problems

As Alzheimer disease progresses to later stages, the person may no longer be able to chew and swallow easily. This is a serious problem. If the person chokes on each bite of food, there is a chance that the food could go into the lungs. This can cause pneumonia, which can lead to death.

The following suggestions may help with swallowing:

- Make sure you cut the food into small pieces, and make it soft enough to eat.

- Grind food or make it liquid using a blender or baby food grinder.

- Offer soft foods, such as ice cream, milkshakes, yogurt, soups, applesauce, gelatin, or custard.

- Don't use a straw; it may cause more swallowing problems. Instead, have the person drink small sips from a cup.

- Limit the amount of milk the person drinks if it tends to catch in the throat.

- Give the person more cold drinks than hot drinks. Cold drinks are easier to swallow.

- Don't give the person thin liquids, such as coffee, tea, water, or broth, because they are hardest to swallow. You can buy Thick-It® at most pharmacies. You add Thick-It® to liquids to make them thicker. You also can use ice cream and sherbet to thicken liquids.

Here are some other ideas to help people swallow:

- Don't hurry the person. She or he needs time to chew and swallow each mouthful before taking another bite.

- Don't feed a person who is drowsy or lying down. She or he should be in an upright, sitting position during the meal and for at least 20 minutes after the meal.

- Have the person keep his or her neck forward and chin down when swallowing.

- Stroke (gently) the person's neck in a downward motion and say "swallow" to remind him or her to swallow.

- Find out if the person's pills can be crushed or taken in liquid form.

Helping the person with AD eat can be exhausting. Planning meals ahead and having the food ready can make this task a little easier for you. Also, remember that people with Alzheimer disease may not eat much at certain times and then feel more like eating at other times. It helps to make mealtime as pleasant and enjoyable as possible. But, no matter how well you plan, the person may not be hungry when you're ready to serve food.

Skin and Foot Problems
Skin Problems

Once the person stops walking or stays in one position too long, she or he may get skin or pressure sores. To prevent skin or pressure sores, you can:

- Move the person at least every two hours if she or he is sitting up.
- Move the person at least every hour if she or he is lying down.
- Put a four-inch foam pad on top of the mattress.
- Check to make sure that the foam pad is comfortable for the person. Some people find these pads too hot for sleeping or may be allergic to them. If the foam pad is a problem, you can get pads filled with gel, air, or water.
- Check to make sure the person sinks a little when lying down on the pad. Also, the pad should fit snugly around his or her body.

To check for pressure sores:

- Look at the person's heels, hips, buttocks, shoulders, back, and elbows for redness or sores.
- Ask the doctor what to do if you find pressure sores.
- Try to keep the person off the affected area.

Foot Care

It's important for the person with AD to take care of his or her feet. If the person can't, you will need to do it. Here's what to do:

- Soak the person's feet in warm water; wash the feet with a mild soap; and check for cuts, corns, and calluses.
- Put lotion on the feet so that the skin doesn't become dry and cracked.
- Cut or file their toenails.
- Talk to a foot care doctor, called a podiatrist, if the person has diabetes or sores on the feet.

401

Body Jerking

Myoclonus is another condition that sometimes happens with AD. The person's arms, legs, or whole body may jerk. This can look like a seizure, but the person doesn't pass out. Tell the doctor right away if you see these signs. The doctor may prescribe one or more medicines to help reduce symptoms.

Chapter 51

Techniques for Communicating with Someone with Alzheimer Disease

Communication is hard for people with Alzheimer disease (AD) because they have trouble remembering things. They may struggle to find words or forget what they want to say. You may feel impatient and wish they could just say what they want, but they can't.

The person with AD may have problems with:

- Finding the right word or losing his or her train of thought when speaking

- Understanding what words mean

- Paying attention during long conversations

- Remembering the steps in common activities, such as cooking a meal, paying bills, or getting dressed

- Blocking out background noises from the radio, TV, or conversations

This chapter includes text excerpted from "Alzheimer's Caregiving: Changes in Communication Skills," National Institute on Aging (NIA), National Institutes of Health (NIH), May 17, 2017.

- Frustration if communication isn't working

- Being very sensitive to touch and to the tone and loudness of voices

Also, AD causes some people to get confused about language. For example, the person might forget or no longer understand English if it was learned as a second language. Instead, she or he might understand and use only the first language learned, such as Spanish.

Help Make Communication Easier

The first step is to understand that the disease causes changes in communication skills. The second step is to try some tips that may make communication easier:

- Make eye contact and call the person by name.

- Be aware of your tone, how loud your voice is, how you look at the person, and your body language.

- Encourage a two-way conversation for as long as possible.

- Use other methods besides speaking, such as gentle touching.

- Try distracting the person if communication creates problems.

To encourage the person to communicate with you:

- Show a warm, loving, matter-of-fact manner.

- Hold the person's hand while you talk.

- Be open to the person's concerns, even if she or he is hard to understand.

- Let her or him make some decisions and stay involved.

- Be patient with angry outbursts. Remember, it's the illness "talking."

To speak effectively with a person who has Alzheimer disease:

- Offer simple, step-by-step instructions.

- Repeat instructions and allow more time for a response. Try not to interrupt.

- Don't talk about the person as if she or he isn't there.

- Don't talk to the person using "baby talk" or a "baby voice."

Be Direct, Specific, and Positive

Here are some examples of what you can say:

- "Let's try this way," instead of pointing out mistakes
- "Please do this," instead of "Don't do this"
- "Thanks for helping," even if the results aren't perfect

You also can:

- Ask questions that require a yes or no answer. For example, you could say, "Are you tired?" instead of "How do you feel?"
- Limit the number of choices. For example, you could say, "Would you like a hamburger or chicken for dinner?" instead of "What would you like for dinner?"
- Use different words if she or he doesn't understand the first time. For example, if you ask the person whether she or he is hungry and you don't get a response, you could say, "Dinner is ready now. Let's eat."
- Try not to say, "Don't you remember?" or "I told you."

If you become frustrated, take a timeout for yourself.

Helping a Person with Memory Loss

Alzheimer disease is being diagnosed at earlier stages. This means that many people are aware of how the disease is affecting their memory. Here are tips on how to help someone who knows that she or he has memory problems:

- Take time to listen. The person may want to talk about the changes she or he is noticing.
- Be as sensitive as you can. Don't just correct the person every time she or he forgets something or says something odd. Try to understand that it's a struggle for the person to communicate.
- Be patient when someone with Alzheimer disease has trouble finding the right words or putting feelings into words.
- Help the person find words to express thoughts and feelings. But be careful not to put words in the person's mouth or "fill in the blanks" too quickly. For example, Mrs. D cried after forgetting her garden club meeting. She finally said, "I wish they stopped."

Her daughter said, "You wish your friends had stopped by for you." Mrs. D nodded and repeated some of the words. Then Mrs. D said, "I want to go." Her daughter said, "You want to go to the garden club meeting." Again, Mrs. D nodded and repeated the words.

• Be aware of nonverbal communication. As people lose the ability to talk clearly, they may rely on other ways to communicate their thoughts and feelings. For example, their facial expressions may show sadness, anger, or frustration. Grasping at their undergarments may tell you they need to use the bathroom.

Chapter 52

Planning the Day for Someone with Dementia

Everyday Care

At some point, people with Alzheimer disease (AD) will need help bathing, combing their hair, brushing their teeth, and getting dressed. Because these are private activities, people may not want help. They may feel embarrassed about being naked in front of caregivers. They also may feel angry about not being able to care for themselves. Below are suggestions that may help with everyday care.

Bathing

Helping someone with AD take a bath or shower can be one of the hardest things you do. Planning can help make the person's bath time better for both of you. The person with AD may be afraid. If so, follow the person's lifelong bathing habits, such as doing the bath or shower in the morning or before going to bed. Here are other tips for bathing.

Safety Tips

- Never leave a confused or frail person alone in the tub or shower.

This chapter includes text excerpted from "Caring for a Person with Alzheimer's Disease," National Institute on Aging (NIA), National Institutes of Health (NIH), January 2017.

- Always check the water temperature before she or he gets in the tub or shower.

- Use plastic containers for shampoo or soap to prevent them from breaking.

- Use a hand-held showerhead.

- Use a rubber bath mat and put safety bars in the tub.

- Use a sturdy shower chair in the tub or shower. This will support a person who is unsteady, and it could prevent falls. You can get shower chairs at drug stores and medical supply stores.

Before a Bath or Shower

- Get the soap, washcloth, towels, and shampoo ready.

- Make sure the bathroom is warm and well lighted. Play soft music if it helps to relax the person.

- Be matter-of-fact about bathing. Say, "It's time for a bath now." Don't argue about the need for a bath or shower.

- Be gentle and respectful. Tell the person what you are going to do, step-by-step.

- Make sure the water temperature in the bath or shower is comfortable.

- Don't use bath oil. It can make the tub slippery and may cause urinary tract infections.

During a Bath or Shower

- Allow the person with AD to do as much as possible. This protects his or her dignity and helps the person feel more in control.

- Put a towel over the person's shoulders or lap. This helps him or her feel less exposed. Then use a sponge or washcloth to clean under the towel.

- Distract the person by talking about something else if she or he becomes upset.

- Give him or her a washcloth to hold. This makes it less likely that the person will try to hit you.

After a Bath or Shower

- Prevent rashes or infections by patting the person's skin with a towel. Make sure the person is completely dry. Be sure to dry between folds of skin.

- If the person has trouble with incontinence, use a protective ointment, such as Vaseline®, around the rectum, vagina, or penis.

- If the person with AD has trouble getting in and out of the bathtub, do a sponge bath instead.

Other Bathing Tips

- Give the person a full bath two or three times a week. For most people, a sponge bath to clean the face, hands, feet, underarms, and genital or "private" area is all you need to do every day.

- Washing the person's hair in the sink may be easier than doing it in the shower or bathtub. You can buy a hose attachment for the sink.

- Get professional help with bathing if it becomes too hard for you to do on your own.

Grooming

For the most part, when people feel good about how they look, they feel better. Helping people with AD brush their teeth, shave, or put on makeup often means they can feel more like themselves. Here are some grooming tips.

Mouth Care

Good mouth care helps prevent dental problems such as cavities and gum disease.

- Show the person how to brush his or her teeth. Go step-by-step. For example, pick up the toothpaste, take the top off, put the toothpaste on the toothbrush, and then brush. Remember to let the person do as much as possible.

- Brush your teeth at the same time.

- Help the person clean his or her dentures. Make sure she or he uses the denture cleaning material the right way.

- Ask the person to rinse his or her mouth with water after each meal and use mouthwash once a day.

- Try a long-handled, angled, or electric toothbrush if you need to brush the person's teeth.

- Take the person to see a dentist. Some dentists specialize in treating people with AD. Be sure to follow the dentist's advice about how often to make an appointment.

Other Grooming Tips

- Encourage a woman to wear makeup if she has always used it. If needed, help her put on powder and lipstick. Don't use eye makeup.

- Encourage a man to shave, and help him as needed. Use an electric razor for safety.

- Take the person to the barber or beauty shop. Some barbers or hairstylists may come to your home.

- Keep the person's nails clean and trimmed.

Dressing

People with AD often need more time to dress. It can be hard for them to choose their clothes. They might wear the wrong clothing for the season. They also might wear colors that don't go together or forget to put on a piece of clothing. Allow the person to dress on his or her own for as long as possible.

Other tips include the following:

- Lay out clothes in the order the person should put them on, such as underwear first, then pants, then a shirt, and then a sweater.

- Hand the person one thing at a time or give step-by-step dressing instructions.

- Put away some clothes in another room to reduce the number of choices. Keep only one or two outfits in the closet or dresser.

- Keep the closet locked if needed. This prevents some of the problems people may have while getting dressed.

- Buy three or four sets of the same clothes, if the person wants to wear the same clothing every day.

- Buy loose-fitting, comfortable clothing. Avoid girdles, control-top pantyhose, knee-high nylons, garters, high heels, tight socks, and bras for women. Sports bras are comfortable and provide good support. Short cotton socks and loose cotton underwear are best. Sweatpants and shorts with elastic waistbands are helpful.

- Use Velcro® tape or large zipper pulls for clothing, instead of shoelaces, buttons, or buckles. Try slip-on shoes that won't slide off or shoes with Velcro® straps.

Adapting Activities for People with Alzheimer Disease

Doing things we enjoy gives us pleasure and adds meaning to our lives. People with AD need to be active and do things they enjoy. However, don't expect too much. It's not easy for them to plan their days and do different tasks.

Here are two reasons:

- They may have trouble deciding what to do each day. This could make them fearful and worried or quiet and withdrawn.

- They may have trouble starting tasks. Remember, the person is not being lazy. She or he might need help organizing the day or doing an activity.

Daily Activities

Plan activities that the person with AD enjoys. She or he can be a part of the activity or just watch. Also, you don't always have to be the "activities director."

Here are things you can do to help the person enjoy an activity:

- Match the activity with what the person with AD can do.

- Choose activities that can be fun for everyone.

- Help the person get started.

- Decide if she or he can do the activity alone or needs help.

- Watch to see if the person gets frustrated.

- Make sure she or he feels successful and has fun.

- Let him or her watch if that is more enjoyable.

411

The person with AD can do different activities each day. This keeps the day interesting and fun. The following pages may give you some ideas.

Household Chores

Doing household chores can boost the person's self-esteem. When the person helps you, don't forget to say "thank you."
The person could:

- Wash dishes, set the table, or prepare food.

- Sweep the floor.

- Polish shoes.

- Sort mail and clip coupons.

- Sort socks and fold laundry.

- Sort recycling materials or other things.

Cooking and Baking

Cooking and baking can bring the person with AD a lot of joy. She or he might help do the following:

- Decide on what is needed to prepare the dish.

- Make the dish.

- Measure, mix, and pour.

- Tell someone else how to prepare a recipe.

- Taste the food.

- Watch others prepare food.

Children

Being around children also can be fun. It gives the person with AD someone to talk with and may bring back happy memories. It also can help the person realize how much she or he still can love others and can still be loved.
Here are some things the person might enjoy doing with children:

- Play a simple board game.

- Read stories or books.

- Visit family members who have small children.

- Walk in the park or around schoolyards.

- Go to sports or school events that involve young people.

- Talk about fond memories from childhood.

Music and Dancing

Music can bring back happy memories and feelings. Some people feel the rhythm and may want to dance. Others enjoy listening to or talking about their favorite music. Even if the person with AD has trouble finding the right words to speak, she or he still may be able to sing songs from the past.

Consider the following musical activities:

- Play CDs, tapes, or records.

- Talk about the music and the singer.

- Ask what she or he was doing when the song was popular.

- Talk about the music and past events.

- Sing or dance to well-known songs.

- Play musical games like "Name That Tune."

- Attend a concert or musical program.

Pets

Many people with AD enjoy pets, such as dogs, cats, or birds. Pets may help "bring them to life." Pets also can help people feel more loved and less worried.

Suggested activities with pets include:

- Care for, feed, or groom the pet.

- Walk the pet.

- Sit and hold the pet.

Gardening

Gardening is a way to be part of nature. It also may help people remember past days and fun times. Gardening can help the person focus on what she or he still can do.

Here are some suggested gardening activities:

- Take care of indoor or outdoor plants.

- Plant flowers and vegetables.

- Water the plants when needed.

- Talk about how much the plants are growing.

Going Out

Early in the disease, people with AD may still enjoy the same kinds of outings they enjoyed in the past. Keep going on these outings as long as you are comfortable doing them.

Plan outings for the time of day when the person is at his or her best. Keep outings from becoming too long. You want to note how tired the person with AD gets after a certain amount of time (1/2 hour, 1 hour, 2 hours, etc.).

The person might enjoy outings to a:

- Favorite restaurant

- Zoo, park, or shopping mall

- Swimming pool (during a slow time of day at the pool)

- Museum, theater, or art exhibits for short trips

Remember that you can use a business-size card, as shown below, to tell others about the person's disease. Sharing the information with store clerks or restaurant staff can make outings more comfortable for everyone.

Eating Out

Going out to eat can be a welcome change. But, it also can have some challenges. Planning can help. You need to think about the layout of the restaurant, the menu, the noise level, waiting times, and the helpfulness of staff. Below are some tips for eating out with the person who has AD.

Before choosing a restaurant, ask yourself:

- Does the person with AD know the restaurant well?

- Is it quiet or noisy most of time?

- Are tables easy to get to? Do you need to wait before you can be seated?

- Is the service quick enough to keep the person from getting restless?

- Does the restroom meet the person's needs?

- Are foods the person with AD likes on the menu?

- Is the staff understanding and helpful?

Before going to the restaurant, decide:

- Is it a good day to go?

- When is the best time to go? Going out earlier in the day may be best, so the person is not too tired. Service may be quicker, and there may be fewer people. If you decide to go later, try to get the person to take a nap first.

- What should you take with you? You may need to take utensils, a towel, wipes, or toilet items that the person already uses. If so, make sure this is OK with the restaurant.

At the restaurant:

- Tell the waiter or waitress about any special needs, such as extra spoons, bowls, or napkins.

- Ask for a table near the washroom and in a quiet area.

- Seat the person with his or her back to the busy areas.

- Help the person choose his or her meal, if needed. Suggest food you know the person likes. Read parts of the menu or show the person a picture of the food. Limit the number of choices.

- Ask the waiter or waitress to fill glasses half full or leave the drinks for you to serve.

- Order some finger food or snacks to hold the attention of the person with AD.

- Go with the person to the restroom. Go into the stall if the person needs help.

Traveling

Taking the person with AD on a trip is a challenge. Traveling can make the person more worried and confused. Planning can make travel easier for everyone. Below are some tips that you may find helpful.

415

Before you leave on the trip:

- Talk with your doctor about medicines to calm someone who gets upset while traveling.

- Find someone to help you at the airport or train station.

- Keep important documents with you in a safe place. These include: insurance cards, passports, doctor's name and phone number, list of medicines, and a copy of medical records.

- Pack items the person enjoys looking at or holding for comfort.

- Travel with another family member or friend.

- Take an extra set of clothing in a carry-on bag.

After you arrive:

- Allow lots of time for each thing you want to do. Do not plan too many activities.

- Plan rest periods.

- Follow a routine like the one you use at home. For example, try to have the person eat, rest, and go to bed at the same time she or he does at home.

- Keep a well-lighted path to the toilet, and leave the bathroom light on all night.

- Be prepared to cut your visit short.

People with memory problems may wander around a place they don't know well.

In case someone with AD gets lost:

- Make sure they wear or have something with them that tells who they are, such as an ID bracelet.

- Carry a recent photo of the person with you on the trip.

Spiritual Activities

Like you, the person with AD may have spiritual needs. If so, you can help the person stay part of his or her faith community. This can help the person feel connected to others and remember pleasant times.

Here are some tips for helping a person with AD who has spiritual needs:

- Involve the person in spiritual activities that she or he has known well. These might include worship, religious or other readings, sacred music, prayer, and holiday rituals.

- Tell people in your faith community that the person has AD. Encourage them to talk with the person and show him or her that they still care.

- Play religious or other music that is important to the person. It may bring back old memories. Even if the person with AD has a problem finding the right words to speak, she or he still may be able to sing songs or hymns from the past.

Holidays

Many caregivers have mixed feelings about holidays. They may have happy memories of the past. But, they also may worry about the extra demands that holidays make on their time and energy.

Here are some suggestions to help you find a balance between doing many holiday-related things and resting:

- Celebrate holidays that are important to you. Include the person with AD as much as possible.

- Understand that things will be different. Be realistic about what you can do.

- Ask friends and family to visit. Limit the number of visitors at any one time. Plan visits when the person usually is at his or her best.

- Avoid crowds, changes in routine, and strange places that may make the person with AD feel confused or nervous.

- Do your best to enjoy yourself. Find time for the holiday activities you like to do. Ask a friend or family member to spend time with the person while you're out.

- Make sure there is a space where the person can rest when she or he goes to larger gatherings such as weddings or family reunions.

Visitors

Visitors are important to people with AD. They may not always remember who visitors are, but they often enjoy the company.

Here are ideas to share with a person planning to visit someone with AD:

- Plan the visit when the person with AD is at his or her best.

- Consider bringing along some kind of activity, such as a well-known book or photo album to look at. This can help if the person is bored or confused and needs to be distracted. But, be prepared to skip the activity if it is not needed.

- Be calm and quiet. Don't use a loud voice or talk to the person as if she or he were a child.

- Respect the person's personal space, and don't get too close.

- Make eye contact and call the person by name to get his or her attention.

- Remind the person who you are if she or he doesn't seem to know you. Try not to say "Don't you remember?"

- Don't argue if the person is confused. Respond to the feelings that they express. Try to distract the person by talking about something different.

- Remember not to take it personally if the person doesn't recognize you, is unkind, or gets angry. She or he is acting out of confusion.

Chapter 53

Safety Issues for People with Alzheimer Disease

Chapter Contents

Section 53.1

Safety at Home

This section contains text excerpted from the following sources:
Text in this section begins with excerpts from "Home Safety and
Alzheimer's Disease," National Institute on Aging (NIA), National
Institutes of Health (NIH), May 18, 2017; Text under the heading
"Home Safety Checklist for Alzheimer Disease" is excerpted from
"Home Safety Checklist for Alzheimer's Disease," National Institute
on Aging (NIA), National Institutes of Health (NIH), May 18, 2017.

Over time, people with Alzheimer disease (AD) become less able
to manage around the house. For example, they may forget to turn
off the oven or the water, how to use the phone during an emergency,
which things around the house are dangerous, and where things are
in their own home.

As a caregiver, you can do many things to make the person's home
a safer place. Think prevention—help avoid accidents by controlling
possible problems.

While some Alzheimer disease behaviors can be managed medically,
many, such as wandering and agitation, cannot. It is more effective to
change the person's surroundings—for example, to remove dangerous
items—than to try to change behaviors. Changing the home environment can give the person more freedom to move around independently
and safely.

Create an Alzheimer-Safe Home

Add the following items to the person's home if they are not already
in place:

- Smoke and carbon monoxide detectors in or near the kitchen and
  in all bedrooms

- Emergency phone numbers (ambulance, poison control, doctors,
  hospital, etc.) and the person's address near all phones

- Safety knobs and an automatic shut-off switch on the stove

- Childproof plugs for unused electrical outlets and childproof
  latches on cabinet doors

You can buy home safety products at stores carrying hardware,
electronics, medical supplies, and children's items.

Lock up or remove these potentially dangerous items from the home:

- Prescription and over-the-counter (OTC) medicines
- Alcohol
- Cleaning and household products, such as paint thinner and matches
- Poisonous plants—contact the National Poison Control Center at 800-222-1222 or www.poison.org to find out which houseplants are poisonous
- Guns and other weapons, scissors, knives, power tools, and machinery
- Gasoline cans and other dangerous items in the garage

Moving around the House

Try these tips to prevent falls and injuries:

- Simplify the home. Too much furniture can make it hard to move around freely.
- Get rid of clutter, such as piles of newspapers and magazines.
- Have a sturdy handrail on stairways.
- Put carpet on stairs, or mark the edges of steps with brightly colored tape so the person can see them more easily.
- Put a gate across the stairs if the person has balance problems.
- Remove small throw rugs. Use rugs with nonskid backing instead.
- Make sure cords to electrical outlets are out of the way or tacked to baseboards.
- Clean up spills right away.

Make sure the person with AD has good floor traction for walking. To make floors less slippery, leave floors unpolished or install nonskid strips. Shoes and slippers with good traction also help the person move around safely.

Minimize Danger

People with Alzheimer disease may not see, smell, touch, hear, and/ or taste things as they used to. You can do things around the house to make life safer and easier for the person.

Seeing

Although there may be nothing physically wrong with their eyes, people with AD may no longer be able to interpret accurately what they see. Their sense of perception and depth may be altered, too. These changes can cause safety concerns.

- Make floors and walls different colors. This creates contrast and makes it easier for the person to see.
- Remove curtains and rugs with busy patterns that may confuse the person.
- Mark the edges of steps with brightly colored tape so people can see the steps as they go up or downstairs.
- Use brightly colored signs or simple pictures to label the bathroom, bedroom, and kitchen.
- Be careful about small pets. The person with AD may not see the pet and trip over it.
- Limit the size and number of mirrors in your home, and think about where to put them. Mirror images may confuse the person with Alzheimer disease.
- Use dishes and placemats in contrasting colors for easier identification.

Touching

People with AD may experience loss of sensation or may no longer be able to interpret feelings of heat, cold, or discomfort.

- Reset your water heater to 120°F to prevent burns.
- Label hot-water faucets red and cold-water faucets blue or write the words "hot" and "cold" near them.
- Put signs near the oven, toaster, iron, and other things that get hot. The sign could say, "Stop!" or "Don't Touch—Very Hot!" Be sure the sign is not so close that it could catch on fire. The person with AD should not use appliances without supervision. Unplug appliances when not in use.
- Pad any sharp corners on your furniture, or replace or remove furniture with sharp corners.
- Test the water to make sure it is a comfortable temperature before the person gets into the bath or shower.

Smelling

A loss of or decrease in smell is common in people with Alzheimer disease.

- Use good smoke detectors. People with AD may not be able to smell smoke.

- Check foods in your refrigerator often. Throw out any that have gone bad.

Tasting

People with AD may not taste as well as before. They also may place dangerous or inappropriate things in their mouths.

- Keep foods like salt, sugar, and spices away from the person if you see him or her using too much.

- Put away or lock up things like toothpaste, lotions, shampoos, rubbing alcohol, soap, perfume, or laundry detergent pods. They may look and smell like food to a person with Alzheimer disease.

- Keep the poison control number (800-222-1222) by the phone.

- Learn what to do if the person chokes on something. Check with your local Red Cross chapter about health or safety classes.

Hearing

People with Alzheimer disease may have normal hearing, but they may lose their ability to interpret what they hear accurately. This loss may result in confusion or overstimulation.

- Don't play the television (TV), compact disc (CD) player, or radio too loudly, and don't play them at the same time. Loud music or too many different sounds may be too much for the person with AD to handle.

- Limit the number of people who visit at any one time. If there is a party, settle the person with AD in an area with fewer people.

- Shut the windows if it's very noisy outside.

- If the person wears a hearing aid, check the batteries and settings often.

It may not be necessary to make all these changes; however, you may want to re-evaluate the safety of the person's home as behavior and abilities change.

Is It Safe to Leave the Person with Alzheimer Disease Alone?

This issue needs careful evaluation and is certainly a safety concern. The following points may help you decide.

Does the person with AD:

- Become confused or unpredictable under stress?

- Recognize a dangerous situation, for example, fire?

- Know how to use the telephone in an emergency?

- Know how to get help?

- Stay content within the home?

- Wander and become disoriented?

- Show signs of agitation, depression, or withdrawal when left alone for any period of time?

- Attempt to pursue former interests or hobbies that might now warrant supervision, such as cooking, appliance repair, or woodworking?

You may want to seek input and advice from a healthcare professional to assist you in these considerations. As Alzheimer disease progresses, these questions will need ongoing evaluation.

Home Safety Checklist for Alzheimer Disease

Use the following room-by-room checklist to alert you to potential hazards and to record any changes you need to make to help keep a person with Alzheimer disease safe. You can buy products or gadgets necessary for home safety at stores carrying hardware, electronics, medical supplies, and children's items.

Keep in mind that it may not be necessary to make all of the suggested changes. This section covers a wide range of safety concerns that may arise, and some modifications may never be needed. It is important, however, to reevaluate home safety periodically as behavior and abilities change.

Throughout the Home

- Display emergency numbers and your home address near all telephones.

- Use an answering machine when you cannot answer phone calls, and set it to turn on after the fewest number of rings possible. A person with Alzheimer disease often may be unable to take messages or could become a victim of telephone exploitation. Turn ringers on low to avoid distraction and confusion. Put all portable and cell phones and equipment in a safe place so they will not be easily lost.

- Install smoke alarms and carbon monoxide detectors in or near the kitchen and all sleeping areas. Check their functioning and batteries frequently.

- Avoid the use of flammable and volatile compounds near gas appliances. Do not store these materials in an area where a gas pilot light is used.

- Install secure locks on all outside doors and windows.

- Install alarms that notify you when a door or window is opened.

- Hide a spare house key outside in case the person with Alzheimer disease locks you out of the house.

- Avoid the use of extension cords if possible by placing lamps and appliances close to electrical outlets. Tack extension cords to the baseboards of a room to avoid tripping.

- Cover unused electrical outlets with childproof plugs.

- Place red tape around floor vents, radiators, and other heating devices to deter the person with AD from standing on or touching them when hot.

- Check all rooms for adequate lighting.

- Place light switches at the top and the bottom of stairs.

- Stairways should have at least one handrail that extends beyond the first and last steps. If possible, stairways should be carpeted or have safety grip strips. Put a gate across the stairs if the person has balance problems.

- Keep all medications (prescription and over-the-counter (OTC)) locked. Each bottle of prescription medicine should be clearly labeled with the person's name, name of the drug, drug strength, dosage frequency, and expiration date. Child-resistant caps are available if needed.

- Keep all alcohol in a locked cabinet or out of reach of the person with AD. Drinking alcohol can increase confusion.

- If the person with Alzheimer disease smokes, remove matches, lighters, ashtrays, cigarettes, and other means of smoking from view. This reduces fire hazards, and with these reminders out of sight, the person may forget the desire to smoke.

- Avoid clutter, which can create confusion and danger. Throw out or recycle newspapers and magazines regularly. Keep all areas where people walk free of furniture.

- Keep plastic bags out of reach. A person with Alzheimer disease may choke or suffocate.

- Remove all guns and other weapons from the home or lock them up. Install safety locks on guns or remove ammunition and firing pins.

- Lock all power tools and machinery in the garage, workroom, or basement.

- Remove all poisonous plants from the home. Check with local nurseries or contact poison control (800-222-1222) for a list of poisonous plants.

- Make sure all computer equipment and accessories, including electrical cords, are kept out of the way. If valuable documents or materials are stored on a home computer, protect the files with passwords and back up the files. Password protect access to the Internet, and restrict the amount of online time without supervision. Consider monitoring computer use by the person with AD, and install software that screens for objectionable or offensive material on the Internet.

- Keep fish tanks out of reach. The combination of glass, water, electrical pumps, and potentially poisonous aquatic life could be harmful to a curious person with Alzheimer disease.

Outside Approaches to the House

- Keep steps sturdy and textured to prevent falls in wet or icy weather.

- Mark the edges of steps with bright or reflective tape.

- Consider installing a ramp with handrails as an alternative to the steps.

- Eliminate uneven surfaces or walkways, hoses, and other objects that may cause a person to trip.

- Restrict access to a swimming pool by fencing it with a locked gate, covering it, and closely supervising it when in use.

- In the patio area, remove the fuel source and fire starters from any grills when not in use, and supervise use when the person with AD is present.

- Place a small bench or table by the entry door to hold parcels while unlocking the door.

- Make sure outside lighting is adequate. Light sensors that turn on lights automatically as you approach the house may be useful. They also may be used in other parts of the home.

- Prune bushes and foliage well away from walkways and doorways.

- Consider a "NO SOLICITING" sign for the front gate or door.

Entryway

- Remove scatter rugs and throw rugs.

- Use textured strips or nonskid wax on hardwood and tile floors to prevent slipping.

Kitchen

- Install childproof door latches on storage cabinets and drawers designated for breakable or dangerous items. Lock away all household cleaning products, matches, knives, scissors, blades, small appliances, and anything valuable.

- If prescription or nonprescription drugs are kept in the kitchen, store them in a locked cabinet.

- Remove scatter rugs and foam pads from the floor.

- Install safety knobs and an automatic shut-off switch on the stove.

- Do not use or store flammable liquids in the kitchen. Lock them in the garage or in an outside storage unit.

- Keep a night-light in the kitchen.

- Remove or secure the family "junk drawer." A person with AD may eat small items such as matches, hardware, erasers, plastics, etc.

- Remove artificial fruits and vegetables or food-shaped kitchen magnets, which might appear to be edible.

- Insert a drain trap in the kitchen sink to catch anything that may otherwise become lost or clog the plumbing.

- Consider disconnecting the garbage disposal. People with AD may place objects or their own hands in the disposal.

Bedroom

- Anticipate the reasons a person with Alzheimer disease might get out of bed, such as hunger, thirst, going to the bathroom, restlessness, and pain. Try to meet these needs by offering food and fluids and scheduling ample toileting.

- Use a night-light.

- Use a monitoring device (like those used for infants) to alert you to any sounds indicating a fall or other need for help. This also is an effective device for bathrooms.

- Remove scatter rugs and throw rugs.

- Remove portable space heaters. If you use portable fans, be sure that objects cannot be placed in the blades.

- Be cautious when using electric mattress pads, electric blankets, electric sheets, and heating pads, all of which can cause burns and fires. Keep controls out of reach.

- If the person with Alzheimer disease is at risk of falling out of bed, placemats next to the bed, as long as they do not create a greater risk of accident.

- Use transfer or mobility aids.

- If you are considering using a hospital-type bed with rails and/ or wheels, read the U.S. Food and Drug Administration's (FDA) safety information.

Bathroom

- Do not leave a severely impaired person with AD alone in the bathroom.

- Remove the lock from the bathroom door to prevent the person with AD from getting locked inside.

- Place nonskid adhesive strips, decals, or mats in the tub and shower. If the bathroom is uncarpeted, consider placing these strips next to the tub, toilet, and sink.

- Use washable wall-to-wall bathroom carpeting to prevent slipping on wet tile floors.

- Use a raised toilet seat with handrails, or install grab bars beside the toilet.

- Install grab bars in the tub/shower. A grab bar in contrasting color to the wall is easier to see.

- Use a foam rubber faucet cover (often used for small children) in the tub to prevent serious injury should the person with Alzheimer disease fall.

- Use a plastic shower stool and a hand-held shower head to make bathing easier.

- In the shower, tub, and sink, use a single faucet that mixes hot and cold water to avoid burns.

- Set the water heater at 120°F to avoid scalding tap water.

- Insert drain traps in sinks to catch small items that may be lost or flushed down the drain.

- Store medications (prescription and nonprescription) in a locked cabinet. Check medication dates and dispose of outdated medications.

- Remove cleaning products from under the sink, or lock them away.

- Use a night-light.

- Remove small electrical appliances from the bathroom. Cover electrical outlets.

- If a man with Alzheimer disease uses an electric razor, have him use a mirror outside the bathroom to avoid water contact.

Living Room

- Clear electrical cords from all areas where people walk.

- Remove scatter rugs or throw rugs. Repair or replace torn carpet.

- Place decals at eye level on sliding glass doors, picture windows, or furniture with large glass panels to identify the glass pane.

- Do not leave the person with Alzheimer disease alone with an open fire in the fireplace. Consider alternative heating sources.

- Keep matches and cigarette lighters out of reach.

- Keep the remote controls for the television, digital video disc (DVD) player, and stereo system out of sight.

Laundry Room

- Keep the door to the laundry room locked if possible.

- Lock all laundry products in a cabinet. Laundry detergent pods can be fatal if eaten by accident.

- Remove large knobs from the washer and dryer if the person with Alzheimer disease tampers with machinery.

- Close and latch the doors and lids to the washer and dryer to prevent objects from being placed in the machines.

Garage / Shed / Basement

- Lock access to all garages, sheds, and basements if possible.

- Inside a garage or shed, keep all potentially dangerous items, such as tools, tackle, machines, and sporting equipment either locked away in cabinets or in appropriate boxes/cases.

- Secure and lock all motor vehicles and keep them out of sight if possible. Consider covering vehicles, including bicycles, that are not frequently used. This may reduce the possibility that the person with AD will think about leaving.

- Keep all toxic materials, such as paint, fertilizers, gasoline, or cleaning supplies, out of view. Either put them in a high, dry place, or lock them in a cabinet.

- If the person with AD is permitted in a garage, shed, or basement, preferably with supervision, make sure the area is well lit and that stairs have a handrail and are safe to walk up and down. Keep walkways clear of debris and clutter, and place overhanging items out of reach.

Section 53.2

Using Medicines Safely

This section includes text excerpted from "Managing Medicines
for a Person with Alzheimer's," National Institute on Aging (NIA),
National Institutes of Health (NIH), May 18, 2017.

People with Alzheimer disease (AD) may take medicines to treat the
disease itself, mood or behavior changes, and other medical conditions.
Caregivers can ensure that medicines are taken safely and correctly.
Here are some tips to help you manage medications for someone with
AD.

People with Alzheimer disease often need help taking their medicine. If the person lives alone, you may need to call and remind him
or her or leave notes around the home. A pillbox allows you to put
pills for each day in one place. Some pillboxes come with alarms that
remind a person to take the medicine.

As Alzheimer disease gets worse, you will need to keep track of the
person's medicines. You also will need to make sure the person takes
the medicines or give the medicines to him or her.

Some people with Alzheimer disease take medicines to treat behavior problems such as restlessness, anxiety, depression, trouble sleeping, and aggression. Experts agree that medicines to treat behavior
problems should be used only after other strategies that don't use
medicine have been tried. Talk with the person's doctor about which
medicines are safest and most effective. With these types of medicines,
it is important to:

- Use the lowest dose possible

- Watch for side effects such as confusion and falls

- Allow the medicine a few weeks to take effect

People with Alzheimer disease should NOT take anticholinergic
drugs. These drugs are used to treat many medical problems such as
sleeping problems, stomach cramps, incontinence, asthma, motion
sickness, and muscle spasms. Side effects, such as confusion, can be
serious for a person with Alzheimer disease. These drugs should NOT
be given to a person with Alzheimer disease. You might talk with the
person's doctor about other options. Examples of these drugs include:

- Atrovent® (ipratropium)

431

- Dramamine® (dimenhydrinate)

- Diphenhydramine—includes brand names such as Benadryl® and Nytol®

Some people, especially those with late-stage Alzheimer disease, may have trouble swallowing pills. In this case, ask the pharmacist if the medicine can be crushed or taken in liquid form. Other ways to make sure medicines are taken safely:

- Keep all medications locked up.

- Check that the label on each prescription bottle has the drug name and dose, patient's name, dosage frequency, and expiration date.

- Call the doctor or pharmacist if you have questions about any medicine.

Section 53.3

Wandering

This section includes text excerpted from "Wandering and Alzheimer's Disease," National Institute on Aging (NIA), National Institutes of Health (NIH), May 17, 2017.

Many people with Alzheimer disease (AD) wander away from their home or caregiver. As the caregiver, you need to know how to limit wandering and prevent the person from becoming lost. This will help keep the person safe and give you greater peace of mind.

First Steps

Try to follow these steps before the person with AD wanders:

- Make sure the person carries some kind of ID or wears a medical bracelet. If the person gets lost and can't communicate clearly, an ID will let others know about his or her illness. It also shows where the person lives.

- Consider enrolling the person in the MedicAlert® + Alzheimer Association Safe Return® Program (call 888-572-8566 to find the program in your area).

- Let neighbors and the local police know that the person with AD tends to wander. Ask them to alert you immediately if the person is seen alone and on the move.

- Place labels in garments to aid in identification.

- Keep an article of the person's worn, unwashed clothing in a plastic bag to aid in finding him or her with the use of dogs.

- Keep a recent photograph or video recording of the person to help police if she or he becomes lost.

Tips to Prevent Wandering

Here are some tips to help prevent the person with AD from wandering away from home:

- Keep the doors locked. Consider a keyed deadbolt, or add another lock placed up high or down low on the door. If the person can open a lock, you may need to get a new latch or lock.

- Use loosely fitting doorknob covers so that the cover turns instead of the actual knob.

- Place "STOP," "DO NOT ENTER," or "CLOSED" signs on doors.

- Divert the attention of the person with Alzheimer disease away from using the door by placing small scenic posters on the door; placing removable gates, curtains, or brightly colored streamers across the door; or wallpapering the door to match any adjoining walls.

- Install safety devices found in hardware stores to limit how much windows can be opened.

- Install an "announcing system" that chimes when a door is opened.

- Secure the yard with fencing and a locked gate.

- Keep shoes, keys, suitcases, coats, hats, and other signs of departure out of sight.

- Do not leave a person with AD who has a history of wandering unattended.

You can also make changes in your home to improve safety for someone who wanders.

Section 53.4

Disaster Preparedness for Patients with Alzheimer Disease Caregivers

This section includes text excerpted from "Disaster Preparedness for Alzheimer's Caregivers," National Institute on Aging (NIA), National Institutes of Health (NIH), May 17, 2017.

People with AD disease can be especially vulnerable during disasters such as severe weather, fires, floods, earthquakes, and other emergency situations. It is important for caregivers to have a disaster plan that includes the special needs of people with AD, whose impairments in memory and reasoning severely limit their ability to act appropriately in crises.

In general, you should prepare to meet the needs of your family for three to seven days, including having supplies and backup options if you lose basic services such as water or electricity. Organizations such as the Federal Emergency Management Agency (FEMA) and the American Red Cross (ARC) provide information about making a general disaster preparedness plan.

Gather Supplies

As you assemble supplies for your family's disaster kit, consider the needs of the person with AD. Be sure to store all supplies in a watertight container. The kit might contain:

- Incontinence undergarments, wipes, and lotions

- Pillow, toy, or something the person can hold onto

- Favorite snacks and high-nutrient drinks

- Physician's name, address, and phone number

- Copies of legal, medical, insurance, and Social Security information
- Ziplock® bags to hold medications and documents
- Recent photos of the person

Other supplies you may need are:

- Warm clothing and sturdy shoes
- Spare eyeglasses and hearing-aid batteries
- Medications
- Flashlights and extra batteries

If You Must Leave Home

In some situations, you may decide to "ride out" a natural disaster at home. In others, you may need to move to a safer place, like a community shelter or someone's home. Relocation may make the person with AD very anxious. Be sensitive to his or her emotions. Stay close, offer your hand, or give the person reassuring hugs.

To plan for an evacuation:

- Know how to get to the nearest emergency shelters.
- If you don't drive or driving is dangerous, arrange for someone to transport your group.
- Make sure the person with AD wears an ID bracelet.
- Take both general supplies and your AD emergency kit.
- Pack familiar, comforting items. If possible, plan to take along the household pet.
- Save emergency numbers in your cell phone, and keep it charged.
- Plan to keep neighbors, friends, and family informed about your location.
- If conditions are noisy or chaotic, try to find a quieter place.

If You Are Separated

It's very important to stay with a person with AD in a disaster. Do not count on the person to stay in one place while you go to get help.

However, the unexpected can happen, so it is a good idea to plan for possible separation:

- Enroll the person in the MedicAlert® + Alzheimer Association Safe Return® Program—an identification and support service for people who may become lost.

- Prepare for wandering. Place labels in garments to aid in identification. Keep an article of the person's clothing in a plastic bag to help dogs find him or her.

- Identify specific neighbors or nearby family and friends who would be willing to help in a crisis. Make a plan of action with them should the person with AD be unattended during a crisis. Tell neighbors about the person's specific disabilities, including inability to follow complex instructions, memory loss, impaired judgment, disorientation, and confusion. Give examples of simple one-step instructions that the person may be able to follow.

- Give someone you trust a house key and list of emergency phone numbers.

- Provide local police and emergency services with photos of the person with AD and copies of his or her medical documents, so they are aware of the person's needs.

Section 53.5

Understanding Elder Abuse

This section contains text excerpted from the following sources: Text in this section begins with excerpts from "How at Risk for Abuse Are People with Dementia?" Administration for Community Living (ACL), 2011. Reviewed December 2018; Text beginning with the heading "What Is the Impact of Elder Abuse?" is excerpted from "What We Do—Research," Administration for Community Living (ACL), May 15, 2008. Reviewed December 2018.

Elder abuse is one of the most overlooked public health hazards in the United States. The National Center on Elder Abuse

(NCEA) estimates that between two to five million elderly Americans suffer from some form of elder abuse each year. The main types of elder abuse are physical abuse, sexual abuse, emotional and psychological abuse, neglect and self-neglect, abandonment, and financial exploitation. Elders with dementia are thought to be at greater risk of abuse and neglect than those of the general elderly population. The following studies looked directly at several questions related to how often people with dementia are abused by their caregivers and what, if any, variables are associated with mistreatment.

- The number of Americans with Alzheimer disease (AD) is expected to grow exponentially in the coming decades.

- At present, approximately 5.3 million Americans of all ages have Alzheimer disease.

- Approximately 7.7 million people will have Alzheimer disease in 2030, and the number will increase to 16 million in 2050.

Do Caregivers Fear Becoming Abusive with Person with Dementia?

In one U.S. study, 20 percent of caregivers expressed fears that they would become violent with the people for whom they cared for.

How Often Are Caregivers Abusive to People with Dementia?

- Three international studies found overall rates of abuse of people with dementia by their caregivers ranging from 34 to 62 percent.

- In a U.S. study, caregiver abuse and neglect of people with dementia was detected in 47.3 percent of the surveyed caregivers.

What Type of Abuse Is Most Reported by U.S. Caregivers of People with Dementia?
Verbal Abuse

One study shows 60 percent of caregivers had been verbally abusive with the person for whom they were providing care.

Physical Abuse

Between 5 and 10 percent of caregivers reported that they were physically abusive toward the care recipients.

Neglect

Fourteen percent of caregivers reported that they were neglectful.

What, If Any, Characteristics Are Associated with Different Kinds and Combinations of Mistreatment of People with Dementia?

Characteristics associated with mistreatment of people with dementia included:

- The caregiver's anxiety, depressive symptoms, social contacts, perceived burden, emotional status, and role limitations due to emotional problems.

- The care recipient's psychological aggression and physical assault behaviors. These behaviors were the best indicators for elder mistreatment as defined by the expert panel convened for this research study.

What Is the Impact of Elder Abuse?

Elder abuse has multitude of negative impacts on both the micro and macro levels including physical, psychological, financial, social, hospitalizations and disability, medical, and others.

Physical

- The most commonly documented physical impacts of elder abuse include: welts, wounds, and injuries (bruises, lacerations, dental problems, head injuries, broken bones, pressure sores); persistent physical pain and soreness; nutrition and hydration issues; sleep disturbances; increased susceptibility to new illnesses (including sexually transmitted diseases); exacerbation of preexisting health conditions; and increased risks for premature death.

- Elders who experienced abuse, even modest abuse, had a 300 percent higher risk of death when compared to those who had not been abused.

Psychological

- Established psychological impacts include levels of psychological distress, emotional symptoms, and depression higher than those observed among elders who have not experienced these exposures.

- One study of older women found that verbal abuse only leads to greater declines in mental health than physical abuse only.

Financial

- Financial exploitation causes large economic losses for businesses, families, elders, and government programs, and increases reliance on federal healthcare programs such as Medicaid.

- Research indicates that those with cognitive incapacities suffer 100 percent greater economic losses than those without such incapacities.

- Financial abuse by itself costs older Americans over $2.6 billion dollars annually.

Social

Social consequences may vary from increased social isolation (due to self-withdrawal or perpetrator imposition) to decreased social resources (social identities, supports, roles in key networks) and increased expenditures on services to compensate for resources lost through exploitation and to identify and rehabilitate elder abuse victims.

Hospitalizations and Disability

- Victims of elder abuse are three times more likely to be admitted to a hospital.

- Elder abuse is predictive of later disability among persons who initially displayed no disability and is associated with increased rates of emergency department (ED) utilization, increased risks for hospitalization, and increased risk for mortality.

Medical Costs

- The direct medical costs of injuries are estimated to contribute more than $5.3 billion to the nation's annual health expenditures.

- Most adverse events in nursing homes—due largely to inadequate treatment, care and understaffing—lead to preventable harm and $2.8 billion per year in Medicare hospital costs alone (excluding additional—and substantial—Medicaid costs caused by the same events).

Other Impacts

- Other societal costs may include expenses associated with the prosecution, punishment, and rehabilitation of elder abuse perpetrators. Estimates of such expenses are not currently available.

- Elder abuse causes victims to be more dependent on caregivers. As a result of providing care, caregivers experience declines in their own physical and mental health and their financial security suffers.

What Types of Interventions Have Been Identified?

Research on elder abuse interventions is a growing area. Below are some examples of interventions both in the community and among professionals that have been identified in academic literature.

Interventions in the Community

- **Social support:** Social support has been acknowledged as a potentially beneficial intervention. Efforts to enhance social support of older adults will have the dual benefit of building mental health resilience in response to extreme stressors and lowering the risk of interpersonal violence against the senior members of our society. One example of social support intervention is as follows:

  - A community-based elder abuse intervention program called "Eliciting Change in At-Risk Elders (ECARE)" assists suspected victims of elder abuse and self-neglect through a partnership with local law enforcement had favorable outcomes. This program involves building alliances with the elder and family members, connecting the elder to supportive services that reduce risk of further abuse, and utilizing motivational interviewing-type skills to help elders overcome ambivalence regarding making difficult life changes. Risk factors of elder abuse decreased over the course of the intervention and nearly three-quarters of participants made progress on their treatment goal. The project's findings suggest that a longer-term, relationship-based intervention for entrenched elders who are reluctant to receive services may be effective, and therefore, worth considering.

- **Education:** Education on elder abuse is another important way to intervene at the community level. Altering attitudes toward elder abuse may impact a persons' behavior toward older adults. The following example illustrates a way in which to provide elder abuse education, particularly to young adults.

  - Hayslip and colleagues examined the effectiveness of educational interventions in altering tolerance for and behavioral intentions of elder abuse among college student young adults. Findings suggested that while specific interventions may reduce elder abuse tolerance, supplemental educational efforts over time may be necessary to maintain intervention-specific gains in intentions and behaviors particular to elder abuse.

Professional Interventions

- **Multidisciplinary teams:** Given the complex nature of elder abuse, inter-professional teams, also referred to as multidisciplinary teams consisting of physicians, social workers, law-enforcement personnel, attorneys, and other community participants working together in a coordinated fashion, have been identified as a possibly successful intervention as no single discipline or sector alone has the resources or expertise needed to address the issue.

- **APS guidelines:** Interventions are also developing in reporting and data collection of elder abuse incidents. Adult Protective Services (APS) systems play a critical role in addressing the abuse, neglect, self-neglect, and financial exploitation of adults. Historically, there has been no federal "home" for APS nor a designated federal appropriation for this critically important service. Instead, states and local agencies have developed a wide variety of APS practices, resulting in significant variations between and sometimes within states. In an effort to support Adult Protective Service (APS) Agencies and enhance elder abuse response, the Administration on Community Living (ACL) has been developing guidelines intended to assist states in developing efficient and effective APS systems.

Chapter 54

Dementia, Caregiving, and Controlling Frustration

Taking care of yourself—physically and mentally—is one of the most important things you can do as a caregiver. This could mean asking family members and friends to help out, doing things you enjoy, or getting help from a home healthcare service. Taking these actions can bring you some relief. It also may help keep you from getting ill or depressed.

Ways to Take Care of Yourself

Here are some ways you can take care of yourself:

- Ask for help when you need it.
- Eat healthy foods.
- Join a caregiver's support group.

This chapter contains text excerpted from the following sources: Text in this chapter begins with excerpts from "Alzheimer's Caregiving: Caring for Yourself," National Institute on Aging (NIA), National Institutes of Health (NIH), May 17, 2017; Text under the heading "Taking Care of Yourself: Tips for Caregivers" is excerpted from "Taking Care of Yourself: Tips for Caregivers," National Institute on Aging (NIA), National Institutes of Health (NIH), May 2, 2017; Text under the heading "Holiday Hints for Alzheimer Disease Caregivers" is excerpted from "Holiday Hints for Alzheimer's Caregivers," National Institute on Aging (NIA), National Institutes of Health (NIH), May 18, 2017.

- Take breaks each day.

- Spend time with friends.

- Keep up with your hobbies and interests.

- Get exercise as often as you can.

- See your doctor on a regular basis.

- Keep your health, legal, and financial information up-to-date.

Asking for Help

Everyone needs help at times. However, many caregivers find it hard to ask for help. They may feel they should be able to do everything themselves, or that it's not all right to leave the person in their care with someone else. Or maybe they can't afford to pay someone to watch the person for an hour or two.

Here are some tips about asking for help:

- Remind yourself that it's okay to ask for help from family, friends, and others. You don't have to do everything yourself.

- Ask people to help out in specific ways, like making a meal, visiting the person, or taking the person out for a short time.

- Call for help from home healthcare or adult day care services when needed. To find providers in your area, contact Eldercare Locator (eldercare.acl.gov/public/Index.aspx).

- Use national and local resources to find out how to pay for some of this help, or get respite care services.

You may want to join a support group of Alzheimer disease (AD) caregivers. These groups meet in person or online to share experiences and tips and give each other support. Ask your doctor, check online, or contact the local chapter of the Alzheimer's Association.

What If Something Happened to You?

It is important to have a plan in case of your own illness, disability, or death.

- Consult a lawyer about setting up a living trust, durable power of attorney for healthcare and finances, and other estate planning tools.

444

- Consult with family and close friends to decide who will take responsibility for the person with AD. You also may want to seek information about your local public guardian's office, mental health conservator's office, adult protective services, or other case management services. These organizations may have programs to assist the person with AD in your absence.

- Maintain a notebook for the responsible person who will assume caregiving. Such a notebook should contain the following information:

  - Emergency phone numbers

  - Current problem behaviors and possible solutions

  - Ways to calm the person with AD

  - Assistance needed with toileting, feeding, or grooming

  - Favorite activities or food

Preview board and care or long-term care facilities in your community and select a few as possibilities. Share this information with the responsible person. If the person with Alzheimer disease is no longer able to live at home, the responsible person will be better able to carry out your wishes for long-term care.

Coping with Emotions and Stress

Caring for a person with AD takes a lot of time and effort. Your job can become even harder when the person gets angry with you, hurts your feelings, or forgets who you are. Sometimes, you may feel discouraged, sad, lonely, frustrated, confused, or angry. These feelings are normal.

Here are some things you can say to yourself that might help you feel better:

- I'm doing the best I can.

- What I'm doing would be hard for anyone.

- I'm not perfect, and that's okay.

- I can't control some things that happen.

- Sometimes, I just need to do what works for right now.

- I will enjoy the moments when we can be together in peace.

445

- Even when I do everything I can think of, the person with Alzheimer disease will still have problem behaviors because of the illness, not because of what I do.

- I will try to get help from a counselor if caregiving becomes too much for me.

Some caregivers find that going to a church, temple, or mosque helps them cope with the daily demands placed on them. For others, simply having a sense that larger forces are at work in the world helps them find a sense of balance and peace.

Getting Professional Help

Mental health professionals and social workers help you deal with any stress you may be feeling. They help you understand feelings, such as anger, sadness, or feeling out of control. They can also help you make plans for unexpected or sudden events.

Mental health professionals charge by the hour. Medicare, Medicaid, and some private health insurance plans may cover some of these costs. Ask your health insurance plan which mental health counselors and services it covers. Then check with your doctor, local family service agencies, and community mental health agencies for referrals to counselors.

More Tips for Self-Care

Here are other things to keep in mind as you take care of yourself:

- Understand that you may feel powerless and hopeless about what's happening to the person you care for.

- Understand that you may feel a sense of loss and sadness.

- Understand why you've chosen to take care of the person with Alzheimer disease. Ask yourself if you made this choice out of love, loyalty, a sense of duty, a religious obligation, financial concerns, fear, a habit, or self-punishment.

- Let yourself feel day-to-day "uplifts." These might include good feelings about the person you care for, support from other people, or time spent on your own interests.

Tips for Caregivers

Taking care of yourself is one of the most important things you can do as a caregiver. Make sure you're eating healthy, being active, and taking time for yourself.

Dealing with Feelings of Frustration and Guilt

Caregiving, especially from a distance, is likely to bring out many different emotions, both positive and negative. Feeling frustrated and angry with everyone, from the care recipient to the doctors, is a common experience. Anger could be a sign that you are overwhelmed or that you are trying to do too much. If you can, give yourself a break: take a walk, talk with your friends, get some sleep—try to do something for yourself.

Although they may not feel as physically exhausted and drained as the primary, hands-on caregiver, long-distance caregivers may still be worried and anxious. Sometimes, long-distance caregivers feel guilty about not being closer, not doing enough, not having enough time with the person, and perhaps even feeling jealous of those who do. Many long-distance caregivers also find that worrying about being able to afford to take time off from work, being away from family, or the cost of travel increases these frustrations. Remember that you are doing the best you can given the circumstances and that you can only do what you can do. It may help to know that these are feelings shared by many other long-distance caregivers—you are not alone in this.

Taking Care of Yourself

Taking care of yourself if one of the most important things you can do as a caregiver. Make sure you are making time for yourself, eating healthy foods, and being active. Consider joining a caregiver support group, either in your own community or online. Meeting other caregivers can relieve your sense of isolation and will give you a chance to exchange stories and ideas. If you need help, don't be afraid to ask for it.

Caregiving is not easy for anyone—not for the caregiver and not for the care recipient. There are sacrifices and adjustments for everyone. When you don't live where the care is needed, it may be especially hard to feel that what you are doing is enough and that what you are doing is important. It often is.

Holiday Hints for Alzheimer Disease Caregivers

Holidays can be meaningful, enriching times for both the person with Alzheimer disease and his or her family. Maintaining or adapting family rituals and traditions helps all family members feel a sense of belonging and family identity. For a person with Alzheimer disease, this link with a familiar past is reassuring.

However, when celebrations, special events, or holidays include many people, this can cause confusion and anxiety for a person with Alzheimer disease. She or he may find some situations easier and more pleasurable than others. The tips below can help you and the person with Alzheimer disease visit and reconnect with family, friends, and neighbors during holidays.

Finding the Right Balance

Many caregivers have mixed feelings about holidays. They may have happy memories of the past, but they also may worry about the extra demands that holidays make on their time and energy.

Here are some ways to balance doing many holiday-related activities while taking care of your own needs and those of the person with Alzheimer disease:

- Celebrate holidays that are important to you. Include the person with Alzheimer disease as much as possible.

- Set your own limits, and be clear about them with others. You do not have to live up to the expectations of friends or relatives. Your situation is different now.

- Involve the person with Alzheimer disease in simple holiday preparations, or have him or her observe your preparations. Observing you will familiarize him or her with the upcoming festivities. Participating with you may give the person the pleasure of helping and the fun of anticipating and reminiscing.

- Consider simplifying your holidays around the home. For example, rather than cooking an elaborate dinner, invite family and friends for a potluck. Instead of elaborate decorations, consider choosing a few select items.

- Encourage friends and family to visit even if it's difficult. Limit the number of visitors at any one time, or have a few people visit quietly with the person in a separate room. Plan visits when the person usually is at his or her best.

- Prepare quiet distractions to use, such as a family photo album, if the person with Alzheimer disease becomes upset or overstimulated.

- Make sure there is a space where the person can rest when she or he goes to larger gatherings.

- Try to avoid situations that may confuse or frustrate the person with Alzheimer disease, such as crowds, changes in routine, and strange places. Also try to stay away from noise, loud conversations, loud music, lighting that is too bright or too dark, and having too much rich food or drink (especially alcohol).
- Find time for holiday activities you like to do. If you receive invitations to celebrations that the person with Alzheimer disease cannot attend, go yourself. Ask a friend or family member to spend time with the person while you're out.

Preparing Guests

Explain to guests that the person with Alzheimer disease does not always remember what is expected and acceptable. Give examples of unusual behaviors that may take place such as incontinence, eating food with fingers, wandering, or hallucinations.

If this is the first visit since the person with Alzheimer disease became severely impaired, tell guests that the visit may be painful. The memory-impaired person may not remember guests' names or relationships but can still enjoy their company.

- Explain that memory loss is the result of the disease and is not intentional.
- Stress that the meaningfulness of the moment together matters more than what the person remembers.

Preparing the Person with Alzheimer Disease

Here are some tips to help the person with Alzheimer disease get ready for visitors:

- Begin showing a photo of the guest to the person a week before arrival. Each day, explain who the visitor is while showing the photo.
- Arrange a phone call for the person with Alzheimer disease and the visitor. The call gives the visitor an idea of what to expect and gives the person with Alzheimer disease an opportunity to become familiar with the visitor.
- Keep the memory-impaired person's routine as close to normal as possible.
- During the hustle and bustle of the holiday season, guard against fatigue and find time for adequate rest.

Chapter 55

Respite Care: Giving Caregivers a Break

Respite care provides short-term relief for primary caregivers. It can be arranged for just an afternoon or for several days or weeks. Care can be provided at home, in a healthcare facility, or at an adult day center.

Respite Care Costs

Respite services charge by the hour or by the number of days or weeks that services are provided. Most insurance plans do not cover these costs. You must pay all costs not covered by insurance or other funding sources. Medicare will cover most of the cost of up to five days in a row of respite care in a hospital or skilled nursing facility for a person receiving hospice care. Medicaid also may offer assistance.

Getting Help with Caregiving

Some caregivers need help when the person is in the early stages of Alzheimer disease (AD). Other caregivers look for help when the person

---

This chapter contains text excerpted from the following sources: Text in this chapter begins with excerpts from "What Is Respite Care?" National Institute on Aging (NIA), National Institutes of Health (NIH), May 1, 2017; Text beginning with the heading "Getting Help with Caregiving" is excerpted from "Caring for a Person with Alzheimer's Disease," National Institute on Aging (NIA), National Institutes of Health (NIH), January 2017.

is in the later stages of AD. It's okay to seek help whenever you need it. As the person moves through the stages of AD, she or he will need more care. One reason is that medicines used to treat AD can only control symptoms; they cannot cure the disease. Symptoms, such as memory loss and confusion, will get worse over time. Because of this, you will need more help. You may feel that asking for help shows weakness or a lack of caring, but the opposite is true. Asking for help shows your strength. It means you know your limits and when to seek support.

Build a Support System

According to many caregivers, building a local support system is a key way to get help. Your support system might include your caregiver support group, the local chapter of the Alzheimer's Association, family, friends, and faith groups.

Call the Alzheimer's Disease Education and Referral (ADEAR) Center at 800-438-4380, the Alzheimer's Association at 800-272-3900, and the Eldercare Locator at 800-677-1116 to learn about where to get help in your community.

Caring for Yourself

Taking care of yourself is one of the most important things you can do as a caregiver. This could mean asking family members and friends to help out, doing things you enjoy, using adult day care services, or getting help from a local home healthcare agency. Taking these actions can bring you some relief. It also may help keep you from getting ill or depressed.

How to Take Care of Yourself

Here are some ways you can take care of yourself:

- Ask for help when you need it.
- Join a caregiver's support group.
- Take breaks each day.
- Spend time with friends.
- Keep up with your hobbies and interests.
- Eat healthy foods.
- Get exercise as often as you can.

- See your doctor on a regular basis.
- Keep your health, legal, and financial.

Getting Help

Everyone needs help at times. It's okay to ask for help and to take time for yourself. However, many caregivers find it hard to ask for help. You may feel:

- You should be able to do everything yourself
- That it's not all right to leave the person with someone else
- No one will help even if you ask
- You don't have the money to pay someone to watch the person for an hour or two

If you have trouble asking for help, try using some of the tips below.

- It's okay to ask for help from family, friends, and others. You don't have to do everything yourself.
- Ask people to help out in specific ways like making a meal, visiting the person, or taking the person out for a short time.
- Join a support group to share advice and understanding with other caregivers.
- Call for help from home healthcare or adult day care services when you need it.
- Use national and local resources to find out how to pay for some of this help, or get respite care services.

You may want to join a support group of AD caregivers in your area or on the Internet. These groups meet in person or online to share experiences and tips and to give each other support. Ask your doctor, check online, or contact a local chapter of the Alzheimer's Association.

If you are a veteran or are caring for one, the Veterans Administration might be of help to you.

Your Emotional Health

You may be busy caring for the person with AD and don't take time to think about your emotional health. But, you need to. Caring for a person with AD takes a lot of time and effort. Your job as caregiver can become even harder when the person you're caring for gets angry with you, hurts your feelings, or forgets who you are. Sometimes, you may feel really discouraged, sad, lonely, frustrated, confused, or angry. These feelings are normal.

Here are some things you can say to yourself that might help you feel better:

- I'm doing the best I can.

- What I'm doing would be hard for anyone.

- I'm not perfect, and that's okay.

- I can't control some things that happen.

- Sometimes, I just need to do what works for right now.

- Even when I do everything I can think of, the person with AD will still have problem behaviors because of the illness, not because of what I do.

- I will enjoy the moments when we can be together in peace.

- I will try to get help from a counselor if caregiving becomes too much for me.

Meeting Your Spiritual Needs

Many of us have spiritual needs. Going to a church, temple, or mosque helps some people meet their spiritual needs. They like to be part of a faith community. For others, simply having a sense that larger forces are at work in the world helps meet their spiritual needs. As the caregiver of a person with AD, you may need more spiritual resources than others do.

Meeting your spiritual needs can help you:

- Cope better as a caregiver

- Know yourself and your needs

- Feel recognized, valued, and loved

- Become involved with others

- Find a sense of balance and peace

Other caregivers made these suggestions to help you cope with your feelings and spiritual needs:

- Understand that you may feel powerless and hopeless about what's happening to the person you care for.

- Understand that you may feel a sense of loss and sadness.

- Understand why you've chosen to take care of the person with AD. Ask yourself if you made this choice out of love, loyalty, a sense of duty, a religious obligation, financial concerns, fear, a habit, or self-punishment.

- Let yourself feel day-to-day "uplifts." These might include good feelings about the person you care for, support from other caring people, or time to spend on your own interests and hobbies.

- Keep a connection to something "higher than yourself." This may be a belief in a higher power, religious beliefs, or a belief that something good comes from every life experience.

Chapter 56

Residential Facilities, Assisted Living, and Nursing Homes

At some point, support from family, friends, and local programs may not be enough. People who require help full-time might move to a residential facility that provides many or all of the long-term care services they need.

Facility-based long-term care services include board and care homes, assisted living facilities, nursing homes, and continuing care retirement communities.

Some facilities have only housing and housekeeping but may also provide personal care and medical services. Many facilities offer special programs for people with Alzheimer disease (AD) and other types of dementia.

Board and Care Homes

Board and care homes, also called residential care facilities or group homes, are small private facilities, usually with 20 or fewer residents. Rooms may be private or shared. Residents receive personal care and

This chapter includes text excerpted from "Residential Facilities, Assisted Living, and Nursing Homes," National Institute on Aging (NIA), National Institutes of Health (NIH), May 1, 2017.

meals and have staff available around the clock. Nursing and medical care usually are not provided on site.

Assisted Living

Assisted living is for people who need help with daily care, but not as much help as a nursing home provides. Assisted living facilities range in size from as few as 25 residents to 120 or more. Typically, a few "levels of care" are offered, with residents paying more for higher levels of care.

Assisted living residents usually live in their own apartments or rooms and share common areas. They have access to many services, including up to three meals a day; assistance with personal care; help with medications, housekeeping, and laundry; 24-hour supervision, security, and on-site staff; and social and recreational activities. Exact arrangements vary from state to state.

Nursing Homes

Nursing homes, also called skilled nursing facilities, provide a wide range of health and personal care services. Their services focus on medical care more than most assisted living facilities. These services typically include nursing care, 24-hour supervision, three meals a day, and assistance with everyday activities. Rehabilitation services, such as physical, occupational, and speech therapy, are also available.

Some people stay at a nursing home for a short time after being in the hospital. After they recover, they go home. However, most nursing home residents live there permanently because they have ongoing physical or mental conditions that require constant care and supervision.

Continuing Care Retirement Communities

Continuing care retirement communities (CCRCs), also called life care communities, offer different levels of service in one location. Many of them offer independent housing (houses or apartments), assisted living, and skilled nursing care all on one campus. Healthcare services and recreation programs are also provided.

In a CCRC, where you live depends on the level of service you need. People who can no longer live independently move to the assisted living facility or sometimes receive home care in their independent living unit. If necessary, they can enter the CCRC's nursing home.

Chapter 57

Choosing a Nursing Home

Steps to Find a Nursing Home

Follow these four steps to find the nursing home that best meets your needs:

Step One: Find Nursing Homes in Your Area

There are many ways you can learn about nursing homes in your area:

- Ask people you trust, like your family, friends, or neighbors.

- Ask your doctor if she or he provides care at any local nursing homes. You may be able to get care from him or her while you're in the nursing home.

- Visit Medicare.gov/nursinghomecompare to find nursing homes in your area.

- Use the Eldercare Locator or an Aging and Disability Resource Center (ADRC).

- Contact your local senior and community activity center.

This chapter includes text excerpted from "Your Guide to Choosing a Nursing Home or Other Long-Term Services and Supports," Centers for Medicare & Medicaid Services (CMS), May 2018.

- If you're in the hospital, ask your social worker about discharge planning as early in your hospital stay as possible. The hospital's staff should be able to help you find a nursing home that meets your needs and help with your transfer when you're ready to be discharged.

Step Two: Compare the Quality of the Nursing Homes You're Considering
Medicare's Nursing Home Compare

Visit Medicare.gov/nursinghomecompare to get information on the quality of every Medicare- and Medicaid-certified nursing home in the country. Consider the information you find on Nursing Home Compare carefully. Use it, along with the other information you gather, to help guide your decision.

There are a variety of resources available to help you choose a nursing home.

- Call your Long-term Care Ombudsman (LTCO).

- Call your state health department or state licensing agency. Look in the blue pages in the phone book or on the Internet. Ask if they have written information on the quality of care given in local nursing homes. You can also ask for a copy of the full survey or the last complaint investigation report.

- Look at survey findings (CMS Form 2567) for the facility. They can be found on Nursing Home Compare at Medicare.gov/nursinghomecompare and in the nursing home.

Step Three: Visit the Nursing Homes You're Interested In, or Have Someone You Trust Visit for You

After you consider what's important to you in a nursing home, visit the nursing homes. It's best to visit the nursing homes that interest you before you make a final decision on which one meets your needs. A visit gives you the chance to see the residents, staff, and the nursing home setting. It also allows you to ask questions of the nursing home staff and talk with residents and their family members. If you can't visit the nursing home yourself, you may want to get a family member or friend to visit you. You can also call for information, however, a visit can help you see the quality of care and life of the actual residents.

Important Things to Know When Visiting Nursing Homes

- Before you go, call and make an appointment to meet with someone on the staff. You're also encouraged to visit the nursing homes at other times without an appointment.

- Don't be afraid to ask questions.

- Ask the staff to explain anything you see and hear that you don't understand.

- Ask who to call if you have further questions, and write down their name and phone number.

- If a resident or a resident's family wishes, you may talk to them about the care offered at the facility and their experience.

- Don't go into resident rooms or care areas without asking the resident and nursing home staff first. Always knock first and ask a resident before entering their room.

- Residents have a right to privacy and can refuse to allow you to come into their rooms.

- After your visit, write down any questions you still have about the nursing home or how the nursing home will meet your needs.

Here are some general things to consider when you visit a nursing home:

- How does the nursing home help you to participate in social, recreational, religious, or cultural activities that are important to you?

- Is transportation provided to community activities?

- What kind of private spaces does the nursing home offer for when you have visitors?

- Who are the doctors that will care for you? Can you still see your personal doctors? If your personal doctors don't visit the nursing home, who will help you arrange transportation if you choose to continue to see them?

- What does the quality of care and staffing information on Nursing Home Compare at Medicare.gov/nursinghomecompare show about how well this nursing home cares for its residents?

- Will the same nursing home staff take care of your day-to-day, or do they change?

- How many residents is a certified nursing assistant (CNA) assigned to work with during each shift (day and night) and during meals?

- What type of therapy is available at this facility? Are therapy staff available?

- What types of meals does the nursing home serve? (**Note**: Ask the nursing home if you can see a menu.)

- How will the nursing home make sure that your dietary needs are met?

- Does the nursing home make sure residents get preventive care to help keep them healthy? Are specialists like eye doctors, ear doctors, dentists, and podiatrists (foot doctors) available to see residents on a regular basis? Does the facility help make arrangements to see these specialists? (Note: Nursing homes must either provide treatment or help you make appointments and arrange transportation for you to see specialists.)

- Does the nursing home have a screening program for vaccinations, like flu (influenza) and pneumonia? (**Note**: Nursing homes are required to provide flu shots each year, but you have the right to refuse if you don't want the shot, have already been immunized during the immunization period, or if the shots are medically contraindicated.)

- How will you get access to oral care in the nursing home?

- How will you get access to mental healthcare in the nursing home?

- What's the nursing home's policy for the use of antipsychotic medication for people with dementia?

Use the "Nursing Home Checklist" When You Visit a Nursing Home

Take a copy of the "Nursing home checklist" when you visit to help you evaluate the quality of a nursing home. Use a new checklist for each nursing home you visit. You can photocopy the checklist or print more copies at Medicare.gov/files/nursing-home-checklist.pdf.

Step Four: Choose the Nursing Home That Meets Your Needs

When you have all the information that's important to you about the nursing homes you're considering, talk with people who understand your personal and healthcare needs. This can include your family, friends, doctor, clergy, spiritual advisor, hospital discharge planner, or social worker.

What If More Than One Nursing Home Meets My Needs?

If you find more than one nursing home you like with a bed available, use the information you gathered to compare them. Trust your senses. If you don't like what you saw on a visit (for example, if the facility wasn't clean or you weren't comfortable talking with the nursing home staff), you may want to choose another nursing home. If you felt that the residents were treated well, the facility was clean, and the staff was helpful, you might feel better about choosing that nursing home.

What If I'm Helping Someone Make a Decision?

If you're helping someone, keep the person you're helping involved in the decision-making process as much as possible. People who are involved from the beginning are better prepared when they move into a nursing home. If the person you're helping isn't alert or able to communicate well, keep his or her values and preferences in mind.

What If I Don't like a Nursing Home I Visit?

If you visit a nursing home that you don't like, look at other options, if available. Your happiness and the quality of your care is important.

What If I'm in the Hospital and Don't like the Nursing Home That Has an Available Bed?

If you're in a hospital and decide not to go to a certain nursing home that has an available bed, talk to the hospital discharge planner or your doctor. They may be able to help you find a more suitable nursing home or arrange for other care, like short-term home healthcare, until a bed is available at another nursing home you choose. However, you may be responsible for paying the bill for any additional days you stay in the hospital.

What If I Don't like a Nursing Home I'm Currently In?

If you don't like the nursing home you're currently living in, you can move to another facility with an available bed. Moving can be difficult, but an extra move may be better for you than choosing to stay at a facility that isn't right for you.

The nursing home you leave may require that you let them know ahead of time that you're planning to leave. Talk to the nursing home staff about their rules for leaving. If you don't follow the rules for leaving, you may have to pay extra fees.

Note: If you want information about living in the community, nursing homes are required to reach out to a local agency that can give you more information. Talk to the nursing home social worker about your plan to transition to the community.

Next Steps: After You've Chosen a Nursing Home

After you choose a nursing home, you'll need to make arrangements to be admitted. When you contact the nursing home office, it's helpful to have this information ready.

Information for the Nursing Home Office Staff

Insurance information: Provide information about any health coverage and long-term care insurance you have that pays for nursing home care, healthcare, or both. This includes the name of the insurance company and the policy number.

Note: If Medicare or Medicaid will cover your nursing home care, the nursing home can't require you to pay a cash deposit. They may ask that you pay your Medicare coinsurance and other charges you would normally have to pay. The nursing home can't require you to pay more than the rates allowed by Medicare or Medicaid for covered services. There may be charges for items or services that Medicare or Medicaid don't cover, but the nursing home can't require that you accept services that Medicare or Medicaid don't cover as a condition of your continued stay.

It's best to pay charges once they're billed to you—not in advance. You may have to pay a cash deposit before you're admitted to a nursing home, if your care won't be covered by either Medicare or Medicaid, and the nursing home isn't limited to the rates allowed by Medicare or Medicaid.

Information for the Nursing Home Medical Staff

- **Information on your medical history:** Your doctor may give the staff some of this information. This includes a list of past health problems, any past surgeries or treatments, any shots you've had, and allergies you may have to food or medicine.

- **Information on your current health status:** Your doctor should give the staff this information, including a list of your current health problems, recent diagnostic test results, and information about any activities of daily living that might be difficult for you to do by yourself.

- **A list of your current medicines:** Include the dose, how often you take it, when you take it, and why you take it.

- **A list of all your healthcare providers:** Include names, addresses, and phone numbers.

- **A list of family members to call in case of an emergency:** Include names, addresses, and phone numbers.

Other Important Information to Have Ready

Healthcare Advance Directives
You may be asked if you have a healthcare advance directive, which is a written legal document that says how you want medical decisions to be made if you become unable to make decisions for yourself. There are two common types of healthcare advance directives:

- **A living will**: A written legal document that shows what type of treatments you want or don't want in case you can't speak for yourself, like whether you want life support. Usually, this document only comes into effect if you're unconscious.

- **A durable power of attorney for healthcare**: A legal document that names someone else to make healthcare decisions for you. This is helpful if you become unable to make your own decisions.

- If you don't have a healthcare advance directive and need help preparing one, or you need more information, talk to a social worker, discharge planner, your doctor, or the nursing home staff. You can use the Eldercare Locator to find out if your state has any legal services that can help you prepare these forms.

Personal Needs Accounts
You may want to open an account managed by the nursing home, although the nursing home can't require this. You can deposit money into the account for personal use. Check with the nursing home to find

out what expenses you can use the account for and how they manage the accounts.

Information the Nursing Home Must Give You

Once you choose a nursing home, they must give you information about how to apply for and use Medicare and Medicaid benefits in a language and format you understand. They must also give you information on how to get refunds for previous payments you may have made that are covered by these benefits.

Chapter 58

Hospitalization and Alzheimer Disease

A trip to the hospital can be stressful for people with Alzheimer disease (AD) or another dementia and their caregivers. Being prepared for emergency and planned hospital visits can relieve some of that stress. This chapter suggests ways to help you prepare and tips for making your visit to the emergency room or hospital easier.

Hospital Emergencies: What You Can Do

A trip to the emergency room (ER) can tire and frighten a person with Alzheimer or other dementia. Here are some ways to cope:

- Ask a friend or family member to go with you or meet you in the ER. She or he can stay with the person while you answer questions.

- Be ready to explain the symptoms and events leading up to the ER visit—possibly more than once to different staff members.

- Tell ER staff that the person has dementia. Explain how best to talk with the person.

This chapter includes text excerpted from "Going to the Hospital: Tips for Dementia Caregivers," National Institute on Aging (NIA), National Institutes of Health (NIH), May 18, 2017.

- Comfort the person. Stay calm and positive. How you are feeling will get absorbed by others.

- Be patient. It could be a long wait if the reason for your visit is not life-threatening.

- Recognize that results from the lab take time.

- Realize that just because you do not see staff at work does not mean they are not working.

- Be aware that emergency room staff have limited training in Alzheimer disease and related dementias, so try to help them better understand the person.

- Encourage hospital staff to see the person as an individual and not just another patient with dementia who is confused and disoriented from the disease.

- Do not assume the person will be admitted to the hospital.

- If the person must stay overnight in the hospital, try to have a friend or family member stay with him or her.

Do not leave the emergency room without a plan. If you are sent home, make sure you understand all instructions for follow-up care.

What to Pack

An emergency bag with the following items, packed ahead of time, can make a visit to the ER go more smoothly:

- Health insurance cards

- Lists of current medical conditions, medicines being taken, and allergies

- Healthcare providers' names and phone numbers

- Copies of healthcare advance directives (documents that spell out a patient's wishes for end-of-life care)

- "Personal information sheet" stating the person's preferred name and language; contact information for key family members and friends; need for glasses, dentures, or hearing aids; behaviors of concern; how the person communicates needs and expresses emotions; and living situation

- Snacks and bottles of water

- Incontinence briefs, if usually worn, moist wipes, and plastic bags
- Comforting objects or music player with earphones
- A change of clothing, toiletries, and personal medications for yourself
- Pain medicine, such as ibuprofen, acetaminophen, or aspirin—a trip to the emergency room may take longer than you think, and stress can lead to a headache or other symptoms
- A pad of paper and pen to write down information and directions given to you by hospital staff
- A small amount of cash
- A note on the outside of the emergency bag to remind you to take your cell phone and charger with you

By taking these steps in advance, you can reduce the stress and confusion that often accompany a hospital visit, particularly if the visit is an unplanned trip to the emergency room.

Before a Planned Hospital Stay

With Alzheimer disease and related dementias, it is wise to accept that hospitalization is a "when" and not an "if" event. Due to the nature of the disease, it is very probable that, at some point, the person you are caring for will be hospitalized. Keep in mind that hospitals are not typically well-designed for patients with dementia. Preparation can make all the difference. Here are some tips.

- Think about and discuss hospitalization before it happens, and as the disease and associated memory loss progress. Hospitalization is a choice. Talk about when hospice may be a better and more appropriate alternative.
- Build a care team of family, friends, and/or professional caregivers to support the person during the hospital stay. Do not try to do it all alone.
- Ask the doctor if the procedure can be done during an outpatient visit. If not, ask if tests can be done before admission to the hospital to shorten the hospital stay.
- Ask questions about anesthesia, catheters, and intravenous (IV). General anesthesia can have side effects, so see if local anesthesia is an option.

- Ask if regular medications can be continued during the hospital stay.

- Ask for a private room, with a reclining chair or bed, if insurance will cover it. It will be calmer than a shared room.

- Involve the person with dementia in the planning process as much as possible.

- Do not talk about the hospital stay in front of the person as if she or he is not there. This can be upsetting and embarrassing.

- Shortly before leaving home, tell the person with dementia that the two of you are going to spend a short time in the hospital.

During the Hospital Stay

While the person with dementia is in the hospital:

- Ask doctors to limit questions to the person, who may not be able to answer accurately. Instead, talk with the doctor in private, outside the person's room.

- Help hospital staff understand the person's normal functioning and behavior. Ask them to avoid using physical restraints or medications to control behaviors.

- Have a family member, trusted friend, or hired caregiver stay with the person with AD at all times if possible—even during medical tests. This may be hard to do, but it will help keep the person calm and less frightened, making the hospital stay easier.

- Tell the doctor immediately if the person seems suddenly worse or different. Medical problems such as fever, infection, medication side effects, and dehydration can cause delirium, a state of extreme confusion and disorientation.

- Ask friends and family to make calls, or use e-mail or online tools to keep others informed about the person's progress.

- Help the person fill out menu requests. Open food containers and remove trays. Assist with eating as needed.

- Remind the person to drink fluids. Offer fluids regularly and have him or her make frequent trips to the bathroom.

- Assume the person will experience difficulty finding the bathroom and/or using a call button, bed adjustment buttons, or the phone.

- Communicate with the person in the way she or he will best understand and respond.

- Recognize that an unfamiliar place, medicines, invasive tests, and surgery will make a person with dementia more confused. She or he will likely need more assistance with personal care.

- Take deep breaths and schedule breaks for yourself!

If anxiety or agitation occurs, try the following:

- Remove personal clothes from sight; they may remind the person of getting dressed and going home.

- Post reminders or cues, like a sign labeling the bathroom door, if this comforts the person.

- Turn off the television, telephone ringer, and intercom. Minimize background noise to prevent overstimulation.

- Talk in a calm voice and offer reassurance. Repeat answers to questions when needed.

- Provide a comforting touch or distract the person with offers of snacks and beverages.

- Consider "unexpressed pain" (i.e., furrowed brow, clenched teeth or fists, kicking). Assume the person has pain if the condition or procedure is normally associated with pain. Ask for pain evaluation and treatment every four hours—especially if the person has labored breathing, loud moaning, crying or grimacing, or if you are unable to console or distract him or her.

- Listen to soothing music or try comforting rituals, such as reading, praying, singing, or reminiscing.

- Slow down; try not to rush the person.

- Avoid talking about subjects or events that may upset the person.

Working with Hospital Staff

Remember that not everyone in the hospital knows the same basic facts about memory loss, Alzheimer disease, and related dementias. You may need to help teach hospital staff what approach works best with the person with Alzheimer disease, what distresses or upsets him or her, and ways to reduce this distress.

You can help the staff by providing them with a personal information sheet that includes the person's normal routine, how she or he prefers to be addressed (e.g., Miss Minnie, Dr. James, Jane, Mr. Miller, etc.) personal habits, likes and dislikes, possible behaviors (what might trigger them and how best to respond), and nonverbal signs of pain or discomfort.

Help staff understand what the person's "baseline" is (prior level of functioning) to help differentiate between dementia and acute confusion or delirium.

You should:

- Place a copy of the personal information sheet with the chart in the hospital room and at the nurse's station.

- With the hospital staff, decide who will do what for the person with Alzheimer disease. For example, you may want to be the one who helps with bathing, eating, or using the bathroom.

- Inform the staff about any hearing difficulties and/or other communication problems, and offer ideas for what works best in those instances.

- Make sure the person is safe. Tell the staff about any previous issues with wandering, getting lost, falls, suspiciousness and/or delusional behavior.

- Not assume the staff knows the person's needs. Inform them in a polite, calm manner.

- Ask questions when you do not understand certain hospital procedures and tests or when you have any concerns. Do not be afraid to be an advocate.

- Plan early for discharge. Ask the hospital discharge planner about eligibility for home health services, equipment, or other long-term care options. Prepare for an increased level of caregiving.

- Realize that hospital staff are providing care for many people. Practice the art of patience.

Chapter 59

Making Decisions about Resuscitation and Tube Feeding

Maybe you are now faced with making end-of-life choices for some-one close to you. You've thought about that person's values and opinions, and you've asked the healthcare team to explain the treatment plan and what you can expect to happen.

But, there are other issues that are important to understand in case they arise. What if the dying person starts to have trouble breathing and a doctor says a ventilator might be needed? Maybe one family member wants the healthcare team to do everything possible to keep this relative alive. What does that involve? Or, what if family members can't agree on end-of-life care or they disagree with the doctor? What happens then?

Here are some other common end-of-life issues. They will give you a general understanding and may help your conversations with the doctors.

This chapter includes text excerpted from "End of Life: Helping with Comfort and Care," National Institute on Aging (NIA), National Institutes of Health (NIH), July 2016.

If We Say Do Everything Possible, What Does That Mean?

This means that if someone is dying, all measures that might keep vital organs working will be tried—for example, using a ventilator to support breathing or starting dialysis for failing kidneys. Such life support can sometimes be a temporary measure that allows the body to heal itself and begin to work normally again. It is not intended to be used indefinitely in someone who is dying.

What Can Be Done If Someone's Heart Stops Beating (Cardiac Arrest)?

CPR (cardiopulmonary resuscitation) can sometimes restart a stopped heart. It is most effective in people who were generally healthy before their heart stopped. During CPR, the doctor repeatedly pushes on the chest with great force and periodically puts air into the lungs. Electric shocks (called defibrillation) may also be used to correct an abnormal heart rhythm, and some medicines might also be given. Although not usually shown on television, the force required for CPR can cause broken ribs or a collapsed lung. Often, CPR does not succeed in older adults who have multiple chronic illnesses or who are already frail.

What If Someone Needs Help Breathing or Completely Stops Breathing (Respiratory Arrest)?

If a patient has very severe breathing problems or has stopped breathing, a ventilator may be needed. A ventilator forces the lungs to work. Initially, this involves intubation, putting a tube attached to a ventilator down the throat into the trachea or windpipe. Because this tube can be quite uncomfortable, people are often sedated with very strong intravenous medicines. Restraints may be used to prevent them from pulling out the tube. If the person needs ventilator support for more than a few days, the doctor might suggest a tracheotomy, sometimes called a "trach" (rhymes with "make").

This tube is then attached to the ventilator. This is more comfortable than a tube down the throat and may not require sedation. Inserting the tube into the trachea is a bedside surgery. A tracheotomy can carry risks, including a collapsed lung, a plugged tracheotomy tube, or bleeding.

How Can I Be Sure the Medical Staff Knows That We Don't Want Efforts to Restore a Heartbeat or Breathing?

Tell the doctor in charge as soon as the patient or person making healthcare decisions decides that CPR or other life-support procedures should not be performed. The doctor will then write this on the patient's chart using terms such as DNR (Do Not Resuscitate), DNAR (Do Not Attempt to Resuscitate), AND (Allow Natural Death), or DNI (Do Not Intubate). DNR forms vary by State and are usually available online.

If end-of-life care is given at home, a special nonhospital DNR, signed by a doctor, is needed. This ensures that if emergency medical technicians (EMTs) are called to the house, they will respect your wishes. Make sure it is kept in a prominent place so EMTs can see it. Without a nonhospital DNR, in many states EMTs are required to perform CPR and similar techniques. Hospice staff can help determine whether a medical condition is part of the normal dying process or something that needs the attention of EMTs.

DNR orders do not stop all treatment. They only mean that CPR and a ventilator will not be used. These orders are not permanent—they can be changed if the situation changes.

What about Pacemakers (Or Similar Devices)— Should They Be Turned Off?

A pacemaker is a device implanted under the skin on the chest that keeps a heartbeat regular. It will not keep a dying person alive. Some people have an implantable cardioverter defibrillator (ICD) under the skin. An ICD shocks the heart back into regular rhythm when needed. The ICD should be turned off at the point when life support is no longer wanted. This can be done at the bedside without surgery.

What If the Doctor Suggests a Feeding Tube?

If a patient can't or won't eat or drink, the doctor might suggest a feeding tube. While a patient recovers from an illness, getting nutrition temporarily through a feeding tube can be helpful. But, at the end of life, a feeding tube might cause more discomfort than not eating. For people with dementia, tube feeding does not prolong life or prevent aspiration.

As death approaches, loss of appetite is common. Body systems start shutting down, and fluids and food are not needed as before.

Some experts believe that at this point few nutrients are absorbed from any type of nutrition, including those received through a feeding tube. Further, after a feeding tube is inserted, the family might need to make a difficult decision about when, or if, to remove it.

If tube feeding will be tried, there are two methods that could be used. In the first, a feeding tube, known as a nasogastric or NG tube, is threaded through the nose down to the stomach to give nutrition for a short time. Sometimes, the tube is uncomfortable. Someone with an NG tube might try to remove it. This usually means the person has to be restrained, which could mean binding his or her hands to the bed.

If tube feeding is required for an extended time, then a gastric or G tube is put directly into the stomach through an opening made in the side or abdomen. This second method is sometimes called a PEG (percutaneous endoscopic gastrostomy) tube. It carries risks of infection, pneumonia, and nausea.

Hand feeding (sometimes called assisted oral feeding) is an alternative to tube feeding. This approach may have fewer risks, especially for people with dementia.

Chapter 60

Caring for Someone near the End of Life

Comfort care is an essential part of medical care at the end of life. It is care that helps or soothes a person who is dying. The goals are to prevent or relieve suffering as much as possible and to improve quality of life (QOL) while respecting the dying person's wishes.

You are probably reading this because someone close to you is dying. You wonder what will happen. You want to know how to give comfort, what to say, what to do. You might like to know how to make dying easier—how to help ensure a peaceful death, with treatment consistent with the dying person's wishes.

A peaceful death might mean something different to you than to someone else. Your sister might want to know when death is near so she can have a few last words with the people she loves and take care of personal matters. Your husband might want to die quickly and not linger. Perhaps your mother has said she would like to be at home when she dies, while your father wants to be in a hospital where he can receive treatment for his illness until the very end.

Some people want to be surrounded by family and friends; others want to be alone. Of course, often one doesn't get to choose. But, avoiding suffering, having your end-of-life wishes followed, and being treated with respect while dying are common hopes.

This chapter includes text excerpted from "End of Life: Helping with Comfort and Care," National Institute on Aging (NIA), National Institutes of Health (NIH), July 2016.

Generally speaking, people who are dying need care in four areas—physical comfort, mental and emotional needs, spiritual issues, and practical tasks. Their families need support as well. In this section, you will find a number of ways you can help someone who is dying. Always remember to check with the healthcare team to make sure these suggestions are appropriate for your situation.

Physical Comfort

There are ways to make a person who is dying more comfortable. Discomfort can come from a variety of problems. For each, there are things you or a healthcare provider can do, depending on the cause. For example, a dying person can be uncomfortable because of:

- **Pain.** Watching someone you love die is hard enough, but thinking that person is also in pain makes it worse. Not everyone who is dying experiences pain, but there are things you can do to help someone who does. Experts believe that care for someone who is dying should focus on relieving pain without worrying about possible long-term problems of drug dependence or abuse.

  Don't be afraid of giving as much pain medicine as is prescribed by the doctor. Pain is easier to prevent than to relieve, and severe pain is hard to manage. Try to make sure that the level of pain does not get ahead of pain-relieving medicines. Tell the doctor or nurse if the pain is not controlled. Medicines can be increased or changed. If this doesn't help, then ask for consultation with a palliative medical specialist who has experience in pain management for seriously ill patients.

  Struggling with severe pain can be draining. It can make it hard for families to be together in a meaningful way. Pain can affect mood—being in pain can make someone seem angry or short-tempered. Although understandable, irritability resulting from pain might make it hard to talk, hard to share thoughts and feelings.

- **Breathing problems.** Shortness of breath or the feeling that breathing is difficult is a common experience at the end of life. The doctor might call this dyspnea. Worrying about the next breath can make it hard for important conversations or connections. Try raising the head of the bed, opening a window, using a humidifier, or having a fan circulating air in the room.

Sometimes, morphine or other pain medications can help relieve the sense of breathlessness.

People very near death might have noisy breathing, sometimes called a death rattle. This is caused by fluids collecting in the throat or by the throat muscles relaxing. It might help to try turning the person to rest on one side. There is also medicine that can be prescribed that may help clear this up. Not all noisy breathing is a death rattle. It may help to know that this noisy breathing is usually not upsetting to the dying person, even if it is to family and friends.

- **Skin irritation.** Skin problems can be very uncomfortable. With age, skin naturally becomes drier and more fragile, so it is important to take extra care with an older person's skin. Gently applying alcohol-free lotion can relieve dry skin and be soothing.

  Dryness on parts of the face, such as the lips and eyes, can be a common cause of discomfort near death. A lip balm could keep this from getting worse. A damp cloth placed over closed eyes might relieve dryness. If the inside of the mouth seems dry, giving ice chips (if the person is conscious) or wiping the inside of the mouth with a damp cloth, cotton ball, or specially treated swab might help.

  Sitting or lying in one position puts constant pressure on sensitive skin, which can lead to painful bed sores (sometimes called pressure ulcers). When a bed sore first forms, the skin gets discolored or darker. Watch carefully for these discolored spots, especially on the heels, hips, lower back, and back of the head.

  Turning the person from side to back and to the other side every few hours may help prevent bed sores. Try putting a foam pad under an area like a heel or elbow to raise it off the bed and reduce pressure. Ask if a special mattress or chair cushion might also help. Keeping the skin clean and moisturized is always important.

- **Digestive problems.** Nausea, vomiting, constipation, and loss of appetite are common issues at the end of life. The causes and treatments for these symptoms are varied, so talk to a doctor or nurse right away. There are medicines that can control nausea or vomiting or relieve constipation, a common side effect of strong pain medications. If someone near death wants to eat but is too tired or weak, you can help with feeding. To address loss of appetite, try gently offering favorite foods in small amounts. Or, try serving frequent, smaller meals rather than three big ones.

You don't have to force a person to eat. Going without food and/or water is generally not painful, and eating can add to discomfort. Losing one's appetite is a common and normal part of dying. Swallowing may also be a problem, especially for people with dementia. A conscious decision to give up food can be part of a person's acceptance that death is near.

- **Temperature sensitivity.** People who are dying may not be able to tell you that they are too hot or too cold, so watch for clues. For example, someone who is too warm might repeatedly try to remove a blanket. You can take off the blanket and try a cool cloth on his or her head.

  If a person is hunching his or her shoulders, pulling the covers up, or even shivering—those could be signs of cold. Make sure there is no draft, raise the heat, and add another blanket. Avoid electric blankets because they can get too hot.

- **Fatigue.** It is common for people nearing the end of life to feel tired and have little or no energy. Keep activities simple. For example, a bedside commode can be used instead of walking to the bathroom. A shower stool can save a person's energy, as can switching to sponging off in bed.

Mental and Emotional Needs

Complete end-of-life care also includes helping the dying person manage mental and emotional distress. Someone who is alert near the end of life might understandably feel depressed or anxious. It is important to treat emotional pain and suffering. Encouraging conversations about feelings might help. You might want to contact a counselor, possibly one familiar with end-of-life issues. If the depression or anxiety is severe, medicine may help.

A dying person may also have some specific fears and concerns. She or he may fear the unknown or worry about those left behind. Some people are afraid of being alone at the very end. This feeling can be made worse by the understandable reactions of family, friends, and even the medical team. For example, when family and friends do not know how to help or what to say, sometimes they stop visiting. Or, someone who is already beginning to grieve may withdraw.

Doctors may feel helpless because they can't cure their patient. Some seem to avoid a dying patient. This can add to a dying person's sense of isolation. If this is happening, discuss your concerns with the family, friends, or the doctor.

The simple act of physical contact—holding hands, a touch, or a gentle massage—can make a person feel connected to those she or he loves. It can be very soothing. Warm your hands by rubbing them together or running them under warm water.

Try to set a comforting mood. Remember that listening and being present can make a difference. For example, Gordon loved a party, so it was natural for him to want to be around family and friends when he was dying. Ellen always liked spending quiet moments with one or two people at a time, so she was most comfortable with just a few visitors.

Some experts suggest that when death is very near, music at a low volume and soft lighting are soothing. In fact, near the end of life, music therapy might improve mood, help with relaxation, and lessen pain. Listening to music might also evoke memories those present can share. For some people, keeping distracting noises like televisions and radios to a minimum is important.

Often, just being present with a dying person is enough. It may not be necessary to fill the time with talking or activity. Your quiet presence can be a simple and profound gift for a dying family member or friend.

Spiritual Issues

People nearing the end of life may have spiritual needs as important as their physical concerns. Spiritual needs include finding meaning in one's life and ending disagreements with others, if possible. The dying person might find peace by resolving unsettled issues with friends or family. Visits from a social worker or a counselor may also help.

Many people find solace in their faith. Others may struggle with their faith or spiritual beliefs. Praying, talking with someone from one's religious community (such as a minister, priest, rabbi, or imam), reading religious texts, or listening to religious music may bring comfort.

Family and friends can talk to the dying person about the importance of their relationship. For example, adult children can share how their father has influenced the course of their lives. Grandchildren can let their grandfather know how much he has meant to them. Friends can relate how they value years of support and companionship. Family and friends who can't be present could send a recording of what they would like to say or a letter to be read out loud.

Sharing memories of good times is another way some people find peace near death. This can be comforting for everyone. Some doctors think it is possible that even if a patient is unconscious, she or he might still be able to hear. It is probably never too late to say how you feel or to talk about fond memories.

Always talk to, not about, the person who is dying. When you come into the room, it is a good idea to identify yourself, saying something like, "Hi, Juan. It's Mary, and I've come to see you." Another good idea is to have someone write down some of the things said at this time—both by and to the person who is dying. In time, these words might serve as a source of comfort to family and friends. People who are looking for ways to help may welcome the chance to aid the family by writing down what is said.

There may come a time when a dying person who has been confused suddenly seems clear-thinking. Take advantage of these moments, but understand that they might be only temporary, not necessarily a sign she or he is getting better. Sometimes, a dying person may appear to see or talk to someone who is not there. Try to resist the temptation to interrupt or say they are imagining things. Give the dying person the space to experience their own reality.

Practical Tasks

Many practical jobs need to be done at the end of life—both to relieve the person who is dying and to support the caregiver. Everyday tasks can be a source of worry for someone who is dying, and they can overwhelm a caregiver. Taking over small daily chores around the house—such as picking up the mail or newspaper, writing down phone messages, doing a load of laundry, feeding the family pet, taking children to soccer practice, or picking up medicine from the pharmacy—can provide a much-needed break for caregivers.

A person who is dying might be worried about who will take care of things when she or he is gone. Offering reassurance—"I'll make sure your African violets are watered," "Jessica has promised to take care of Bandit," "Dad, we want Mom to live with us from now on"—might provide a measure of peace. Reminding the dying person that his or her personal affairs are in good hands can also bring comfort.

Everyone may be asking the family, "What can I do for you?" It helps to make a specific offer. Say to the family, "Let me help with . . . " and suggest something like bringing meals for the caregivers, paying bills, walking the dog, or babysitting. If you're not sure what to offer, talk to someone who has been through a similar situation. Find out what kind of help was useful.

If you want to help but can't get away from your own home, you could schedule other friends or family to help with small jobs or to bring in meals. This can allow the immediate family to give their full attention to the person who is dying. If you are the primary caregiver, ask for help when you need it and accept help when it's offered. Don't hesitate to suggest a specific task to someone who offers to help. Friends and family are probably anxious to do something for you and/ or the person who is dying, but they may be reluctant to repeatedly offer when you are so busy. Keeping close friends and family informed can feel overwhelming. Setting up an outgoing voicemail message, a blog, an e-mail list, a private Facebook page, or even a phone tree can reduce the number of calls you have to make. Some families create a blog or website to share news, thoughts, and wishes.

Chapter 61

What Happens When Someone Dies

When death comes suddenly, there is little time to prepare. In contrast, watching an older person become increasingly frail may mean that it's hard to know when the end of life begins because changes can happen so slowly. But, if you do know death is approaching and understand what will happen, then you do have a chance to plan. Listen carefully to what doctors and nurses are saying. They may be suggesting that death could be soon. You might also ask—how much time do you think my loved one has left, based on your experience with other patients in this condition?

Just as each life is unique, so is each death. But, there are some common experiences very near the end:

- Shortness of breath, known as dyspnea

- Depression

- Anxiety

- Tiredness and sleepiness

This chapter includes text excerpted from "End of Life: Helping with Comfort and Care," National Institute on Aging (NIA), National Institutes of Health (NIH), July 2016.

- Mental confusion or reduced alertness

- Refusal to eat or drink

Each of these symptoms, taken alone, is not a sign of death. But, for someone with a serious illness or declining health, these might suggest that the person is nearing the end of life.

In addition, when a person is closer to death, the hands, arms, feet, or legs may be cool to the touch. Some parts of the body may become darker or blue-colored. Breathing and heart rates may slow. In fact, there may be times when the person's breathing becomes abnormal, known as Cheyne-Stokes breathing. Some people hear a death rattle, noisy breathing that makes a gurgling or rattling sound. The chest stops moving, no air comes out of the nose, and there is no pulse. Eyes that are open can seem glassy.

After death, there may still be a few shudders or movements of the arms or legs. There could even be an uncontrolled cry because of muscle movement in the voice box. Sometimes there will be a release of urine or stool, but usually only a small amount since so little has probably been eaten in the last days of life.

Should There Always Be Someone in the Room with a Dying Person?

Staying close to someone who is dying is often called keeping a vigil. It can be comforting for the caregiver to always be there, but it can also be tiring and stressful. Unless your cultural or religious traditions require it, do not feel that you must stay with the person all the time. If there are other family members or friends around, try taking turns sitting in the room. Some people almost seem to prefer to die alone. They appear to slip away just after visitors leave.

Call 911 or Not?

When there is a medical emergency, such as a heart attack, stroke, or serious accident, we know to call 911. But, if a person is dying at home and does not want CPR (cardiopulmonary resuscitation), calling 911 is not necessary. In fact, a call to 911 could cause confusion. Many places require EMTs (emergency medical technicians) who respond to 911 calls to perform CPR if someone's heart has stopped.

Consider having a nonhospital DNR (Do Not Resuscitate order) if the person is dying at home. Ask your doctor or the hospice care team who you should call at the time of death.

Things to Do after Someone Dies

Nothing has to be done immediately after a person's death. Take the time you need. Some people want to stay in the room with the body; others prefer to leave. You might want to have someone make sure the body is lying flat before the joints become stiff and cannot be moved. This rigor mortis begins sometime during the first hours after death.

After the death, how long you can stay with the body may depend on where death happens. If it happens at home, there is no need to move the body right away. This is the time for any special religious, ethnic, or cultural customs that are performed soon after death. If the death seems likely to happen in a facility, such as a hospital or nursing home, discuss any important customs or rituals with the staff early on, if possible. That will allow them to plan so you can have the appropriate time with the body.

If the death seems likely to happen in a facility, such as a hospital or nursing home, discuss any important customs or rituals with the staff early on, if possible. That will allow them to plan so you can have the appropriate time with the body.

Some families want time to sit quietly with the body, console each other, and maybe share memories. You could ask a member of your religious community or a spiritual counselor to come. If you have a list of people to notify, this is the time to call those who might want to come and see the body before it is moved.

As soon as possible, the death must be officially pronounced by someone in authority like a doctor in a hospital or nursing facility or a hospice nurse. This person also fills out the forms certifying the cause, time, and place of death. These steps will make it possible for an official death certificate to be prepared. This legal form is necessary for many reasons, including life insurance and financial and property issues.

If hospice is helping, a plan for what happens after death is already in place. If death happens at home without hospice, try to talk with the doctor, local medical examiner (coroner), your local health department, or a funeral home representative in advance about how to proceed. Arrangements should be made to pick up the body as soon as the family is ready and according to local laws. Usually, this is done by a funeral home. The hospital or nursing facility, if that is where the death took place, may call the funeral home for you. If at home, you will need to contact the funeral home directly or ask a friend or family member to do that for you.

The doctor may ask if you want an autopsy. This is a medical procedure conducted by a specially trained physician to learn more about what caused the death. For example, if the person who died was believed to have Alzheimer disease (AD), a brain autopsy will allow for a definitive diagnosis. If your religion or culture objects to autopsies, talk to the doctor. Some people planning a funeral with a viewing worry about having an autopsy, but the physical signs of an autopsy are usually hidden by clothing.

Organ Donation

At some time before death or right after it, the doctor may ask about donating organs such as the heart, lungs, pancreas, kidneys, cornea, liver, and skin. Organ donation allows healthy organs from someone who died to be transplanted into living people who need them. People of any age can be organ donors.

The person who is dying may have already said that she or he would like to be an organ donor. Some states list this information on the driver's license. If not, the decision has to be made quickly. There is no cost to the donor's family for this gift of life. If the person has requested a do not resuscitate (DNR) order but wants to donate organs, she or he might have to indicate that the desire to donate supersedes the DNR. That is because it might be necessary to use machines to keep the heart beating until the medical staff is ready to remove the donated organs.

Part Seven

Additional Help and Information

Chapter 62

Glossary of Terms Related to Alzheimer Disease and Dementia

acetylcholine: A neurotransmitter that plays an important role in many neurological functions, including learning and memory.

Alzheimer disease: A progressive, irreversible disease characterized by degeneration of the brain cells and serve loss of memory, causing the individual to become dysfunctional and dependent upon others for basic living needs.

amygdala: An almond-shaped structure involved in processing and remembering strong emotions such as fear. It is part of the limbic system and located deep inside the brain.

amyloid: A protein that's found in the brains of people with Alzheimer disease. It builds up into a "plaque" or "tangles."

amyloid plaques: A largely insoluble deposit found in the space between nerve cells in the brain. Plaques are made of beta-amyloid, other molecules, and different kinds of nerve and nonnerve cells.

antidepressant: Medication used to treat depression and other mood and anxiety disorders.

This glossary contains terms excerpted from documents produced by several sources deemed reliable.

apolipoprotein E (APOE): A gene that has been linked to an increased risk of Alzheimer disease. People with a variant form of the gene, called APOE epsilon 4, have about 10 times the risk of developing Alzheimer disease.

assisted living facility: A residential care setting that combines housing, support services, and healthcare for people in the early or middle stages of a disabling disease, such as Alzheimer disease.

ataxia: A loss of muscle control.

atherosclerosis: A blood vessel disease characterized by the buildup of plaque, or deposits of fatty substances and other matter in the inner lining of an artery.

axon: The long extension from a neuron that transmits outgoing signals to other cells.

beta-amyloid: A part of the amyloid precursor protein found in plaques, the insoluble deposits outside neurons.

Binswanger disease: A rare form of dementia characterized by damage to small blood vessels in the white matter of the brain. This damage leads to brain lesions, loss of memory, disordered cognition, and mood changes.

brain stem: The portion of the brain that connects to the spinal cord and controls automatic body functions, such as breathing, heart rate, and blood pressure.

care plan: Written document which outlines the types and frequency of the long-term care services that a consumer receives. It may include treatment goals for him or her for a specified time period. Also called service plan or treatment plan.

cerebral cortex: The outer layer of nerve cells surrounding the cerebral hemispheres.

cerebral hemispheres: The largest portion of the brain, composed of billions of nerve cells in two structures connected by the corpus callosum. The cerebral hemispheres control conscious thought, language, decision making, emotions, movement, and sensory functions.

cerebrospinal fluid: The fluid found in and around the brain and spinal cord. It protects these organs by acting like a liquid cushion and by providing nutrients.

cholinesterase inhibitors: Drugs that slow the breakdown of the neurotransmitter acetylcholine.

chromosomes: A threadlike structure in the nucleus of a cell that contains DNA. DNA sequences make up genes. Most human cells have 23 pairs of chromosomes containing approximately 30,000 genes.

chronic traumatic encephalopathy: A form of dementia caused by repeated traumatic brain injury.

clinical trial: A research study involving humans that rigorously tests safety, side effects, and how well a medication or behavioral treatment works.

cognition: Conscious mental activities (such as thinking, communicating, understanding, solving problems, processing information and remembering) that are associated with gaining knowledge and understanding.

cognitive behavioral therapy (CBT): CBT helps people focus on how to solve their current problems. The therapist helps the patient learn how to identify distorted or unhelpful thinking patterns, recognize and change inaccurate beliefs, relate to others in more positive ways, and change behaviors accordingly.

cognitive functions: All aspects of conscious thought and mental activity, including learning, perceiving, making decisions, and remembering.

cognitive impairment: Deterioration or loss of intellectual capacity which requires continual supervision to protect the insured or others, as measured by clinical evidence and standardized tests that reliably measure impairment in the area of short or long-term memory, orientation as to person, place and time, or deductive or abstract reasoning.

cognitive training: A type of training in which patients practice tasks designed to improve mental performance. Examples include memory aids, such as mnemonics and computerized recall devices.

computed tomography (CT) scan: A diagnostic procedure that uses special X-ray equipment and computers to create cross-sectional pictures of the body.

concussion: Injury to the brain caused by a hard blow or violent shaking, causing a sudden and temporary impairment of brain function, such as a short loss of consciousness or disturbance of vision and equilibrium.

corticobasal degeneration: A progressive disorder characterized by nerve cell loss and atrophy in multiple areas of the brain.

Creutzfeldt-Jakob disease: A rare, degenerative, fatal brain disorder believed to be linked to an abnormal form of a protein called a prion.

dementia: Term which describes a group of diseases (including Alzheimer disease) which are characterized by memory loss and other declines in mental functioning.

dementia with Lewy bodies: A type of Lewy body dementia that is a common form of progressive dementia.

dendrite: Branch-like extension of a neuron that receives messages from other neurons.

do not resuscitate (DNR) form: Document that tells healthcare staff that the person with AD does not want them to try to return the heart to a normal rhythm if it stops or is beating unevenly.

dopamine: A chemical messenger, deficient in the brains of people with Parkinson disease, that transmits impulses from one nerve cell to another.

Down syndrome: Many people with Down syndrome develop early-onset AD, with signs of dementia by the time they reach middle age.

dyskinesias: Abnormal involuntary twisting and writhing movements that can result from long-term use of high doses of levodopa.

dystonia: Involuntary muscle contractions that cause slow repetitive movements or abnormal postures.

early-onset Alzheimer disease: A rare form of AD that usually affects people between ages 30 and 60. It is called familial AD (FAD) if it runs in the family.

electroencephalogram (EEG): A medical procedure that records patterns of electrical activity in the brain.

entorhinal cortex: An area deep within the brain where damage from AD often begins.

free radical: A highly reactive molecule (typically oxygen or nitrogen) that combines easily with other molecules because it contains an unpaired electron. The combination with other molecules sometimes damages cells.

frontotemporal disorders: A group of dementias characterized by degeneration of nerve cells, especially those in the frontal and temporal lobes of the brain.

gene: The biologic unit of heredity passed from parent to child. Genes are segments of DNA and contain instructions that tell a cell how to make specific proteins.

genetic mutation: A permanent change in a gene that can be passed on to children. The rare, early-onset familial form of Alzheimer disease is associated with mutations in genes on chromosomes 21, 14, and 1.

genetic risk factor: A variant in a cell's DNA that does not cause a disease by itself but may increase the chance that a person will develop a disease.

genetic variant: A difference in a gene that may increase or decrease a person's risk of developing a disease or condition.

genome: An organism's complete set of DNA, including all of its genes. Each genome contains all of the information needed to build and maintain that organism.

genome-wide association study (GWAS): A study approach that involves rapidly scanning the genomes of many individuals to find genetic variations associated with a particular disease.

geriatrician: Physician who is certified in the care of older people.

Gerstmann-Straussler-Scheinker disease (GSS): Symptoms include a loss of coordination (ataxia) and dementia that begin when people are 50 to 60 years old.

glial cell: A specialized cell that supports, protects, or nourishes nerve cells.

hippocampus: A structure in the brain that plays a major role in learning and memory and is involved in converting short-term to long-term memory.

HIV-associated dementia: A dementia that results from infection with the human immunodeficiency virus that causes AIDS.

Huntington disease: A degenerative hereditary disorder caused by a faulty gene for a protein called huntingtin. The disease causes degeneration in many regions of the brain and spinal cord and patients eventually develop severe dementia.

hypersexuality: Condition in which people with AD become overly interested in sex.

hypertension: High blood pressure has been linked to cognitive decline, stroke, and types of dementia that affect the white matter regions of the brain.

hypothalamus: A structure in the brain under the thalamus that monitors activities such as body temperature and food intake.

inpatient: A person who has been admitted at least overnight to a hospital or other health facility (which is, therefore, responsible for his or her room and board) for the purpose of receiving diagnostic treatment or other health services.

late-onset Alzheimer disease: The most common form of AD. It occurs in people aged 60 and older.

Lewy body dementia: One of the most common types of progressive dementia, characterized by the presence of abnormal structures called Lewy bodies in the brain.

magnetic resonance imaging (MRI): A diagnostic and research technique that uses magnetic fields to generate a computer image of internal structures in the body. MRIs are very clear and are particularly good for imaging the brain and soft tissues.

Medicaid: Federal and state-funded program of medical assistance to low-income individuals of all ages.

meningitis: Inflammation of the three membranes that envelop the brain and spinal cord, collectively known as the meninges; the meninges include the dura, pia mater, and arachnoid.

mental illness/impairment: A deficiency in the ability to think, perceive, reason, or remember, resulting in loss of the ability to take care of one's daily living needs.

microtubule: An internal support structure for a neuron that guides nutrients and molecules from the body of the cell to the end of the axon.

mild cognitive impairment (MCI): A condition in which a person has memory problems greater than those expected for his or her age, but not the personality or cognitive problems that characterize AD.

mixed dementia: Dementia in which one form of dementia and another condition or dementia cause damage to the brain, for example, Alzheimer disease and small vessel disease or vascular dementia.

multi-infarct dementia: A type of vascular dementia caused by numerous small strokes in the brain.

mutation: A permanent change in a cell's DNA that can cause a disease.

myelin: A whitish, fatty layer surrounding an axon that helps the axon rapidly transmit electrical messages from the cell body to the synapse.

myoclonus: Condition that sometimes happens with AD, in which a person's arms, legs, or whole body may jerk. It can look like a seizure, but the person doesn't pass out.

neural stem cells: Cells found only in adult neural tissue that can develop into several different cell types in the central nervous system.

neurodegenerative disease: A disease characterized by a progressive decline in the structure, activity, and function of brain tissue. These diseases include AD, Parkinson disease, frontotemporal lobar degeneration, and dementia with Lewy bodies. They are usually more common in older people.

neurofibrillary tangles: Bundles of twisted filaments found in nerve cells in the brains of people with Alzheimer disease. These tangles are largely made up of a protein called tau.

neuron: A nerve cell that is one of the main functional cells of the brain and nervous system.

neurotransmitter: A chemical messenger between neurons. These substances are released by the axon on one neuron and excite or inhibit activity in a neighboring neuron.

nucleus: The structure within a cell that contains the chromosomes and controls many of its activities.

plaques: Unusual clumps of material found between the tissues of the brain in Alzheimer disease.

plasticity: Ability of the brain to adapt to deficits and injury.

positron emission tomography (PET): An imaging technique using radioisotopes that allows researchers to observe and measure activity in different parts of the brain by monitoring blood flow and concentrations of substances such as oxygen and glucose, as well as other specific constituents of brain tissues.

progressive dementia: A dementia that gets worse over time, gradually interfering with more and more cognitive abilities.

receptor: Proteins that serve as recognition sites on cells and cause a response in the body when stimulated by chemicals called neurotransmitters. They act as on-and-off switches for the next nerve cell.

rigidity: A symptom of the disease in which muscles feel stiff and display resistance to movement even when another person tries to move the affected part of the body, such as an arm.

schizophrenia: A severe mental disorder that appears in late adolescence or early adulthood. People with schizophrenia may have hallucinations, delusions, loss of personality, confusion, agitation, social withdrawal, psychosis, and/or extremely odd behavior.

secondary dementia: A dementia that occurs as a consequence of another disease or an injury.

seizures: Abnormal activity of nerve cells in the brain causing strange sensations, emotions, and behavior, or sometimes convulsions, muscle spasms, and loss of consciousness.

single photon emission computed tomography (SPECT): An imaging technique that allows researchers to monitor blood flow to different parts of the brain.

subdural hematoma: Bleeding confined to the area between the dura and the arachnoid membranes.

support groups: Groups of people who share a common bond (e.g., caregivers) who come together on a regular basis to share problems and experiences.

synapse: The tiny gap between nerve cells across which neurotransmitters pass.

tau: A protein that helps the functioning of microtubules, which are part of the cell's structural support and help deliver substances throughout the cell. In Alzheimer disease, tau twists into filaments that become tangles. Disorders associated with an accumulation of tau, such as frontotemporal dementia, are called tauopathies.

thalamus: A small structure in the front of the cerebral hemispheres that serves as a way station that receives sensory information of all kinds and relays it to the cortex; it also receives information from the cortex.

trait: Any genetically determined characteristic.

tremor: Shakiness or trembling, often in a hand, which in Parkinson disease is usually most apparent when the affected part is at rest.

vascular dementia: A medical condition caused by strokes or changes in the brain's blood supply. Signs can appear suddenly. These signs include changes in memory, language, thinking skills, and mood.

ventricle: A cavity within the brain that is filled with cerebrospinal fluid.

ventriculostomy: A surgical procedure that drains cerebrospinal fluid from the brain by creating an opening in one of the small cavities called ventricles.

X-ray: A type of high-energy radiation. In low doses, X-rays are used to diagnose diseases by making pictures of the inside of the body.

Chapter 63

Directory of Resources for People with Dementia and Their Caregivers

Government Organizations

Administration for Community Living (ACL)
One Massachusetts Ave. N.W.
Washington, DC 20001
Phone: 202-619-0724
Fax: 202-357-3555
Website: acl.gov
E-mail: aoainfo@aoa.hhs.gov

Agency for Healthcare Research and Quality (AHRQ)
Office of Communications and Knowledge Transfer
5600 Fishers Ln.
Rockville, MD 20857
Phone: 301-427-1104
Website: www.ahrq.gov

Resources in this chapter were compiled from several sources deemed reliable; all contact information was verified and updated in December 2018.

Centers for Disease Control and Prevention (CDC)
1600 Clifton Rd.
Atlanta, GA 30329-4027
Toll-Free: 800-CDC-INFO
(800-232-4636)
Phone: 404-639-3311
Toll-Free TTY: 888-232-6348
Website: www.cdc.gov
E-mail: cdcinfo@cdc.gov

Eldercare Locator
Toll-Free: 800-677-1116
Website: www.eldercare.acl.gov
E-mail: eldercarelocator@n4a.org

Healthfinder®
National Health Information
Center (NHIC)
200 Independence Ave. S.W.
Washington, DC 20201
Website: www.healthfinder.gov
E-mail: healthfinder@hhs.gov

National Cancer Institute (NCI)
9609 Medical Center Dr.
Bethesda, MD 20892-9760
Toll-Free: 800-422-6237
Toll-Free TTY: 800-332-8615
Website: www.cancer.gov
E-mail: cancergovstaff@mail.nih.gov

National Center for Complementary and Integrative Health (NCCIH)
National Institutes of Health
(NIH)
9000 Rockville Pike
Bethesda, MD 20892
Toll-Free: 888-644-6226
Toll-Free TTY: 866-464-3615
Toll-Free Fax: 866-464-3616
Website: www.nccih.nih.gov
E-mail: info@nccih.nih.gov

National Center for Health Statistics (NCHS)
1600 Clifton Rd.
Atlanta, GA 30329-4027
Toll-Free: 800-CDC-INFO
(800-232-4636)
Toll-Free TTY: 888-232-6348
Website: www.cdc.gov
E-mail: cdcinfo@cdc.gov

National Center on Elder Abuse
University of Delaware
University of Southern
California Keck School of
Medicine, Department of Family
Medicine and Geriatrics
1000 S. Fremont Ave.
Unit 22 Bldg. A-6
Alhambra, CA 91803
Toll-Free: 855-500-3537
Fax: 626-457-4090
Website: www.ncea.acl.gov
E-mail: ncea-info@aoa.hhs.gov

National Institute of Mental Health (NIMH)
Office of Science Policy,
Planning, and Communications
6001 Executive Blvd.
Rm. 6200 MSC 9663
Bethesda, MD 20892-9663
Toll-Free: 866-615-6464
Phone: 301-443-4513
Toll-Free TTY: 866-415-8051
Fax: 301-443-4279
Website: www.nimh.nih.gov
E-mail: nimhinfo@nih.gov

National Institute of Neurological Disorders and Stroke (NINDS)
NIH Neurological Institute
P.O. Box 5801
Bethesda, MD 20824
Toll-Free: 800-352-9424
Phone: 301-496-5751
TTY: 301-468-5981
Website: www.ninds.nih.gov
E-mail: braininfo@ninds.nih.gov

National Institute on Alcohol Abuse and Alcoholism (NIAAA)
5635 Fishers Ln.
Bethesda, MD 20892-9304
Toll-Free: 888-696-4222
Phone: 301-443-3860
Toll-Free TTY: 800-222-4225
Website: www.niaaa.nih.gov
E-mail: niaaaweb-r@exchange.
nih.gov

National Institute on Disability, Independent Living, and Rehabilitation Research (NIDILRR)
Administration for Community
Living (ACL), U.S. Department
of Health and Human Services
(HHS)
330 C St. S.W.
Washington, DC 20201
Toll-Free: 800-872-5327
Phone: 202-401-4634
Fax: 202-205-0392
Website: acl.gov

National Institutes of Health (NIH)
9000 Rockville Pike
Bethesda, MD 20892
Phone: 301-496-4000
TTY: 301-402-9612
Website: www.nih.gov
E-mail: nihinfo@od.nih.gov

National Women's Health Information Center (NWHIC)
Office on Women's Health
(OWH)
200 Independence Ave. S.W.
Rm. 712 E
Washington, DC 20201
Toll-Free: 800-994-9662
Phone: 202-690-7650
Toll-Free TTY: 888-220-5446
Fax: 202-205-2631
Website: www.womenshealth.
gov

U.S. Food and Drug Administration (FDA)
10903 New Hampshire Ave.
Silver Spring, MD 20993
Toll-Free: 888-INFO-FDA
(888-463-6332)
Website: www.fda.gov

U.S. National Library of Medicine (NLM)
8600 Rockville Pike
Bethesda, MD 20894
Toll-Free: 888-346-3656
Phone: 301-594-5983
Toll-Free TDD: 800-735-2258
Fax: 301-402-1384
Website: www.nlm.nih.gov

Private Organizations

AARP
601 E. St. N.W.
Washington, DC 20049
Toll-Free: 888-OUR-AARP
(888-687-2277)
Phone: 202-434-3525
Toll-Free TDD: 877-434-7598
Website: www.aarp.org
E-mail: member@aarp.org

Alzheimer Society of Canada
20 Eglinton Ave. W.
16th Fl.
Toronto, ON M4R 1K8
Toll-Free: 800-616-8816 (Canada only)
Phone: 416-488-8772
Fax: 416-322-6656
Website: alzheimer.ca
E-mail: info@alzheimer.ca

Alzheimer's Association
225 N. Michigan Ave.
17th Fl.
Chicago, IL 60601-7633
Toll-Free: 800-272-3900
Phone: 312-335-8700
TDD: 312-335-5886
Toll-Free Fax: 866-464-3616
Website: www.alz.org
E-mail: info@alz.org

Alzheimer's Australia
P.O. Box 4194
Kingston, ACT 2604
Phone: 026-278-8900
Fax: 039-816-5733
Website: fightdementia.org.au
E-mail: nat.admin@alzheimers.org.au

Alzheimer's Disease International (ADI)
64 Great Suffolk St.
London, SE1 0BL
Phone: 44-20-79810880
Fax: 44-20-79282357
Website: www.alz.co.uk
E-mail: info@alz.co.uk

Alzheimer's Drug Discovery Foundation (ADDF)
57 W. 57th St.
Ste. 904
New York, NY 10019
Phone: 212-901-8000
Website: www.alzdiscovery.org
E-mail: info@alzdiscovery.org

Alzheimer's Foundation of America (AFA)
322 Eighth Ave.
Seventh Fl.
New York, NY 10001
Toll-Free: 866-232-8484
Phone: 646-638-1542
Fax: 646-638-1546
Website: www.alzfdn.org
E-mail: info@alzfdn.org

Alzheimer's Society UK
43-44 Crutched Friars
London, EC3N 2AE
Phone: 330-333-0804
Website: alzheimers.org.uk
E-mail: enquiries@alzheimers.
org.uk

American Academy of Neurology (AAN)
201 Chicago Ave.
Minneapolis, MN 55415
Toll-Free: 800-879-1960
Phone: 612-928-6000
Fax: 612-454-2746
Website: www.aan.com
E-mail: memberservices@aan.
com

American Association for Clinical Chemistry (AACC)
900 Seventh St. N.W.
Ste. 400
Washington, DC 20001
Toll-Free: 800-892-1400
Phone: 202-857-0717
Fax: 202-887-5093
Website: www.aacc.org
E-mail: custserv@aacc.org

American Association for Geriatric Psychiatry (AAGP)
6728 Old McLean Village Dr.
McLean, VA 22101
Phone: 703-556-9222
Fax: 703-556-8729
Website: www.aagpgpa.org
E-mail: main@aagponline.org

American Medical Association (AMA)
330 N. Wabash Ave.
Ste. 39300
Chicago, IL 60611-5885
Toll-Free: 800-621-8335
Phone: 312-464-4430
Website: www.ama-assn.org

American Pain Society (APS)
8735 W. Higgins Rd.
Ste. 300
Chicago, IL 60631
Phone: 847-375-4715
Toll-Free Fax: 866-574-2654
Website: www.ampainsoc.org
E-mail: info@
americanpainsociety.org

American Parkinson Disease Association (APDA)
135 Parkinson Ave.
Staten Island, NY 10305-1425
Toll-Free: 800-223-2732
Phone: 718-981-8001
Fax: 718-981-4399
Website: www.apdaparkinson.
org
E-mail: apda@apdaparkinson.
org

American Psychiatric Association (APA)
800 Maine Ave. S.W.
Ste. 900
Washington, DC 20024
Toll-Free: 888-357-7924
Phone: 202-559-3900
Website: www.psych.org
E-mail: apa@psych.org

American Psychological Association (APA)
750 First St. N.E.
Washington, DC 20002-4242
Toll-Free: 800-374-2721
Phone: 202-336-5500
TDD/TTY: 202-336-6123
Website: www.apa.org

American Society on Aging (ASA)
575 Market St.
Ste. 2100
San Francisco, CA 94105-2869
Toll-Free: 800-537-9728
Phone: 415-974-9600
Fax: 415-974-0300
Website: www.asaging.org
E-mail: info@asaging.org

Assisted Living Federation of America (ALFA)
1650 King St.
Ste. 602
Alexandria, VA 22314
Phone: 703-894-1805
Website: www.alfa.org

Association for Frontotemporal Degeneration (AFTD)
Radnor Stn Bldg. #2
Ste. 320
Radnor, PA 19087
Toll-Free: 866-507-7222
Phone: 267-514-7221
Website: www.theaftd.org
E-mail: info@theaftd.org.

Bachmann-Strauss Dystonia & Parkinson Foundation
P.O. Box 38016.
Albany, NY 12203
Phone: 212-509-0995
Fax: 212-682-6156
Website: www.dystonia-parkinsons.org

Brain Injury Association of America, Inc. (BIAA)
1608 Spring Hill Rd.
Ste. 110
Vienna, VA 22182
Toll-Free: 800-444-6443
Phone: 703-761-0750
Fax: 703-761-0755
Website: www.biausa.org
E-mail: braininjuryinfo@biausa.org

Brain Trauma Foundation (BTF)
Website: www.braintrauma.org

BrightFocus Foundation
22512 Gateway Center Dr.
Clarksburg, MD 20871
Toll-Free: 800-437-2423
Phone: 301-948-3244
Website: www.brightfocus.org
E-mail: info@brightfocus.org

*Brookdale Department
of Geriatrics and Adult
Development*
One Gustave L. Levy Place
New York, NY 10029-6574
Phone: 212-241-6500
Fax: 212-241-5977
Website: icahn.mssm.edu

*Caregiving, Palliative Care,
and Hospice Information*
Caring Connections
Unit 15 Ashcroft Centre,
Ashcroft Rd.
Kirkby Industrial Estate, L33
7TW
Toll-Free: 800-658-8898
Phone: 151-289-2761
Website: www.
caringconnections.org.uk
E-mail: admin@
caringconnections.org.uk

Caring.com
2600 S. El Camino Real
Ste. 300
San Mateo, CA 94403
Toll-Free: 800-973-1540
Phone: 650-312-7100
Website: www.caring.com

CJD Aware!
2527 S. Carrollton Ave.
New Orleans, LA 70118-3013
Phone: 504-861-4627
Website: www.cjdaware.com
E-mail: info@cjdaware.com

Cleveland Clinic
9500 Euclid Ave.
Cleveland, OH 44195
Toll-Free: 800-223-2273
TTY: 216-444-0261
Website: my.clevelandclinic.org

*Creutzfeldt-Jakob Disease
Foundation Inc. (CJA)*
3610 W. Market St., Ste. 110
Akron, OH 44333
Toll-Free: 800-659-1991
Fax: 234-466-7077
Website: www.cjdfoundation.org
E-mail: help@cjdfoundation.org

*CurePSP: Foundation for
Progressive Supranuclear
Palsy, Corticobasal
Degeneration, and Related
Brain Diseases*
1216 Bdwy.
Second Fl.
New York, NY 10001
Toll-Free: 800-457-4777
Phone: 347-294-2873
Fax: 410-785-7009
Website: www.curepsp.org
E-mail: info@curepsp.org

*Dana Alliance for Brain
Initiatives (DABI)*
505 Fifth Ave.
Sixth Fl.
New York, NY 10017
Phone: 212-223-4040
Fax: 212-317-8721
Website: www.dana.org
E-mail: dabiinfo@dana.org

Davis Phinney Foundation
4730 Table Mesa Dr., Ste. J-200
Boulder, CO 80305
Toll-Free: 866-358-0285
Phone: 303-733-3340
Fax: 303-733-3350
Website: www.
davisphinneyfoundation.org
E-mail: contact@dpf.org

The Empire State Building
Society of Certified Senior
Advisors (CSA)
720 S. Colorado Blvd., Ste. 750 N.
Denver, CO 80246
Toll-Free: 800-653-1785
Website: www.csa.us
E-mail: Society@csa.us

**Family Caregiver Alliance
(FCA)**
101 Montgomery St.
Ste. 2150
San Francisco, CA 94104
Toll-Free: 800-445-8106
Phone: 415-434-3388
Website: www.caregiver.org

**Fisher Center for Alzheimer's
Research Foundation**
110 E. 42nd St.
16th Fl.
New York, NY 10017
Toll-Free: 800-259-4636
Fax: 212-915-1319
Website: www.alzinfo.org
E-mail: info@alzinfo.org

**Hospice Foundation of
America (HFA)**
1707 L St. N.W., Ste. 220
Washington, DC 20036
Toll-Free: 800-854-3402
Phone: 202-457-5811
Fax: 202-457-5815
Website: www.
hospicefoundation.org
E-mail: hfaoffice@
hospicefoundation.org

**Huntington's Disease Society
of America (HDSA)**
505 Eighth Ave., Ste. 902
New York, NY 10018
Toll-Free: 800-345-4372
Phone: 212-242-1968
Fax: 212-239-3430
Website: www.hdsa.org
E-mail: hdsainfo@hdsa.org

**Lewy Body Dementia
Association (LBDA)**
912 Killian Hill Rd. S.W.
Lilburn, GA 30047
Toll-Free: 800-539-9767
Phone: 404-935-6444
Fax: 480-422-5434
Website: www.lbda.org
E-mail: lbda@lbda.org

**Meals-on-Wheels Association
of America (MOWAA)**
1550 Crystal Dr.
Ste. 1004
Arlington, VA 22202
Toll-Free: 888-998-6325
Phone: 703-548-5558
Fax: 703-548-5274
Website: www.mowaa.org
E-mail: mowaa@mowaa.org

Mental Health America (MHA)
500 Montgomery St.
Ste. 820
Alexandria, VA 22314
Toll-Free: 800-969-6642
Phone: 703-684-7722
Fax: 703-684-5968
Website: www.
mentalhealthamerica.net

Michael J. Fox Foundation for Parkinson's Research
P.O. Box 4777
New York, NY 10163-4777
Toll-Free: 800-708-7644
Phone: 212-509-0995
Website: www.michaeljfox.org

National Academy of Elder Law Attorneys (NAELA)
1577 Spring Hill Rd.
Ste. 310
Vienna, VA 22182
Toll-Free: 800-677-1116
Phone: 703-942-5711
Fax: 703-563-9504
Website: www.naela.org
E-mail: naela@naela.org

National Adult Day Services Association (NADSA)
11350 Random Hills Rd.
Ste. 800
Fairfax, VA 22030
Toll-Free: 877-745-1440
Fax: 919-825-3945
Website: www.nadsa.org
E-mail: info@nadsa.org

National Alliance for Caregiving (NAC)
4720 Montgomery Ln.
Ste. 205
Bethesda, MD 20814
Phone: 301-718-8444
Fax: 301-951-9067
Website: www.caregiving.org
E-mail: info@caregiving.org

National Association for Continence (NAFC)
P.O. Box 1019
Charleston, SC 29402-1019
Toll-Free: 800-252-3337
Phone: 843-377-0900
Fax: 843-377-0905
Website: www.nafc.org
E-mail: memberservices@nafc.
org

National Association of Professional Geriatric Care Managers (NAPGCM)
3275 W. Ina Rd.
Ste. 130
Tucson, AZ 85741-2198
Phone: 520-881-8008
Fax: 520-325-7925
Website: www.healthfinder.gov

National Down Syndrome Society (NDSS)
8 E 41st St.
Eight Fl.
New York, NY 10017
Toll-Free: 800-221-4602
Fax: 646-870-9320
Website: www.ndss.org
E-mail: info@ndss.org

National Gerontological Nursing Association (NGNA)
446 E. High St.
Ste. 10
Lexington, KY 40507
Phone: 859-977-7453
Website: www.ngna.org
E-mail: info@ngna.org

National Hospice and Palliative Care Organization (NHPCO)
1731 King St.
Alexandria, VA 22314
Toll-Free: 800-658-8898
Phone: 703-837-1500
Fax: 703-837-1233
Website: www.nhpco.org
E-mail: nhpco_info@nhpco.org

National Organization for Rare Disorders (NORD)
55 Kenosia Ave.
Danbury, CT 06810-1968
Toll-Free: 800-999-6673
Phone: 203-744-0100
Fax: 203-263-9938
Website: www.rarediseases.org
E-mail: orphan@rarediseases.org

National Palliative Care Research Center (NPCRC)
Brookdale Department of Geriatrics and Palliative Medicine, Icahn School of Medicine
One Gustave L. Levy Place
P.O. Box 1070
New York, NY 10029
Phone: 212-241-7447
Fax: 212-241-5977
Website: www.npcrc.org
E-mail: npcrc@mssm.edu

National Parkinson Foundation
1501 N.W. Ninth Ave.
Bob Hope Rd.
Miami, FL 33136-1494
Toll-Free: 800-327-4545
Phone: 305-243-6666
Fax: 305-243-5595
Website: www.parkinson.org
E-mail: contact@parkinson.org

National Rehabilitation Information Center (NRIC)
8400 Corporate Dr., Ste. 500
Landover, MD 20785
Toll-Free: 800-346-2742
Phone: 301-459-5900
Fax: 301-459-4263
Website: www.naric.com
E-mail: naricinfo@heitechservices.com

National Respite Network and Resource Center
Website: www.archrespite.org

National Senior Citizens Law Center (NSCLC)
1444 Eye St. N.W., Ste. 1100
Washington, DC 20005
Phone: 202-289-6976
Fax: 202-289-7224
Website: www.nsclc.org

National Stroke Association
9707 E. Easter Ln.
Ste. B
Centennial, CO 80112-3747
Toll-Free: 800-787-6537
Phone: 303-649-9299
Fax: 303-649-1328
Website: www.stroke.org
E-mail: info@stroke.org

Palliative Care Policy Center
2000 M St. N.W.
Ste. 520
Washington, DC 20036
Website: www.medicaring.org
E-mail: info@medicaring.org

Parkinson Alliance
P.O. Box 308
Kingston, NJ 08528-0308
Toll-Free: 800-579-8440
Phone: 609-688-0870
Fax: 609-688-0875
Website: www.
parkinsonalliance.org
E-mail: contact@
parkinsonalliance.org

Parkinson's Action Network (PAN)
1025 Vermont Ave. N.W., Ste. 1120
Washington, DC 20005
Toll-Free: 800-850-4726
Phone: 202-638-4101
Fax: 202-638-7257
Website: www.parkinsonsaction.
org
E-mail: info@parkinsonsaction.
org

Parkinson's Disease Foundation
1359 Bdwy., Ste. 1509
New York, NY 10018
Toll-Free: 800-457-6676
Phone: 212-923-4700
Fax: 212-923-4778
Website: www.pdf.org
E-mail: info@pdf.org

Parkinson's Institute and Clinical Center
675 Almanor Ave.
Sunnyvale, CA 94085
Toll-Free: 800-655-2273
Phone: 408-734-2800
Fax: 408-734-8522
Website: www.thepi.org
E-mail: info@thepi.org

PsychCentral
55 Pleasant St., Ste. 207
Newburyport, MA 01950
Website: www.psychcentral.com
E-mail: talkback@psychcentral.com

Society Foundation for Health in Aging
40 Fulton St.
18th Fl.
New York, NY 10038
Toll-Free: 800-563-4916
Phone: 212-308-1414
Fax: 212-832-8646
Website: www.healthinaging.org

Visiting Nurses Associations of America (VNAA)
900 19th St. N.W., Ste. 200
Washington, DC 20006
Phone: 202-384-1420
Fax: 202-384-1444
Website: www.vnaa.org
E-mail: vnaa@vnaa.org

Well Spouse Association
63 W. Main St., Ste. H
Freehold, NJ 07728
Toll-Free: 800-838-0879
Phone: 732-577-8899
Fax: 732-577-8644
Website: www.wellspouse.org
E-mail: info@wellspouse.org

Index

Index

Page numbers followed by 'n' indicate a footnote. Page numbers in *italics* indicate a table or illustration.